Mauro Pittiruti, Giancarlo Scoppettuolo

THE GAVeCeLT MANUAL OF PICC AND MIDLINE

Indications, insertion, management

edra

Original title of the work:
Manuale GAVeCeLT dei PICC e dei Midline. Indicazioni, impianto, gestione

ISBN: 978-88-214-3926-1
eISBN: 978-88-214-3927-8

Translation from italian language, on behalf of Edra S.p.A., by: Priscilla De Angelis, Nick Skidmore

Publishing Manager: Costanza Smeraldi
Senior Editor: Alessandra Mutignani

Production Manager: Matteo Brambilla
Books Project Manager: Chiara Cucinella

Paper, Print and Binding Manager: Michele Ribatti

Cover: Paolo Ballerini

ISBN: 978-88-214-4741-9
eISBN: 978-88-214-4399-2

Edra S.p.A.
Via G. Spadolini 7, 20141 Milano
Tel. 02 881841
www.edizioniedra.it

Printed in Italy
Printed in May 2017 by "Rotomail Italia" S.p.A., Vignate (MI)

(*) Edra S.p.A. is part of LSWR GROUP

Authors

Mauro Pittiruti
Dipartimento di Scienze Chirurgiche
Università Cattolica del Sacro Cuore, Roma

Giancarlo Scoppettuolo
Unità di Consulenza Infettivologica Integrata
Fondazione Policlinico Universitario "A. Gemelli", Roma

This volume was produced with the collaboration of the Venous Access Team of Fondazione Policlinico Universitario "A. Gemelli" (Roma):

Daniele G. Biasucci, Serena Cappuccio, Davide Celentano, Chiara Chiarini, Laura Dolcetti, Alessandro Emoli, Antonio La Greca, Bruno Marche, Ivano Migliorini, Alessandro Mitidieri, Andrea Musarò, Cristina Taraschi

Contents

INTRODUCTION

Definitions

Definition of PICC

PICC (Peripherally Inserted Central Catheters) are devices for venous access made up of a catheter in biocompatible material that after being inserted in a peripheral vein (in most cases, in the upper limb) reaches a "central" position, that is, the transition zone between the superior vena cava and the right atrium.
Under this definition, the term "PICC" covers a wide range of devices, some of which are obsolete, which have been used throughout the history of venous access, from the first central venous access developed by Forssmann in 1929 to the central venous access by peripheral route in 1970s and 1980s, such as Cavafix or Drum Cartridges. As a matter of fact, PICCs as we know them today, at least in terms of calibre and materials, were marketed in the 1990s; these were small-calibre venous catheters (mostly 4 Fr or 5 Fr), in silicone or polyurethane, that were inserted by direct puncture of the superficial veins of the antecubital zone (typically, the cephalic vein or the communicating vein between the cephalic and basilic vein, or the basilic vein itself) as long as they were accessible and identifiable by visualisation or palpation; the catheter was introduced into a short cannula placed in the vein by directly puncturing the skin with a needle. These devices did not reach optimal clinical performance because of the exit site in the antecubital area (an uncomfortable area, due to constant mobility) and because the insertion in superficial veins of the antecubital fussa was associated with high incidence of thrombotic and infective complications, short duration of the device and poor patient compliance.
It was not until the start of this century that the ultrasound guided venipuncture method became part of clinical practice. This revolutionised every field of central venous access and had a particularly significant impact on PICCs. Associating the ultrasound method with two other crucial technological developments, that is, the technique of micro introduction and the development of new, highly reliable and biocompatible materials, such as third-generation polyurethanes, finally led to the PICCs we know today: central venous catheters in biocompatible material that are inserted under ultrasound guidance and the support of micro introduction kits in the deep veins of the

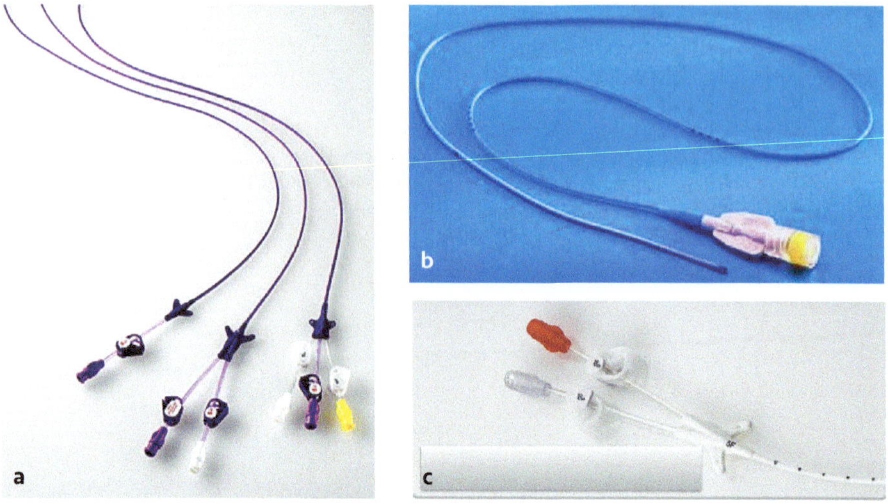

Figure 1

arm (typically, brachial vein or basilic vein) (Figure 1). The ultrasound method and the micro introduction technique (covered in detail in Chapter 2 of this manual) have profoundly changed PICCs in the last century, transforming them into a new venous access device with broader indications, longer duration, less frequent complications and greater patient comfort. Unlike PICCs of the 20th century, the PICCs used in the 21st century (which perhaps deserve to be called "ultrasound PICCs" or "echo-PICCS" to distinguish them from their predecessors) can be inserted in almost all patients, since the deep veins of the arm can be identified and punctured with ultrasound guidance in almost any clinical setting; moreover, the exit site at mid-arm greatly reduces the risk of infections and the risk of thrombosis and displacement thanks to the greater stability of the medication, with a longer duration of the devices as a consequence.The location of the exit site, not secondary in importance, is also associated with greater comfort for the patient.

The adoption of PICCs as the preferred central venous device in most patients in hospital or at home was mainly supported by the introduction of these new "echo-PICCs". For the purposes of this manual, any further reference will therefore indicate these PICCs.

In order to clarify the incorporation of currently employed PICCs in the field of devices for venous access, it is advisable to present a rational classification of all venous access devices taking into account four crucial features: (1) tip position; (2) insertion technique, (3) cannulated vein; (4) exit site. This classification, compared to traditional classifications based on the assumed duration of the system (Table 1) or the location of use (Table 2), has the advantage of classifying the device more accurately on the basis of the associated complication risk.

Table 1 Traditional classification of venous access (according to duration)

- Short term access
  - peripheral needle cannulas in Teflon
  - "long" peripheral cannulas ("mini-Midlines")
  - non-tunneled CICCs in polyurethane
  - non-tunneled catheters for dialysis
- Medium term access (<3-4 months)
  - peripheral Midline catheters
  - peripherally inserted central catheters - PICC
  - non-tunneled CICCs in silicone - Hohn
- Long term access (>3-4 months)
  - tunneled cuffed catheters (TCC) - Groshong, Hickman, Broviac, Leonard, cuffed catheters for dialysis, Pro-Line
  - totally implantable systems – port and PICC-port

Table 2 Classification of venous access according to location of use

- Access for in-hospital use
  - peripheral needle cannulas in Teflon
  - "long" peripheral cannulas
  - non-tunneled CICCs in polyurethane
  - peripheral Midline catheters
  - peripherally inserted central catheters - PICC
  - non-tunneled catheters for dialysis
- Access for use outside the hospital
  - peripheral Midline catheters
  - peripherally inserted central catheters - PICC
  - non-tunneled CICCs in silicone - Hohn
  - TCC - Groshong, Hickman, Broviac, Leonard, cuffed catheters for dialysis, Pro-Line
  - totally implantable systems – port

Traditional classifications (Tables 1 and 2) are based on the international guidelines and distinguish between short term access (peripheral cannulas and centrally inserted central venous access, or CICC), medium term access (PICC and Midline) and long term access (i.e. devices equipped with stabilisation systems, such as tunneled with fully implantable cuff or reservoir). PICCs are widely considered to be medium term access, as ratified by the recent EPIC guidelines of 2014 and, as such, are approved both for in-hospital and extra-hospital use, while short term devices are only meant to be used in a hospital setting and long term devices are for extra-hospital use only (hospice, day hospital, home, clinic). It is important to underline that, in this text, we will adopt the nomenclature recently proposed by WoCoVA, which describes the traditional central venous catheters inserted in veins in the infra- or supraclavicular, or traditional central venous catheters (CVC), as CICC. As a matter of fact, the term CVC is strongly ambiguous, since PICCs are, for all intents and purposes, central venous catheters. The CVC category therefore includes both PICCs (brachially inserted) and CICCs (centrally inserted), as well as FICCs (femorally inserted catheters) with certain reservations that will be illustrated later in the text. Although the classifications reported in Tables 1 and 2 may be useful in guiding device choice, they do not sufficiently define the specifications, risks and opportunities of clinical use, that are, on the other hand, illustrated in the following classifications.

Tip position (Table 3)

Devices can be classified as central – if the tip is in the superior vena cava (SVC) or in the right atrium, preferably close to the cavoatrial junction (i.e., in the lower third of the superior vena cava or in the upper third of the right atrium) - or peripheral (in all other cases). The salient feature of central access (a term that includes, for example, both PICCs and CICCs) is its ability of being used for any type of infusion, irrespective of pH, osmolarity or potentially harmful effects on the endothelium, as well as for haemodynamic monitoring (with particular reference to the detection of central venous pressure and oxygen saturation of mixed venous blood). Devices with tips positioned in other parts of the venous system are defined as peripheral: they cannot be used for haemodynamic monitoring and should not be used for the infusion of intravenous solutions that are too acidic (pH >5), too alkaline (pH >9), hyperosmolar (above 800 mOsm/L), vesicant or irritant (i.e., potentially associated with damage to the endothelium). Venous catheters inserted by femoral and saphenous route (FICC) and whose tip is positioned in the inferior vena cava (IVC), are one exception: these devices, even if not truly central (they cannot be used for haemodynamic monitoring), can be considered central for infusion purposes, since the blood flow of the inferior vena cava enables the administration of any intravenous solution. The inappropriate use of peripheral venous catheters bears a high risk of catheter-related venous thrombosis.

Table 3 Classification of venous access according to tip position

- Proper central venous catheters
  - any catheter whose tip is in SVC/right atrium (catheters inserted in the SVC region: basilica, brachial, cephalic, axillary, external jugular, subclavian, internal jugular, innominate)
- Venous catheters that can be used as central for infusion purposes, but not for monitoring
  - any catheter whose tip is in IVC (catheters inserted in the femoral or saphenous)
- Peripheral venous catheters
  - any catheter whose tip is not in SVC, right atrium or IVC (irrespective of the cannulated vein)

Insertion technique (Table 4)

Insertion technique of devices for venous access include: "direct" venipuncture of visible and/or palpable superficial veins, "blind" venipuncture using anatomical markers (certain deep veins of the neck or groin region), ultrasound-guided venipuncture (superficial and deep veins in patients of any age), surgical venous cutdown (deep or superficial veins, mostly in newborns), and enhanced visualisation with near-infrared technology (NIR) (superficial veins, mostly in newborns). The insertion technique may be more or less traumatic and more or less accurate, thereby decisively influencing the likelihood of success of the cannulation, the incidence of insertion-related complications and the risk of catheter-related venous thrombosis.

Cannulated vein (Table 5)

We can distinguish between devices inserted in superficial and deep veins in the upper limb (cephalic, brachial, basilic, antecubital, axillary in the brachial tract), devices inserted in superficial and deep veins of the neck and thorax (external jugular, internal jugular, innominate, subclavian, axillary in its thoracic tract, cephalic in its infraclavicular tract), and devices inserted in superficial and deep veins of the lower limb (saphenous, femoral). Although the choice of cannulated vein deeply influences the catheter calibre that can be inserted in it (cannulation of a vein that is too small for the size of the catheter leads to an increased risk of venous thrombosis), it has no direct impact on the indications for use of the device, which depend on the final position of the tip. Choosing the inappropriate vein can, however, significantly influence the risk of failure of the manoeuvre or complications at insertion.

Exit site (Table 6)

We can distinguish between exit sites in the arm (after cannulation of superficial or deep veins of the upper limb), the infraclavicular region (after cannulation of the subclavian or axillary), the supraclavicular region (after cannulation of the subclavian or the

Table 4 Classification of venous access according to the insertion technique
• Catheters inserted by means of venous cutdown – saphenous, internal jugular etc., mostly in newborns • Catheters inserted by means of "direct" venipuncture – catheters in the superficial veins (visible and palpable) of the arm • Catheters inserted by means of "blind" venipuncture – catheters inserted in the internal jugular, subclavian and femoral • Catheters inserted by means of ultrasound-guided venipuncture – any vein, superficial or profound, in patients of any age • Catheters inserted by means of NIR technique – superficial veins, mostly in newborns

Table 5 Classification of venous access according to the cannulated vein

- Catheters inserted in the upper limbs
  - needle cannulas, "long" peripheral cannulas, Midlines, PICCs, PICC-port etc., inserted in the brachial, basilica, cephalic and axillary (brachial tract)
- Catheters inserted in the veins of the thorax and the neck
  - CICCs, catheters for dialysis, ports, catheters for cuffed tunnelled, etc., inserted in the cephalic and axillary (subclavian tract), external jugular, internal jugular, subclavian, innominate
- Catheters inserted in the veins of the lower limb
  - FICC, catheters for dialysis, Broviac, etc., inserted in the femoral or saphenous

Table 6 Classification of venous access according to the *exit site*

- *Exit site* in the arm
  - catheters in the brachial, basilica, cephalic, axillary
- *Exit site* in the infraclavicular area
  - catheters in the axillary (ultrasound-guided) and subclavian (without ultrasound-guide)
- *Exit site* in the supraclavicular area
  - catheters in the subclavian (ultrasound-guided), internal jugular and innominate
- *Exit site* in the neck
  - catheters in the internal jugular
- *Exit site* in the inguinal region
  - catheters in the femoral (non-tunnelled)

internal jugular or innominate), the neck (after cannulation of the internal jugular), or the inguinal region (after cannulation of the femoral). The exit site does not exactly correspond to the puncture and cannulation site of the vein since it is possible to tunnel the catheters in the subcutaneous tissue for a greater or lesser length in order to obtain, for example, an exit site that is more appropriate to dressing stability or comfort.

From this new classification of devices for venous access based on these four fundamental characteristics, it is possible to anticipate the risk of potential complications associated with each device: the risk of complication in the insertion will depend primarily on the chosen vein and the implantation technique; the risk of venous thrombosis from catheters will depend on tip position, chosen vein and insertion technique; the choice of a given exit site will impact on the risk of complications from infections, thrombophlebitis and dislocations. The PICCs discussed in this manual may, therefore, be classified as central venous catheters (tip position close to the cavoatrial junction), inserted by means of ultrasound-guided venipuncture in deep veins of the arm, with an exit site in the middle third of the upper arm (i.e., halfway between the elbow and the axillary cavity). As will be further illustrated in the following chapters, PICCs are currently available in various materials and with various technical and structural specifications, different calibres (between 3 Fr and 6 Fr) and numbers of lumens (between 1 and 3).

Definition of Midline

The term "Midline" was coined about two decades ago to indicate venous catheters inserted in the arm, whose length was "halfway" between the length of a needle cannula (3-5 cm) and a PICC (around 30-50 cm or, in any case, of sufficient length to reach the cavoatrial junction from the arm). They were made in polyurethane or silicone, a material similar to that of PICCs. At the time, these devices were 20-25 cm long and were positioned by "direct" insertion technique (by visual inspection and/or palpation) in visible or palpable veins of the antecubital zone: in an adult of average size, the tip reached the brachial tract of the axillary vein. From the outset, therefore, these were peripheral venous catheters (since the tip did not reach a central site).

The same technological evolution that led to the creation of the new PICCs also changed the practice of Midline catheters at the beginning of this century: the use of ultrasound-guided venipuncture and the micro introduction technique led to a change in the cannulation site, from the antecubital fossa to the middle third of the arm, with undoubted advantages in terms of increased success of the procedure, reduction of early and delayed complications and increase in patient comfort. Moving the exit site about 10 cm proximally implied that Midline catheter tips – currently placed at mid-arm - are now placed in the thoracic tract of the axillary vein or even in the subclavian vein, therefore close to the middle portion of the clavicle (hence the term *midclavicular*). This improves the performance in terms of flow, while remaining a peripheral venous access device.

In recent times, new devices for peripheral venous access have been marketed, the length of which is greater than the short cannulas, but shorter than traditional midlines: these "long peripheral cannulas" are 8-10 cm long catheters in polyurethane or polyethilene that can be positioned both in superficial veins (with the direct technique) or in deep veins (with the ultra-sound guided technique). Unlike traditional midlines and PICCs, they are introduced with the direct Seldinger technique rather than with the modified Seldinger technique. The introduction of these devices created some terminological confusion, especially since international associations have proposed to define as Midlines all peripheral insertion devices with lengths greater than 6 cm, the tips of which are positioned no further than the brachial tract of the axillary vein. This definition therefore leaves out most of the "old" Midlines, whose tip is often positioned in the midclavicular position. To avoid such confusion, in this manual we shall distinguish between three types of peripheral venous catheters that can be inserted in the superficial or deep veins of the upper limb (Table 7):

- short peripheral cannulas (Figure 2): <6 cm long cannulas, usually in Teflon or polyurethane and positioned in the superficial veins of the forearm or the arm with direct technique (rarely, in deep veins with the ultrasound-guided technique);

Table 7 Peripheral venous access for intravenous treatments			
	Needle cannulas	**Long cannulas**	**Midline**
Length	3-6 cm	6-15 cm	>15 cm
Material	Teflon	Polyurethane	Polyurethane
Insertion	By sight	Also ultrasound-guided	Also ultrasound-guided
Technique	Direct	Simple Seldinger	Modified Seldinger
Urgent positioning	Yes	Yes	No
Duration	Few days	1-2 weeks	Months
Power injectable	If 20 G or >	Yes	No
Use outside the hospital	No	For short periods	Yes

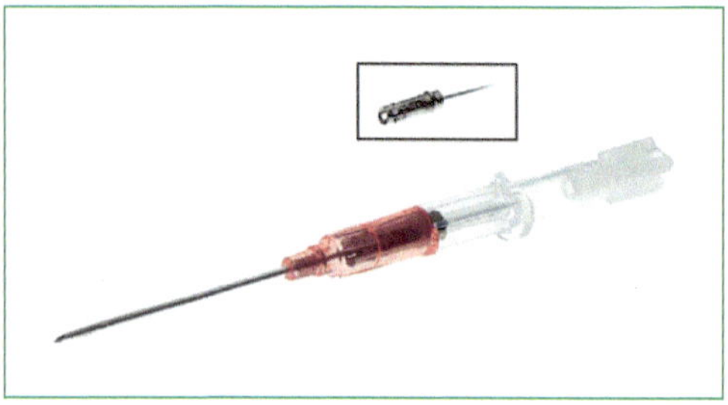

Figure **2**

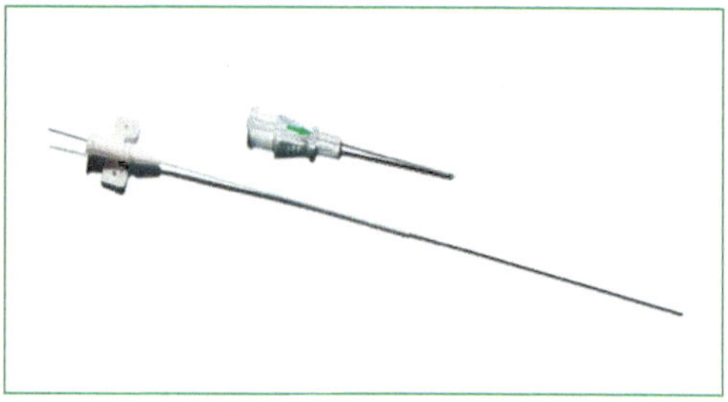

Figure **3**

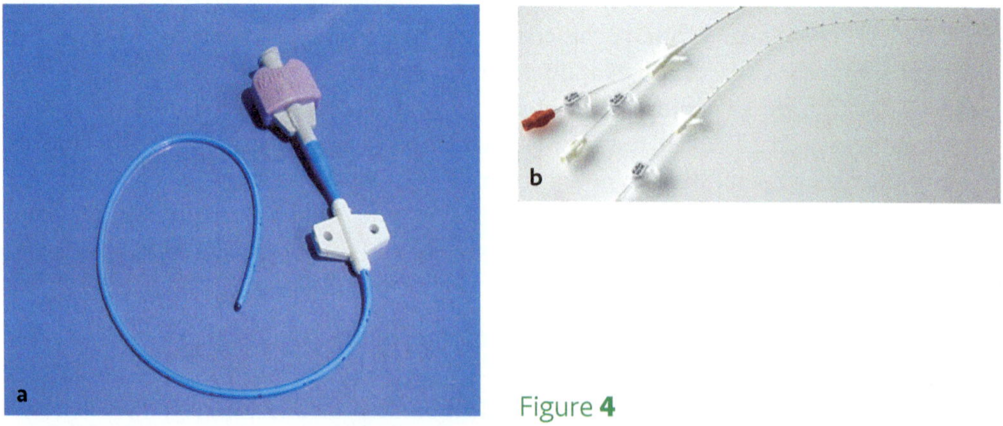

Figure **4**

- long peripheral cannulas (or mini-Midlines, as defined at times) (Figure 3): 8-10 cm long cannulas, usually in polyurethane, placed in the superficial veins of the forearm or the arm with direct technique or in deep veins of the arm with ultrasound-guided technique, the tip of which does not reach beyond the axillary cavity.
- "true" Midline catheters (or midclavicular) (Figure 4): 20-25 cm long, in polyurethane or silicone, positioned in the deep veins of the arm with ultrasound-guided technique, the tip of which is usually positioned in the thoracic tract of the axillary vein or in the subclavian vein.

Unless otherwise indicated, in this text, we shall refer to Midlines in this latter sense.

CHAPTER 1

Indications

Choosing between PICCs and Midlines: central access *versus* peripheral access

It must be stated from the outset that, as with the selection of an appropriate device in general, the choice between PICCs and Midlines for patients requiring venous access is essentially based on access purpose (drug infusion or parenteral nutrition, repeated sampling, haemodynamic monitoring, dialysis or apheresis procedures, etc.), type of drugs or solutions to be infused intravenously, access environment of use (in-hospital or extra-hospital setting) and expected duration. The substantially different indications for PICCs (Peripherally Inserted Central Catheters) and Midlines are based primarily on the fact that the PICC is a central venous access while Midline is a peripheral access (Figure 1.1).

As mentioned in the Introduction, central venous access is the proper description for all intravascular devices whose tip lies close to the junction between the superior vena cava and the right atrium (i.e., in the lower third of the superior vena cava or in the upper third of the right atrium) (Figure 1.2). This is considered the ideal position for safely infusing solutions of any pH and any osmolarity: this site can be used for the safe infusion of vesicant or irritant agents, since the blood flow of the superior vena cava (around 2 L/min in adult patients) dilutes their potential harm to the endothelium. Positioning the tip at this level also enables the catheter to lie on the same axis as the blood flow so that the solutions in question do not directly permeate the venous wall. This position is also considered ideal for haemodynamic monitoring (detection of central venous pressure and oxygen saturation of mixed venous blood) and for exchange procedures (dialysis and apheresis), which require abundant incoming and outgoing flows. Examples of central venous access include PICCs but also centrally inserted central catheters (CICC), ports, catheters for dialysis inserted in veins tributary to the superior vena cava, etc.; among these central devices, the only ones appropriate for exchange procedures (dialysis and apheresis) are the rigid double lumen catheters designed specifically for this purpose.

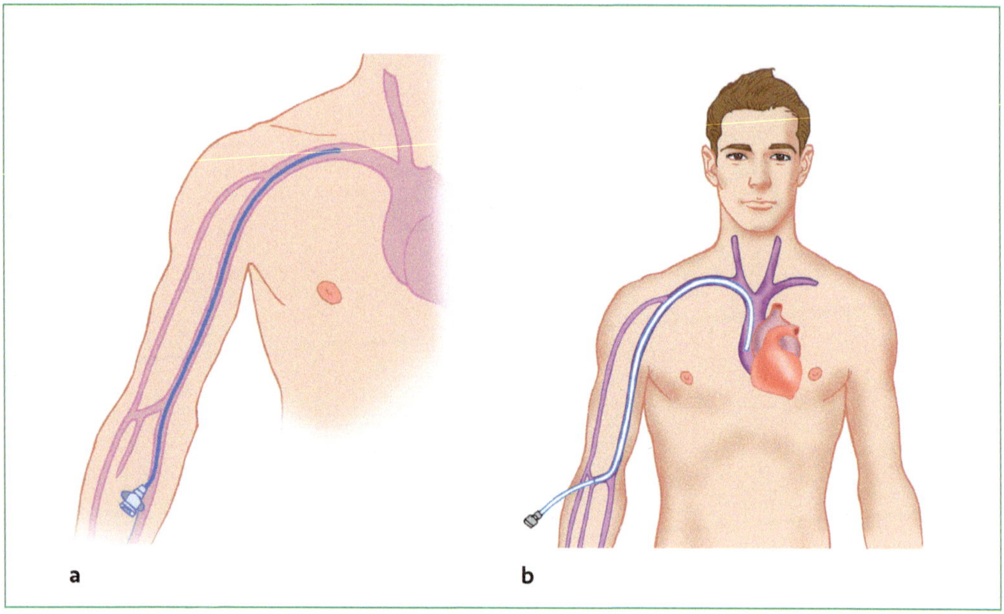

Figure **1.1**

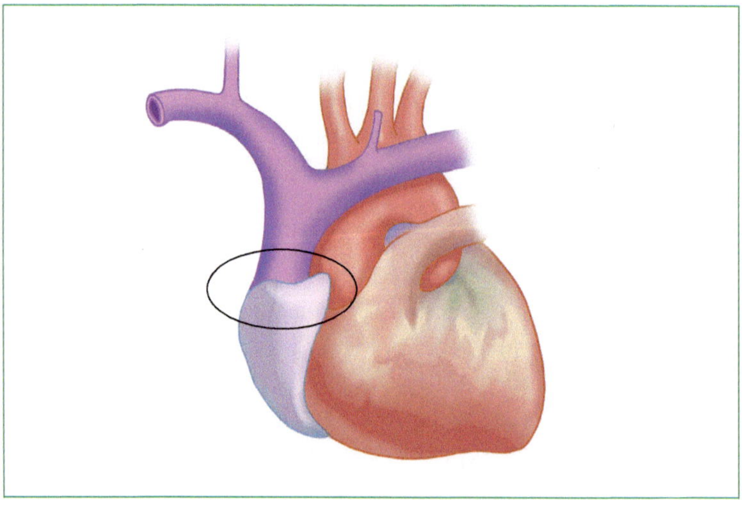

Figure **1.2**

Positioning the tip in the inferior vena cava creates a venous access similar to central venous access in some aspects (the safest position seems to be in the middle part of the inferior cava, above the common iliac veins but below the renal veins). Such access enables the infusion of any drug or solution, as well as exchange procedures (dialysis/apheresis), while excluding haemodynamic monitoring.

Examples of venous access devices are catheters inserted in the femoral vein for infusion, haemodialysis or apheresis purposes. The use of PICCs for femoral access has entered

clinical practice, even though it should probably be regarded as off-label and will be discussed later. Any venous access where the tip is not located in the two positions above described must be considered as peripheral access. This is the case with Midlines, whose tip is positioned in the axillary vein or even in the subclavian vein, as already described. According to national and international guidelines, drugs or solutions with pH <5 or >9 should not be infused through such devices. The same applies to vesicant drugs or solutions with osmolarity >750-850 mOsm/L, as well as to drugs or solutions that, with any other mechanism, could be associated with a high risk of phlebitis. A table of drugs identifying those who are compatible or incompatible with safe peripheral intravenous infusion is given in Appendix 1. In addition to Midline catheters, examples of peripheral venous access are traditional needle cannulas (up to 6 cm long) and long venous cannulas (8-10 cm). The use of these devices for the infusing drugs that are potentially harmful to the endothelium should be discouraged since it is associated with a high risk of thrombophlebitic complications and extravasation.
It is therefore clear that the proper indication for a PICC-type central venous access corresponds to the following cases:

- need for infusing drugs with pH <5 or >9 or vesicant or irritant agents (see Appendix I);
- the need for parenteral nutrition (with the possible exception of short treatments with lipid-based parenteral nutrition with osmolarity <800 mOsm/L);
- the need for repeated blood sampling;
- the need for haemodynamic monitoring.

In the first three settings, a PICC that is not truly central but whose tip is in the inferior vena cava can be utilized (*off-label* use). The use of PICCs for haemodynamic monitoring mainly includes the measurement of central venous pressure (a *power injectable,* non-valved PICC in polyurethane is recommended in this case) and of oxygen saturation in the mixed venous blood (which involves the withdrawal of atrial blood and therefore the use of a PICC whose tip is in the upper third of the right atrium rather than in the superior vena cava). The use of PICCs for dialysis or apheresis is associated with some technical difficulties, however, and can only be carried out in certain selected cases: as such, it is not generally recommended in clinical practice.
Finally, a frequent indication for PICC-type central venous access is a long expected device duration, even in those settings that would theoretically allow the use of a Midline-type peripheral catheter.

Choosing between PICCs and Midlines: field of use

Another important element to take into consideration when choosing the proper venous access is the setting in which it will be used, including hospital settings or situations that can be classified as extra-hospital settings (a patient at home or in a hospice, clinic or day-hospital).
For in-hospital venous access, only short-term (needle cannulas, long peripheral cannulas, non-tunneled CICC) or medium-term (Midline catheters, PICCs, uncuffed-tunneled

CICCs) venous access are considered appropriate. The choice between peripheral and central is therefore based on the aforementioned criteria. An important distinction between short-term systems (needle cannula, non-tunneled CICC etc.) and medium-term systems (PICCs, Midlines etc.) is that the former are not considered appropriate for extra-hospital use, which is the reason why a patient cannot be discharged with a short-term access, but can keep a medium-term access (for example, a PICC or a Midline), should venous infusions still be required at home or as part of a day-hospital regime. Appendix II illustrates an example of an algorithm for choosing the right type of venous access based on setting (in-hospital or extra-hospital) and the duration of use.

PICCs and Midlines in hospitalised patients

The choice of a certain peripheral venous access (when the peripheral route is compatible with the requirements for use) for hospitalised patients is based on the assumed duration of the treatment and the availability of visible or palpable superficial veins in the upper limbs. In the case of emergency peripheral venous access or, in any event, access intended for a duration of less than 5-6 days, usually needle cannulas are used. They are of various sizes (from 24 G to 14 G), with a length between 35 mm and 52 mm, are usually made of Teflon but occasionally in silicone or polyurethane. These needle cannulas are typically inserted through direct cannulation of visible or palpable superficial veins. The use of metal needles (so-called *butterfly*) for prolonged infusion purposes must be absolutely avoided due to the high risk of complications.

If the peripheral venous access is expected to last longer than 5-6 days and/or visible/palpable superficial veins are not available, either long peripheral cannulas (in polyethylene or polyurethane, 18 G or 20 G, 8 or 10 cm long) (Figure 1.3) or Midline catheters (in polyurethane, 4 Fr, 20-25 cm long) will be indicated for insertion. The use of Midline

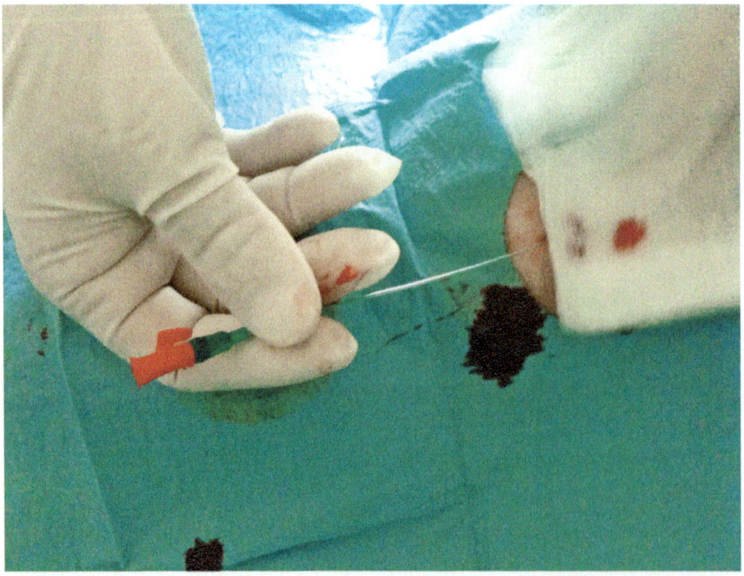

Figure **1.3**

catheters in silicone is not recommended, given their fragility and the consequent risk of ruptures, while the use of valved Midline catheters is not recommended due to the high incidence of malfunctions. Both long peripheral cannulas and Midline catheters are preferably positioned by ultrasound guidance in the deep veins of the arm (basilic, brachial), employing the direct Seldinger method or the modified Seldinger method. The expected duration of long cannulas is two weeks while Midlines, if used appropriately, can be used for months; moreover, since Midlines are medium-term systems, patients could potentially be discharged with this access in place. In all cases, the use of these peripheral accesses must be carefully supervised: their improper use (for example, infusion of hyperosmolar or irritant solutions) can lead to the occurrence of deep vein thrombosis in the arm or in the axillary-subclavian tract. Health operators should be adequately warned – especially in the case of Midlines – that a given access is a peripheral route (*midline)* and not a central one (PICC) to avoid erroneous use (Figure 1.4). In hospitalised patients, the central *venous* access of first choice should be a PICC, that is, an ultrasound-guided, peripherally inserted central venous catheter in a deep vein of the arm (basilic or brachial). The use of power injectable PICCs in high-resistance polyurethane is recommended, since these have optimal stability specifications and enable the infusion of abundant flows (up to 5 mL/sec) (Figure 1.5); the use of other, more fragile materials (especially silicone) is not recommended. The use of PICCs with valves (proximal or distal) is not advisable since convincing scientific evidence on the valve benefits is lacking

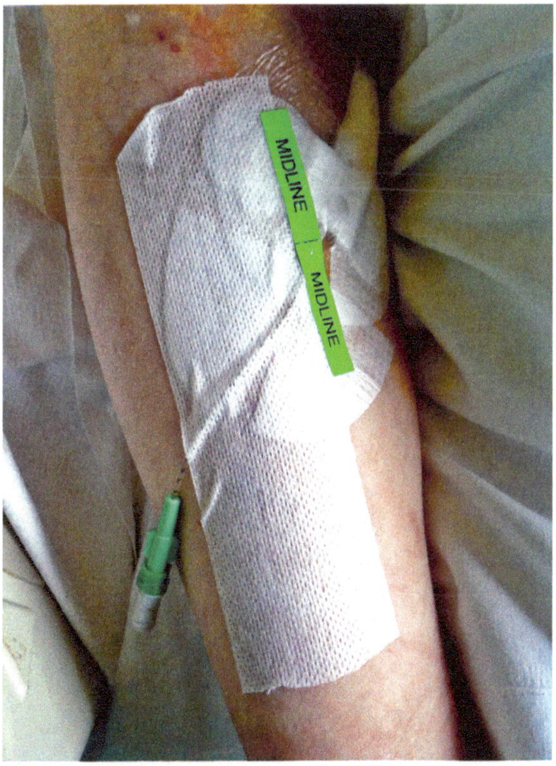

Figure **1.4**

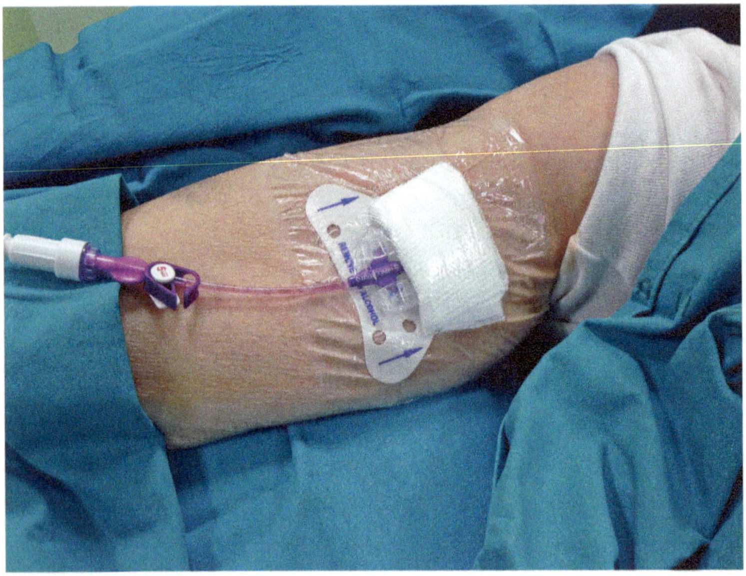

Figure **1.5**

and it is associated with a greater risk of malfunctions and a higher device cost. Power injectable PICCs are available in different calibres: 3 Fr single lumen and 4 Fr double lumen (ideal for pediatric patients), 4 Fr or 5 Fr single lumen, 5 Fr double lumen, and 6 Fr triple lumen. If several incompatible concomitant infusions are needed (for example, when one of these infusions is parenteral nutrition), double or triple lumen PICCs must be used. Triple lumen PICCs are especially indicated for patients in intensive care.

While it is true that PICCs are typically inserted in a basilic or brachial vein, it is equally true that, should these veins prove too small for the calibre of the planned catheter, the PICC can be inserted in the axillary vein (in the brachial tract). In this case, as the venipuncture site will be too close to the axilla, a short tunneling will be necessary to move the catheter's exit site distally (see Chapters 2 and 5 for more details about this technique).

In morbidly obese patients, it is often appropriate to avoid placing the PICC in the deep veins of the arm (basic, brachial, axillary) since the brachial tract of the cephalic vein (a superficial vein that may be the only one easily accessible in very obese patients) is preferred.

While it is true that PICCs should be considered the central venous access of first choice in hospitalised patients, it is also true that certain clinical situations require the insertion of a CICC, that is a central venous catheter inserted by ultrasound-guided puncture of the central veins of the infra/supraclavicular region and the neck (axillary, subclavian, internal jugular and innominate veins) (Figure 1.6); the most frequent of these conditions are:

- bilateral presence of contraindications to the placement of a PICC in the brachial site (previous axillary lymph node drainage, osteoarticular or skin changes, chronic paralysis of the arm, lack of availability of veins of sufficient calibre, venous thrombosis in the basilic-axillary-subclavian axis, etc.):

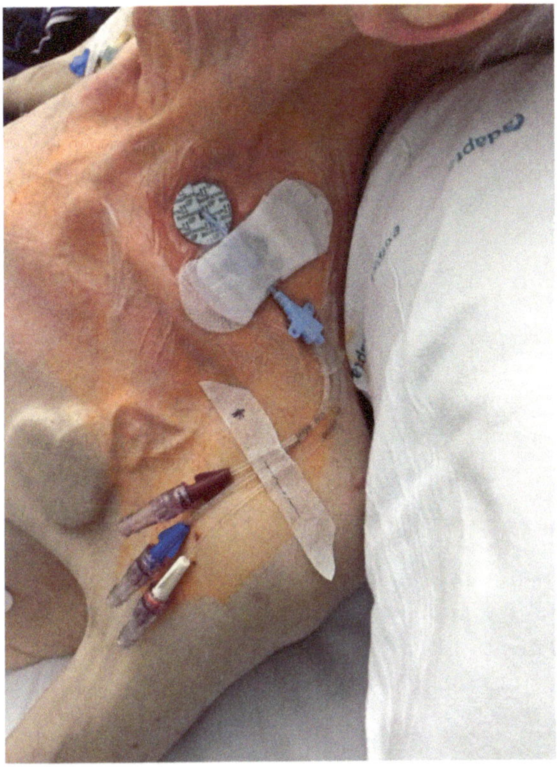

Figure **1.6**

- presence of chronic renal failure in patient receiving haemodialysis or candidate for haemodialysis (chronic renal failure stages 3b – 4-5);
- need for emergency venous access, such as in haemodynamically unstable patients (typically: urgent need for central access in the emergency room, the operating theatre or the intensive care unit);
- indication for a four or five lumen central venous access placement;
- indication for an antimicrobial-coated central venous access (i.e., coated with chlorhexidine or antibiotics) placement, where only antimicrobial-coated CICCs are available.

Placing a venous access by ultrasound-guided venipuncture and cannulation of the femoral vein (Femorally Inserted Central Catheter, FICC) may be strongly indicated in the following cases:

- patients with obstruction/compression of the superior vena cava (superior cava syndrome);
- emergency venous access;
- need for short-term venous access for haemodialysis or apheresis procedures in patients in whom it is advisable to save the superior caval region for other venous accesses.

A central venous access via the veins of the supra/infraclavicular area and the neck or via the femoral vein can be obtained either using a CICC-type catheter or a PICC (off-label).

Using a PICC for this purpose can have the following benefits:

- the PICC's micro-introduction kit (echogenic 21 G needle, micro-introducer, soft-tip metallic guide, without J – "*floppy straight tip*" – and a small calibre, 0.018"), ensures less trauma and easier, safer insertion;
- power injectable PICCs are made of higher quality material (third-generation polyurethane) with better biocompatibility than most CICCs and enable high pressure infusion of contrast medium;
- the specific PICCs length makes them particularly suitable to be tunneled (a very important aspect in femoral insertion, where the exit site should not be positioned in the inguinal fold).

The extreme versatility of PICCs makes them suitable for use as CICCs inserted in the axillary vein (Figure 1.7), the subclavian vein (Figure 1.8), the internal jugular vein or the innominate vein (Figure 1.9). Their length makes them particularly suitable to be inserted as FICCs in the femoral vein, with tunneling to the abdomen (Figure 1.10) or the knee (Figure 1.11), depending on the patient's condition.
It is also true that the emergency placement of a femoral catheter in a patient in hemorrhagic shock for example, would require the preferential use of a CICC rather than a PICC. Moreover, in that case the placement of a catheter in the inferior vena cava for dialysis or apheresis purposes would require the use of a rigid double lumen catheter specifically designed for dialysis.

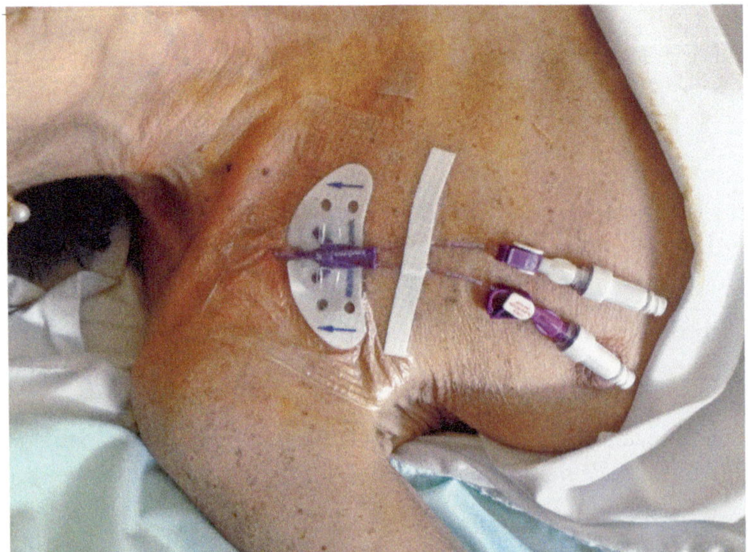

Figure **1.7**

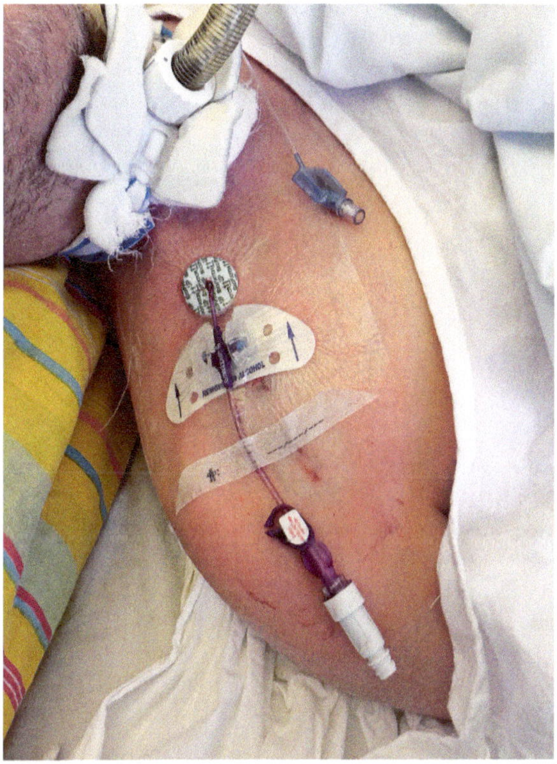

Figure **1.8**

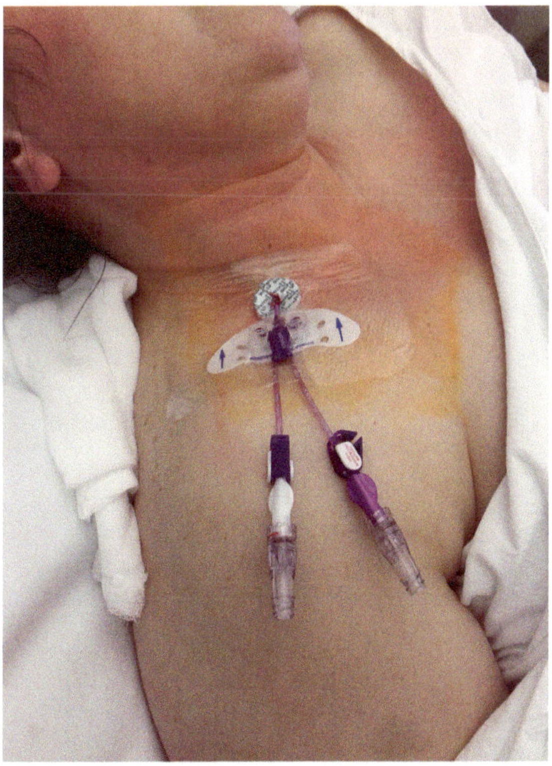

Figure **1.9**

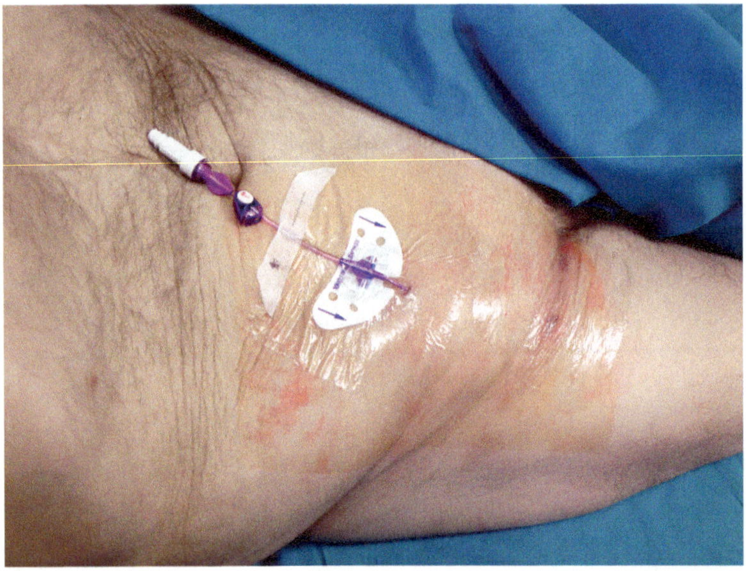

Figure **1.10**

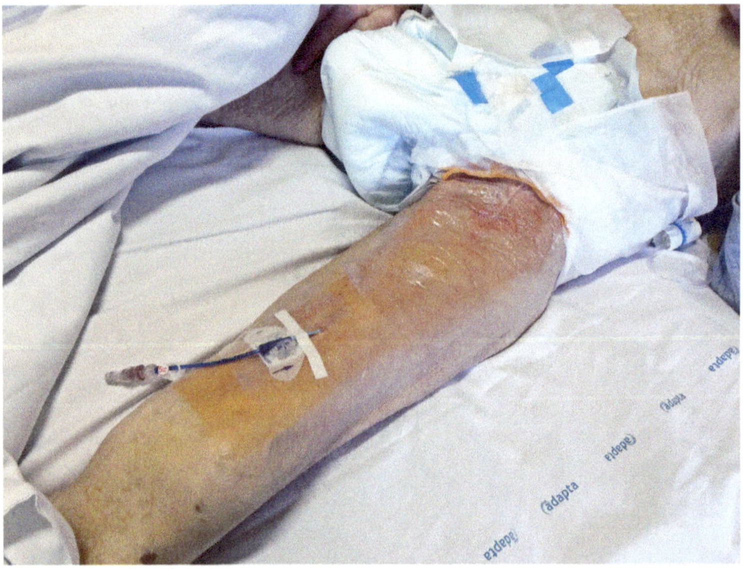

Figure **1.11**

PICCs and Midlines in intensive care patients

Most patients in intensive care require central venous access, for various indications:

- intravenous infusion of drugs and solutions that often have a pH >9 or <5, or osmolarity >600 mOsm/L (vasoactives, anticonvulsants, antibiotics, potassium, etc.);
- administration of parenteral nutrition with osmolarity often >800 mOsm/L;

- need for repeated sampling;
- rapid intravenous infusion of fluids for re-hydration purposes (requiring a device suitable for high flows);
- haemodynamic monitoring (central venous pressure, oxygen saturation in mixed venous blood);
- dialysis/apheresis/dialfiltration procedures.

The use of Midlines is therefore usually inappropriate and insufficient for the performance required in critically ill patients. Their indication is conceivable only in special cases (septic patients in whom the placement of a central catheter could be associated with its rapid colonisation; stable patients on enteral nutrition who also require intravenous treatments that can be safely administered by a peripheral route, etc.).

In most cases, infusion therapies and blood sampling can be carried out with a CICC (Figure 1.12), a catheter in the femoral vein (FICC) or a PICC (as long as the PICC is made of polyurethane, power injectable - with the consequent guarantee of high flows - and preferably non-valved) (Figure 1.13). Haemodynamic monitoring is only feasible with CICCs and PICCs and not with femoral catheters. For the correct detection of central venous pressure, however, that the PICCs should be made in polyurethane, non-valved, and preferably power injectable.

Blood exchange procedures like haemodialysis, apheresis, ultrafiltration, etc., require a double lumen CICC or a FICC of appropriate calibre and material. Little experience has been gathered on the use of PICCs for plasmapheresis or dialysis, and mostly in pediatric patients where flows of around 10-40 mL/min are sufficient. For ultrafiltration in adults (for example, to remove fluids from heart failure patients), the required flows of 10-25 mL/min required can be obtained using double lumen 5 Fr power injectable PICCs. However, the experience in this field is still very limited.

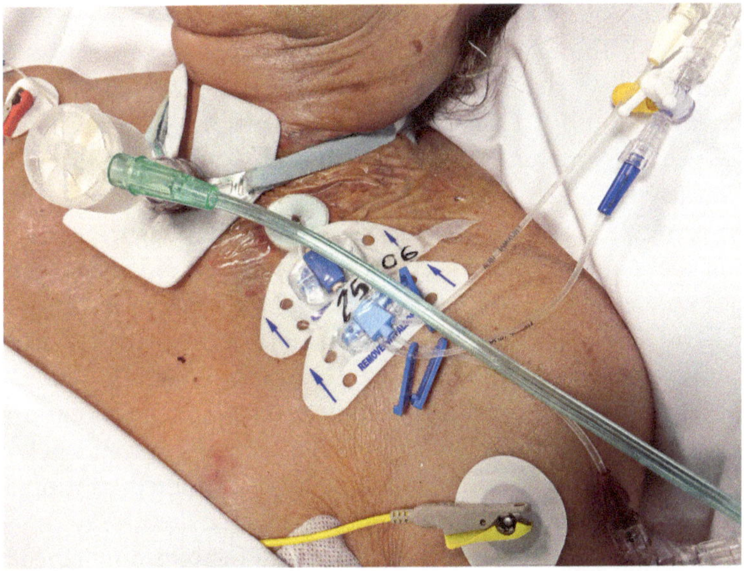

Figure **1.12**

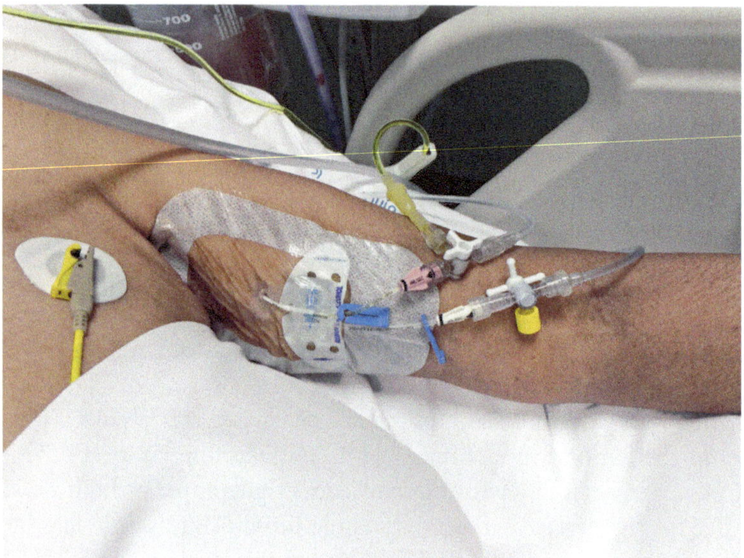

Figure **1.13**

Apart from this latter aspect, in many different situations either a PICC or a CICC can theoretically be used in intensive care patients. To properly identify the correct indications for one or the other, it is advisable to compare their features:

- *Catheter material:* most CICCs are made of first-generation polyurethane and are not power injectable, while the PICCs used today are usually made of more biocompatible and technologically-advanced material; the best material is third-generation polyurethane, equivalent to silicone and old polyurethanes in terms of infection and thrombosis risks, but superior in clinical performance and mechanical resistance. The greater biocompatibility of PICC materials implies that they are more suitable for longer use (it is no coincidence they are described as "medium-term devices"; see EPIC 2014 guidelines). This means they are indicated for long hospital stays in intensive care unit and for being left *in situ* during transfer to a post-intensive care unit. The only current limit of PICCs in terms of material is that, as mentioned, polyurethane PICCs coated with antibiotics or chlorhexidine are not consistently available in all countries.
- *Power injectability*: currently, many PICCs but few CICCs on sale are certified as power injectable. As mentioned, power injectable devices were introduced in clinical practice to tolerate the high pressures associated with the infusion of contrast medium during CT and MRI scans; this represents a significant problem in patients in intensive care units, for they are often subject to contrast imaging.
- *Number of lumina:* the PICCs currently on sale are single lumen, double lumen or triple lumen, unlike CICCs, which can have up to five lumina. It is therefore clear that, should a central access with more than four lumina be required, as it often is the case with critically ill patients, a CICC must be used. The need for multiple lumina in intensive care clearly arises from the requirement to avoid simultaneous

Table 1.1 Safe insertion of a central access (SICA Protocol, GAVeCeLT 2012)
1. Rational selection of the vein by systematic ultrasound examination (RaCeVA)
2. Appropriate aseptic technique: hand hygiene, maximum barrier precautions and skin antisepsis with 2% chlorhexidine
3. Use of ultrasound for ultrasound-guided venipuncture of the selected vein and for the subsequent ultrasound monitoring of the correct guide direction and the absence of pneumothorax
4. Intraprocedural verification of the central position of the tip using the intracavitary ECG technique
5. Protection of the exit site against the risk of bleeding (by means of hystoacryl glue) and/or the risk of contamination (by means of chlorhexidine sponge dressings)
6. Proper stabilisation of the catheter by means of a *sutureless* device and transparent, semipermeable membrane

administration of incompatible drugs. In this regard, the most recent guidelines (see EPIC 2014 guidelines) recommend the use of devices with the least number of lumina possible even though parenteral nutrition should always be administered through a dedicated lumen. Most PICCs in intensive care will necessarily be double lumen (4 Fr or 5 Fr) or triple lumen (6 Fr) and in power injectable polyurethane: in fact, when catheters with small calibre lumina are used, the power injectable PICC must be necessarily used, for its ability to guarantee good flows (from 1 mL/sec up to 5 mL/sec for each lumen, depending on PICC type).

- *Staff assigned to the insertion:* CICCs should be inserted by specifically trained personnel, as should PICCs. The placement by nursing personnel represents a potential advantage of PICCs over CICCs, in terms of human resource optimisation.
- *Insertion protocols:* although specific insertion protocols may exist for CICCs, such as the one developed by GAVeCeLT (SICA protocol, Table 1.1), often these central accesses are inserted in inappropriate ways that do not comply with any protocol or international guideline recommendation and may include deficient asepsis, irregular use of the maximum barrier protections or ultrasound-guided venipuncture, lack of attention to the position of the tip and securement with stitches instead of sutureless devices. On the contrary, the insertion of PICCs is often assigned to dedicated teams and thus carried out in a rather consistent fashion, following the evidence-based recommendations of the guidelines (SIP protocol of GAVeCeLT, Table 1.2). This has a significant impact on the risk of complications. In other words, if CICCs are often associated with immediate, early or delayed complications, this is in large part due to the lack of a defined insertion policy *(*bundle insertion*)* or more precisely to the inability or disinterest towards adopting defined insertion protocols (such as, for example, the SICA protocol) shown by the personnel in charge of inserting CICC. Such disinterest derives from the fact that many CICCs are inserted by "occasional" users, who practice this manoeuvre episodically, rather than by "dedicated" uses, such as clinicians in hospital teams dedicated to central

Table 1.2 Safe insertion of PICCs (SIP Protocol, GAVeCeLT 2010)
1. Hand hygiene, aseptic technique and maximum barrier precautions
2. Ultrasound exploration of all the veins of the arm and neck
3. Selection of the most appropriate vein in terms of calibre, position and depth
4. Clear ultrasound identification of the median nerve and the brachial artery
5. Ultrasound-guided venipuncture
6. Ultrasound control of the internal jugular vein during catheter progressionUse of intracavity ECG method for checking tip positionSecurement of the catheter by means of a *sutureless device*

accesses or anaesthesiologists who work in intensive care units with high volumes of central access practices.

- *Insertion times:* CICC deployment is faster than PICCs, because the direct Seldinger technique is used rather than the modified Seldinger technique, and the central positioning of the tip is simpler and more rapid. This makes PICCs unsuitable in emergency/urgent care situations where venous accesses are to be placed as quickly as possible. The PICC placement manoeuvre in clinical practice should always be planned and performed as a non-emergency manoeuvre. In many situations, the emergency indication for venous access is related to the need to immediately administer certain drugs or fluids to restore blood volume: in this case, the most appropriate access is a peripheral route, such as large calibre needle cannulas (14 G or 16 G); if the peripheral veins are not available, the best (and fastest) choice is the placement of a venous access by the femoral route (FICC), as recommended by ATLS protocols, for example. It must be underlined that, according to international guidelines, any venous access inserted in emergency settings should be removed within 48 hours: the insertion of a PICC would not therefore be cost-effective.
- *Limits to the possibility of insertion:* CICCs can be placed in almost any patient, especially if using the appropriate method under ultra-sound guidance: an adequate rapid ultrasound scan of the central veins (so-called RaCeVA, Rapid Central Vein Assessment) enables to identify the available options to be considered (internal jugular, innominate, subclavian, axillary veins) and to choose the easiest and most suitable vein for each situation. The possibility of inserting a PICC may be limited by the presence of systemic contraindications (chronic renal failure stage 3b, 4 or 5, i.e. patients with arteriovenous fistula for haemodialysis or potential candidates to a fistula) or by local contraindications (skeletal, skin and lymphatic alterations of the arm; absence of veins of an appropriate diameter). The temporary immobility of the upper limb consequent to the pharmacological sedation of the patient is not a contraindication for the placement of a PICC (especially if the patient is passively mobilised); a neurologically based paralysis of the limb (paraplegia, ALS etc.) is,

however, a contraindication for a PICC, especially if long standing (paralysis associated with muscular atrophy leads to hypoplasia of the deep veins of the arm with venous stasis, and therefore to a greater risk of thrombosis). Another important limit is represented by the diameter of the available veins; as will be explained more in depth in Chapter 2, PICCs should be inserted in veins with an internal diameter at least equal to three times the external diameter of the catheter. For example, if a 5 or 6 Fr catheter is to be used, a vein with an internal diameter (assessed by ultrasound) equal to 15 Fr (= 5 mm) or 18 Fr (= 6 mm) will be required. In the absence of deep veins with appropriate diameter in the middle third of the arm, it is possible to puncture and cannulate veins in the proximal third (Dawson's "yellow zone", see Appendix III), tunneling the PICC subcutaneously in order to obtain the exit site in the middle third (Dawson's "green zone", see Appendix III). The tunneling technique, which will be explained in detail in Chapter 5, increases the indications for PICCs by allowing safe insertion in patients who do not have veins of the appropriate diameter in the traditional area of venipuncture (i.e. the middle third of the arm).

- *Complications on insertion:* CICCs show a significant incidence of insertion-related complications that can, however, be minimised by consistently using ultrasound guidance; PICCs have no or negligible insertion-related complications. Specifically, notwithstanding the use of ultrasound guidance, the risk of hemorrhagic complications during CICC insertion is considered prohibitive in patients with severe abnormalities of coagulation. According to BCSH 2007 guidelines (Appendix IV) in patients with a platelet count <9000 or with INR >3, only PICCs should be considered as central access option (FICCs and CICCs are contraindicated).
- *Exit site:* CICC exit site lies in the cervical, supraclavicular or infraclavicular area, depending on the venous approach selected, whereas PICC exit site lies in the middle third of the arm (Dawson's "green zone", Appendix III). This is a significant difference: as described above, the exit site has significant impact on the risk of infective, thrombotic or mechanical complications; as a result, the preferable exit sites are placed in the middle third of the arm or in the infraclavicular area, since they are associated with a lower risk of contamination by pathogenic bacteria (minimal for the exit in the arm), higher catheter stability and greater ease in dressing management (Figure 1.14). In intensive care units, the placement of a central venous access with exit site in the middle third of the arm (i.e., a PICC) can be especially indicated in patients with tracheotomy or injuries, infections or other diseases of the head and neck, patients with neck collars, Halo-type orthopaedic devices, helmets for non-invasive mechanical ventilation (NIV) and other conditions that make access to the neck or base of the neck difficult.
- *Infective risk:* the majority of the most recent literature data suggest that CICCs have a higher risk of catheter-related bacteraemic infections than PICCs; although this statement cannot be generalised, it appears to be true, especially in tracheotomy patients or when the CICC exit site is in the middle or upper cervical region, and/or especially when the CICC is positioned without following the international recommendations for infection prevention (2% chlorhexidine, maximum barrier

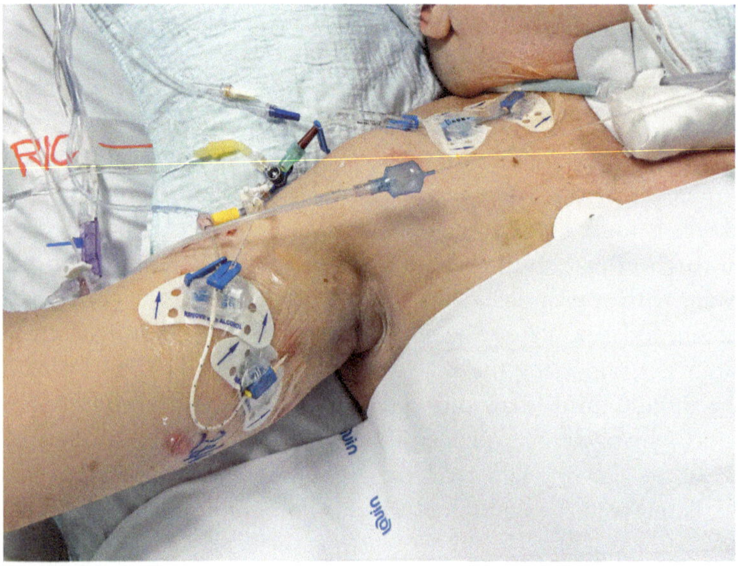

Figure **1.14**

precautions, ultrasound guidance, sutureless securement; see SICA protocol, Table 1.1). It is no coincidence that the recent EPIC 2014 guidelines (see Appendix IV), focused on the prevention of infective complications, recommend (a) to consider the potential infective risk associated with certain sites when choosing the central access exit site, (b) to use PICCs as the first option, rather than CICCs.

- *Thrombotic risk:* the majority of the most recent literature data suggest that PICCs show a higher risk of venous thrombosis on average than CICCs, especially in onco-haematological patients and when the PICC is positioned without following the international recommendations for the prevention of venous thrombosis (appropriate ratio between the catheter's diameter and the diameter of the vein, use of ultrasound guidance, appropriate positioning of the tip, adequate catheter stabilisation at the exit site; see SIP protocol, Table 1.2).

From the foregoing comparative considerations, some conclusions can be drawn on the indications for PICCs (rather than CICCs) in patients in intensive care:

- When considering infective risk, PICCs seem to be preferred to CICCs, while CICCs seem to be preferred to PICCs as far as thrombotic risk is concerned. However, the adoption of a correct insertion protocol (for example, SIP protocol and SICA protocol) is likely to minimise or erase these differences.
- In intensive care, specific clinical situations call for a preferential (and sometimes mandatory) indication for PICCs: the presence of a tracheotomy; the high infective risk of an exit site in the cervical or supra-/infraclavicular region; a compromised coagulation state; the forecast of a prolonged stay in intensive care; practical obstacles in

using the cervical/clavicular area due to the presence of special devices (collars, NIV helmets etc.).

- On the other hand, the placement of a PICC is certainly contraindicated and a CICC (or FICC) is undoubtedly preferred in other clinical situations: the need for a central venous access in emergency/urgent care conditions; the expected need for central access with more than 3 lumina; the existence of specific systemic or local contra-indications to PICC placement (structural alterations of the limb; unavailability of veins with suitable calibres; paraplegia; chronic renal failure with arteriovenous fistula already in place or expected); the need to carry out blood/plasma exchange procedures (haemodialysis, apheresis, diafiltration, etc.); the indication for a catheter coated with antiseptics or antibiotics.

PICCs and Midlines in pediatric patients

PICC and Midline-type peripherally inserted venous accesses became part of pediatric clinical practice only very recently and, specifically, after the advent of ultrasound guidance technology (that is, what we named as "echo-PICC"). Firstly, it is essential to distinguish between proper PICCs – as defined in the introduction to this manual – and the peripherally inserted central catheters that have long been used in newborns and that should, more appropriately, be called "Epicutaneo-Caval Catheters", or ECC. The placement of a PICC in the arm of a pediatric patient is only possible in the presence of a vein having a diameter of at least 3 mm (as explained in Chapter 2, the PICC receiving vein should have an internal diameter at least three times the external diameter (i.e., the calibre) of the catheter: therefore, since the smallest catheters that can currently be inserted by the ultrasound-guided technique are 3 Fr in calibre, a vein of at least 9 Fr = 3 mm must be available). In the vast majority of cases, the occurrence of a vein larger than 3 mm in the arm of a newborn or infant is rare and that makes the option of inserting a PICC by ultrasound guidance in this age range unlikely. In newborns, however, EECs are currently used, typically in intensive care and generally for purely infusion purposes. In practice, ECCs and PICCs are quite dissimilar devices for venous access (Table 1.3):

- ECCs are inserted by direct sight (or with the aid of Near-Infrared technologies that highlight veins running a few millimetres below the surface) into the superficial veins of the limbs or scalp; these are small calibre catheters (from 1 to 2.7 Fr) and, as such, do not allow for high flows and are unsuitable for blood sampling and haemodynamic monitoring; the final position of the tip is often not really central;
- PICCs, as explained above, are inserted by means of ultrasound-guided venipuncture with the indirect Seldinger technique in the deep veins of the arm; these are catheters with a diameter of 3 Fr and more, the tip of which should be strictly central (or close to the cavoatrial junction) and are ideal for high-flow infusions, blood sampling and haemodynamic monitoring, especially if they are power injectable.

The use of PICCs and Midlines is ideal in patients of pediatric age, since such patients limit the possibility of imaging and cannulating the superficial veins and require an appropriate use of techniques to position central venous access with minimum or zero risk.

Table 1.3 ECC vs PICC

Epicutaneo-Caval Catheters (ECC)	Echo-PICC
• Newborns • Direct insertion or NIR • Superficial veins • Tip not always central • 1-2.7 Fr calibre • Low flows • Not suitable for haemodynamic monitoring • Not suitable for blood sampling	• Children • Ultrasound guidance • Deep veins of the arm • Tip at the cavoatrial junction • 3 Fr calibre or higher • High flows (power injectable) • Suitable for haemodynamic monitoring • Suitable for blood sampling

PICC field of use covers hospitalised pediatric patients (in intensive care, pediatric surgery, pediatric onco-haematology, etc.), those at home (on home parenteral nutrition for gastrointestinal diseases) and those treated in day-hospital setting for oncological diseases of various types.

In acutely ill patients, in the emergency/urgent phase the necessity for rapid fluid infusion may require the placement of a device for intraosseous infusion or a peripheral venous access (needle cannula) placed in a superficial vein directly or with the help of Near-Infrared technology or, at the most, of a femoral venous access placed by ultrasound guidance. Nevertheless, once the general conditions have been stabilised and the child is in the intensive care unit, a PICC type central access is the ideal solution, especially if power injectable PICCs are chosen, since they allow high velocity fluid infusion (1-2 mL/sec for each lumen), reliable measurement of the central venous pressure, repeated execution of blood sampling and use of double lumen devices. 3 Fr single lumen PICCs (Figure 1.15) and 4 Fr double lumen PICCs (Figure 1.16) are the most frequently used devices in pediatric patients and their insertion requires deep veins of the arm having a calibre greater than 3 mm and 4 mm, respectively. The manoeuvre can often be carried out without sedation (in teenagers) or under light sedation (in younger children), without necessarily resorting to a full general anesthesia. The indication for peripherally inserted central venous access becomes mandatory in pediatric patients (for example, with haematological diseases) with thrombocytopenia. The presence of a tracheotomy is another firm indication for the use of a PICC rather than a CICC in a acutely ill pediatric patient.

In pediatric intensive care, there are few indications for Midlines. They can be useful in relatively stable patients with no indication for haemodynamic monitoring or the need for repeated blood samples, but needing a stable peripheral venous access. As it is always the case with Midlines, this device should not be used for parenteral nutrition infusions, especially if highly hyperosmolar (>800 mOsm/L), drugs with a pH greater than 9 or less than 5 or drugs considered vesicant or irritants for the endothelium (see Appendix I for the drugs most commonly used intravenously in relation to their phlebitic risk). The use of power injectable PICCs is mandatory in critically ill pediatric patients and in

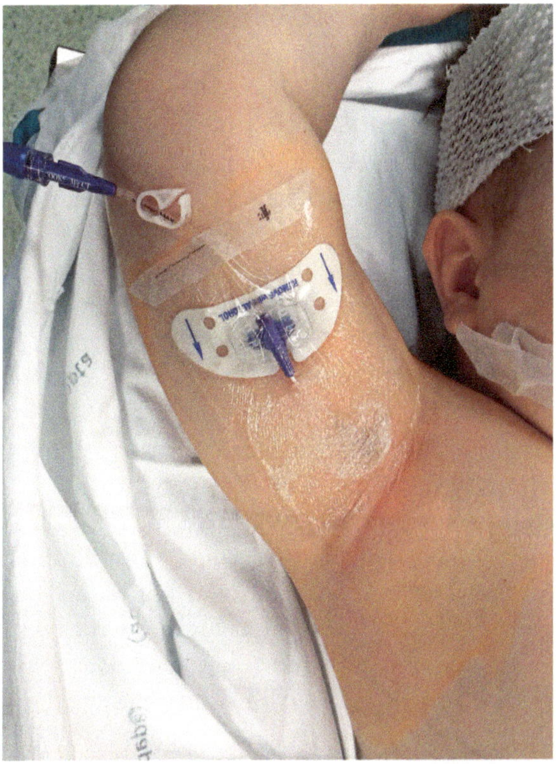

Figure **1.15**

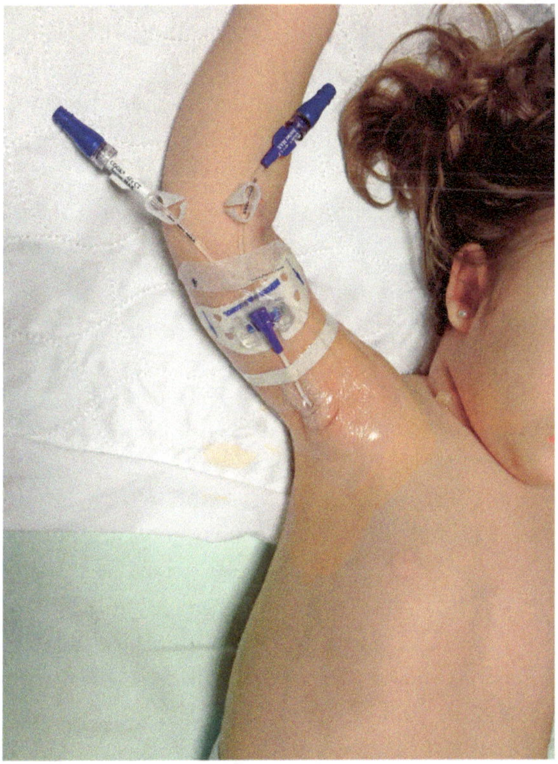

Figure **1.16**

children candidates for radiological examinations with intravenous contrast medium, the injection of which is carried out by pumps that generate high pressures (so-called *power injectors)*.

For children hospitalised in non-intensive department, PICCs have now become the preferred central access, typically indicated in children with chronic, neurologic or oncologic diseases who need central access for parenteral nutrition, chemotherapy or antibiotic treatment with irritant drugs. The use of power injectable non-valved PICCs (made of third-generation polyurethane) is also highly recommended in these categories of non-critical patients. It must be noted that, especially in pediatric patients, it is important to use power injectable PICCs, as they have a low risk of displacement or obstruction and are particularly resistant to mechanical trauma.

As previously mentioned, another important indication for PICCs in pediatric age patients is the need for venous access, either continuous (such as, for example, home parenteral nutrition) or discontinuous (such as, for example, children treated on a day-hospital basis for oncological and haematological diseases) outside the hospital. In this field, PICCs have proved particularly suitable as medium-term access (for months): the need for long-term venous access leads, on the other hand, to an indication for a tunneled-cuffed catheter (TCC) in the case of relatively frequent access (more than once a week) or for a port, i.e a totally implanted venous access device, in the case of relatively episodic access (less than once a week). As with adults, TCCs can be inserted in a central vein, in the femoral vein or in a vein in the arm: in the latter case, this would be a tunneled-cuffed PICC. When access is very frequent, such as, for example, with home parenteral nutrition, the presence of a catheter in the arm (PICC, tunneled PICC and tunneled-cuffed PICC) will have both benefits and disadvantages: the main disadvantage is the possible interference with the child's physical activities, while the main benefit is the greater ease in managing dressing changes and personal hygiene compared to central catheters positioned in central veins.

The PICC insertion technique in pediatric patients does not substantially differ from the technique we will describe below for adult patients. Such technique is based on ultrasound examination of the veins before the manoeuvre, ultrasound-guided puncture and cannulation of a deep vein in the arm (basilic, brachial or axillary), intraprocedural verification of the tip position by intracavitary ECG technique and adequate external stabilisation of the catheter, preferably using *sutureless* devices, adhesive transparent membrane and histoacryl glue. The adoption of the intracavitary ECG technique is particularly important, given the unreliability of the skin markers in establishing the length of the catheter in children and considering the need of avoiding fluoroscopy, which implies x-ray exposure. On the other hand, the intracavitary ECG method has great accuracy in pediatric patients and is always feasible (given the rarity of cardiac diseases in children that can impede the visualisation of the P wave).

It is underlined that contraindications for the PICC placement in children are the same as in adults: emergency venous access insertion, bilateral absence of deep veins of sufficient calibre in the arm, presence of bilateral alterations of the limb (burns, fractures etc.).

A particular aspect of PICCs in pediatric patients is represented by the off -label use of

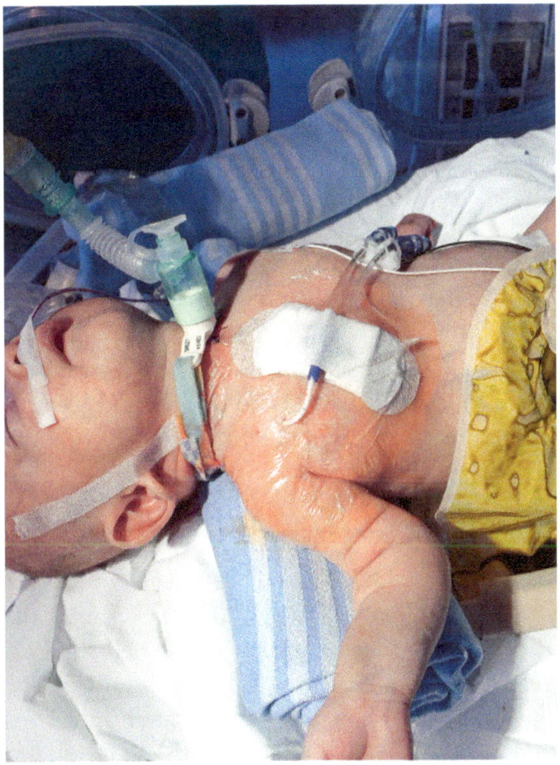

Figure **1.17**

this device as a central venous catheter in central veins (axillary, internal jugular, external jugular, innominate and subclavian) (Figure 1.17): this will be dealt with below (in Chapter 5). For now, it will be sufficient to underline that the particularly biocompatible material, the power injectability, the versatility in terms of length, the possibility of tunneling, the lesser trauma associated with the micro-introducer technique and the modified Seldinger technique make PICCs preferable by a long way to the catheters currently sold as pediatric CICCs.

PICCs and Midlines in patients in home care

National and international guidelines unanimously advise against the use of short-term venous access devices (needle cannulas, non-tunneled CICCs) in home care – or, in any event, outside hospital – due to the special surveillance required by these types of devices and by the high risk of complications (infective, thrombotic, occlusive, mechanical) which is associated with their use in the extra-hospital setting.
The only appropriate venous access devices for use outside the hospital (home, hospice, outpatient clinic, day hospital) are medium-term (Midlines, PICCs, uncuffed-tunneled CICC) and long-term devices (cuffed-tunneled central venous catheters; ports) (Table 1.4).

The low usage versatility limits the use of Midlines outside the hospital. The insertion and management of a Midline at home are undoubtedly feasible and bear minimum risk for the patient, but do require for healthcare personnel to pay extra care to the type of drugs and solutions infused through the device. For example, a Midline placed for the administration of home parenteral nutrition with solutions <800 mOsm/L may become dangerous if a change in the patient's clinical conditions requires a different nutritional solution of greater osmolarity (and therefore unsuitable for peripheral access). It should be noted that the position of the Midline's tip (which necessarily lies in the axillary and subclavian veins) is associated with thrombotic complications in case of inappropriate infusions and such complications are more severe than the thrombosis caused by other shorter peripheral venous access devices (such as needle cannulas or long peripheral cannulas). Moreover, Midlines as a form of peripheral access are not considered ideal for blood sampling. Their role is therefore limited to home care patients who do not require antiblastic chemotherapy, parenteral nutrition or intravenous infusion of irritant drugs (such as many antibiotics, anticonvulsants, vasoactives, etc.), but only hydration and/or administration of analgesics, preferably for limited periods of time. One potential advantage of Midlines compared to PICCs is the relatively simpler insertion, that does not require to assess the tip position; from an economic standpoint, however, the total cost of insertion (including the need for specially-trained insertion personnel) does not differ significantly from the cost of inserting a PICC. In substance, therefore, for most venous accesses at home or in day hospitals, a central line is preferable. In such situations, choosing the most appropriate central venous access device is based on the duration and frequency of use.

Table 1.4 Appropriate devices for use outside the hospital

	Tipo di dispositivo	Posizione della punta
Medium-term access	Midline	Peripheral
	PICC	Central
	Tunneled PICC	Central
	Tunneled CICC	Central
	Tunneled FICC	In inferior vena cava
	Hohn	Central
Long-term access	Central port	Central
	Brachial port (PICC-port)	Central
	Cuffed tunneled CICC	Central
	Cuffed tunneled PICC	Central
	Cuffed tunneled FICC	In inferior vena cava

For periods of time limited to a few months, most guidelines suggest the use of medium-term central venous access devices (PICCs, tunneled CICCs, Hohn). PICC is actually the ideal central venous access for administering intravenous treatments for weeks or months (up to 4-5 months) in extra-hospital settings, both in its classic definition (insertion in a deep vein of the arm) and in its off-label use (insertion in the axillary, subclavian, internal jugular, innominate or femoral vein). In many of these situations (and mandatorily in the case of the femoral approach), it will be appropriate to tunnel the PICC to move the exit site to a more adequate location. Tunneling has a positive effect (direct and indirect) in protecting the catheter from potential bacterial contamination, and this can theoretically prolong the expected duration of the device. PICCs, tunneled or non-tunneled, will therefore be the ideal medium-term venous access, for example, for oncological patients in palliative care.

The use of Hohn catheters (CICCs made of silicone) as medium-term central venous access has been gradually abandoned due to their high incidence of mechanical complications (displacement and ruptures) and their low cost-effectiveness.

In the case of central venous access required for months or years and, in any case, for periods >4-5 months, long-term venous access devices, such as tunneled-cuffed catheters (TCC) or ports, must be used. In the case of frequency of use equal to or less than once a week, the ideal access will be a port, which can be inserted in a vein in the infra/supraclavicular area (chest port) (Figure 1.18) or – more rarely, in special clinical situations – in a deep vein of the arm (brachial port or PICC-port) (Figure 1.19). In the case of chest ports, the reservoir (usually connected with a 6-7 Fr catheter in silicone) is placed in the infraclavicular area; in the case of PICC-ports, the reservoir is smaller, connected with a

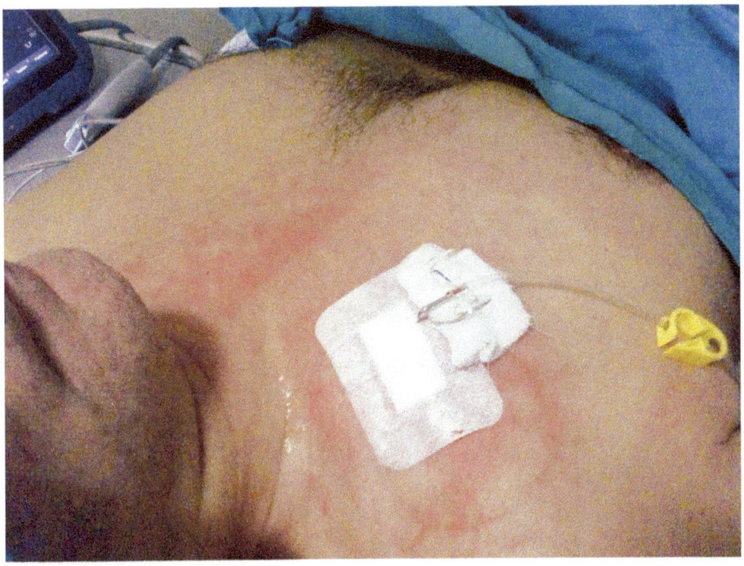

Figure **1.18**

4-5 Fr catheter (preferably in polyurethane), and is placed above the biceps muscle. The use of ports for chemotherapy is ideal in outpatient clinics or day-hospitals, when discontinuous treatments (typically, every 15-20 days) are expected to last for at least 6 months. If the expected use is more frequent than once a week, it is advisable to insert a tunneled-cuffed central catheter (TCC) by ultrasound-guided puncture of a vein in the infra/supraclavicular area (with exit site also below the clavicle) (Figure 1.20), of a deep vein of the arm (exit site at midarm) or of a femoral vein (exit site in the abdominal region or close to the knee). Tunneling provides direct and indirect protection from the risk of bacterial contamination; the presence of the cuff stabilises the catheter. TCCs in power injectable polyurethane (Pro-Line type) are preferable to silicone TCCs (Groshong, Hickman or Broviac): silicone has no advantages over power injectable polyurethane in terms of risk of infective or thrombotic complications but certainly does present a higher risk of mechanical complications (displacements, ruptures, tip migration) due to the greater fragility of the material. The use of TCCs is typical for patients who are candidates for indefinite home parenteral nutrition for benign diseases. As mentioned, it is possible to insert tunneled cuffed catheters in the arm (cuffed PICCs) and they will offer, to all intents and purposes, long-term access to prolonged periods and/or indefinitely.

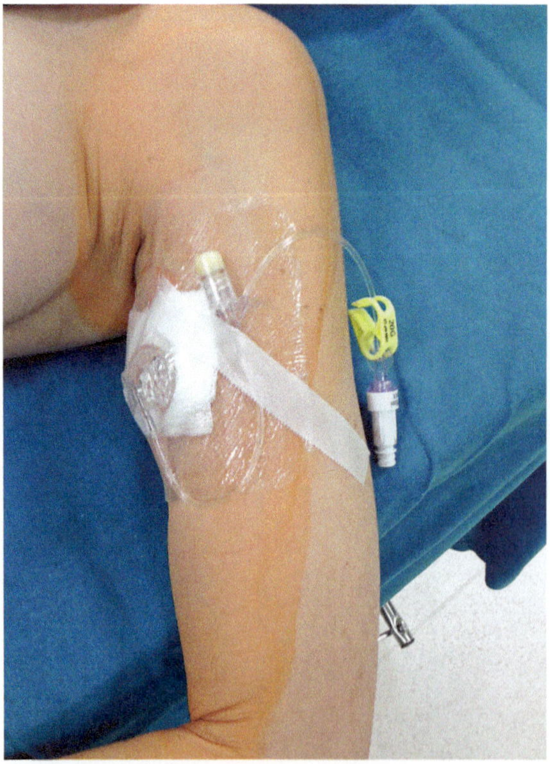

Figure **1.19**

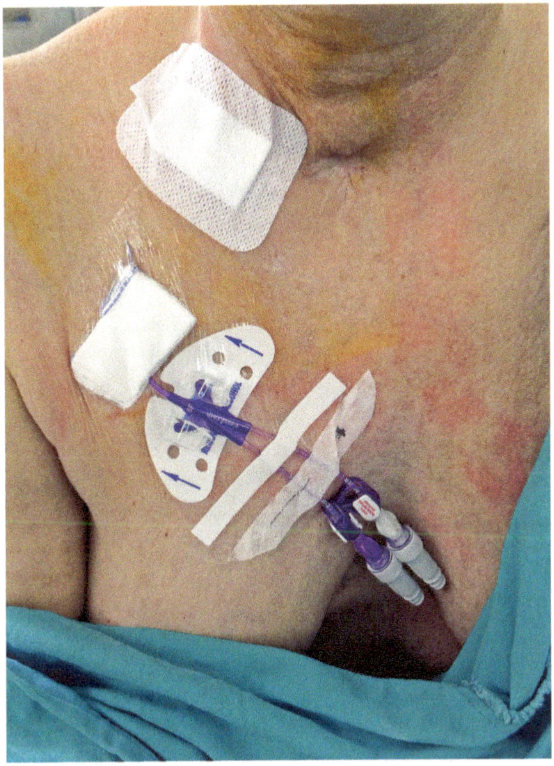

Figure **1.20**

Table 1.4 shows a possible classification of extra-hospital venous accesses compared to the expected duration.

A complete algorithm for the appropriate choice of venous accesses both inside and outside the hospital is given in Appendix II.

Cost-effectiveness of PICCs and PICC Team

The high cost-effectiveness of PICCs is perhaps the major reason for their success in clinical practice. Before analysing this point, it is necessary to clarify the meaning of cost-effectiveness.

A device can be considered effective when it reaches the clinical goal for which it is designated and used; it is efficient when it reaches the set clinical goal with limited resource use or, in any event, without wasting any resources; it is cost-effective when it offers an advantage in terms of the ratio between the resources used and the clinical goal reached. Clearly, cost-effectiveness and efficiency are not the primary objectives of our clinical practice: patient's safety comes first, of course. It is also true that these goals are not in conflict: devices associated with greater safety for the patient actually reduce the risk of complications, which constitute the true "cost" of venous access, and therefore generally increase cost-effectiveness.

By examining the factors that influence device cost-effectiveness, we can schematically list three kinds of problems: (1) resources used for its insertion (in terms of materials, time, location, equipment, human resources, etc.); (2) resources used for its management (again, in terms of materials, time, human resources, etc.); (3) costs of "expected" complications both at the time of insertion and during management, estimated on the basis of the percentage risk taken from the literature. From this, it is clear that it is wrong to compare two devices only in terms of their mere cost, since it is not related to the actual "cost" for the insertion (which depends on many other factors), nor is it linked to the real overall "cost" of the device in terms of use. Pharmacoeconomics compare different clinical "strategies", not different devices.

Actually, the cost for the device for venous access is included in the costs for the insertion, to which, however, it is necessary to add the costs for other materials required, the equipment deemed appropriate or necessary (ultrasound, fluoroscopy, ECG monitor, etc.), human resources (variable, depending on whether the person who carries out the insertion is a nurse, a surgeon, a radiologist or an anesthesiologist, etc.), as well as the cost of the location where the device is inserted (in fact, the cost of a bedside insertion greatly differs from an insertion that requires a dedicated location, or even an operating theatre or X-ray room).When comparing two different devices, the costs for their management should also be taken into account: that is, the cost for the materials required (dressing change kit, etc.), the frequency and type of management required for that device (weekly or multi-weekly frequency of dressing change and flushing, etc.) and the human resources required for the management (nurse, doctor, caregiver, etc.). Finally, the costs for "expected" insertion-related complications, both immediate (arrhythmias, failure of the procedure, prolonged time of the procedure, waste of material, etc.) and delayed (venous thrombosis, pinch-off, displacement, etc.), must be added to "expected" management-related complications (infections, lumen occlusions, displacement, ruptures, etc.). It is advisable to spend some time analysing this point. A cost-effectiveness analysis must add to the real complications (objective risks for the patient) those undesired events that, although not harmful to patients, are associated with excessive costs for a hospital or, in any event, with an anomalous cost-effectiveness ratio or with poor results in terms of the ratio between resource use and hospital efficiency.

Examples of true clinical complications following the placement of a central venous access are pneumothorax (typically by accidental puncture of the pleura during "blind" subclavian venipuncture by infraclavicular route while placing a CICC), multiple and repeated attempts to venipuncture (with the consequent potential increase of the infective and haemorrhagic risk, plus the discomfort for the patient from the manoeuvre), accidental arterial puncture (with the potential risk of haematoma or even haemothorax in the case of a CICC), accidental nerve puncture with the possibility of transient or permanent damage (possible injury to the median nerve when inserting a PICC or to the brachial plexus when inserting a CICC), arrhythmias (typically during manoeuvres with the metallic guidewire), pain during insertion or in the first 48 hours (due to repeated punctures, inappropriate anaesthesia, etc.), the occurrence of early post-insertion infection (often due to improper asepsis during the procedure), *pinch-off* syndrome (which typically arises some time after the insertion of a port or a TCC with silicone catheter by means of "blind" infraclavicular puncture of the subclavian vein, and which causes device malfunction, catheter injury and sometimes embolization of a fragment of the catheter), the so-called "complex regional pain syndrome" (CRPS, typically after difficult venous cannulations and repeated punctures), catheter-related venous thrombosis (secondary to tip malposition, i.e. when the catheter tip is not positioned close to the cavoatrial junction, or to the improper choice of a catheter too large if compared to the calibre of the vein).
Alongside these objective risks for the patient, which may vary depending on the choice of the device and the insertion method, for example, other undesired events occurring may cause excessive costs for the health service or result in an irregular cost-effectiveness ratio. Such circumstances include: the inappropriate choice of a certain device (for example, the choice of a long-term device in a patient who needs a short-term access or the insertion of a device with a high risk of infection in an immunosuppressed patient), the long waiting list for insertion (for example, a long waiting list for long-terms access, which may delay the start of chemotherapy or the transfer of the patient to a hospice or homecare), the excessive cost of the insertion manoeuvre (due to an inappropriate location choice, such as, for example, the use of an operating theatre for a device that can be inserted at the bedside, or prolonged insertion times, typically from difficulties arising during "blind" venipuncture without ultrasound, or an excessive consumption of material for repeated attempts and/or failure of the manoeuvre, with the consequent waste of needle and guidewire and/or use of an additional kit), the failure of the procedure itself (which leads to the need for rescheduling and delays the beginning of the therapy), the early displacement of the device due to inappropriate stabilisation (as for TCCs when the cuff is positioned too close to the skin or for non-tunneled PICCs and CICCs when the securement is insufficient), the need for early replacement and/or removal of the device due to malpositioning or malfunctioning (primary tip malpositioning, external tract kinking, errors during tunneling, etc.).
It is therefore clear, that, in order to optimise the cost-effectiveness of a device, a multimodal strategy is required:

- selection of materials and methods that increase patient safety while reducing complications;

- appropriate choice of the device type;
- use of the operating theatre only for insertions that mandatorily require general anaesthesia and/or fluoroscopy;
- consistent adoption of equipments that make the procedure easier, quicker and safer;
- definition of a specific group of professionals for CICC and PICC insertion in hospitalised patients (dedicated team);
- definition of a specific procedure for implementing medium to long-term access (PICC, TCC and ports) in candidates to treatment in day-hospital, hospice or home care (for each procedure, specific policies are warranted to define reference team, waiting list method, place designed for the insertion, insertion team, place and team designed for handling post-insertion complications, etc.);
- appropriate training of all physicians and nurses in charge of inserting and managing central venous access devices.

In particular, it is therefore possible to optimise the overall cost-effectiveness of PICCs by applying the following strategies:

1. *Appropriate choice of the specific PICC:* the market offers PICCs in various materials but power injectable PICCs made of third-generation polyurethane are preferable, since they cost less than silicone, are more versatile to use and cause fewer potentially expensive complications (such as ruptures, lumen occlusions, displacements, etc.); the use of PICCs with proximal or distal valves is not recommended, since there is no scientific evidence that any valve may be effective in reducing complications, even though it increases the device cost by 50-150%; finally, the micro-introduction kit quality is also relevant, since this is probably the major factor determining the success of the manoeuvre.
2. *Choice of the appropriate insertion technique:* scientific literature indicates as fundamental points for optimising the cost-effectiveness of the insertion (a) an aseptic technique based on the use of 2% chlorhexidine and maximum barrier precautions (for the purpose of minimising the risk of infections), (b) the use of ultrasound for venipuncture and the control of the catheter progression (to reduce the risk of failures and/or repeated punctures), (c) the use of the intracavitary ECG method (to exclude the risk of primary tip malposition), (d) the appropriate catheter securement by means of sutureless devices, transparent membranes, etc. (for the purpose of reducing the risk of displacements). All such recommendations should be included in an insertion bundle such as the one proposed by GAVeCeLT as "SIP protocol" (see Table 1.2).
3. *Appropriate choice of the insertion site:* PICCs attain the maximum cost-effectiveness when inserted bedside or in a dedicated, low-cost location (outpatient room, day-hospital room, etc.); the programmatic choice of inserting PICCs in the operating theatre or in the radiology suite does not increase the insertion safety while greatly reducing its cost-effectiveness.
4. *Appropriate choice of the professional figure dedicated to insertion:* PICCs show maximum cost-effectiveness when the insertion is mainly assigned to professional nurses rather than physicians, anesthesiologists or radiologists, and preferably

when the inserters are structured as a "PICC Team" (see later in this chapter); obviously, the cost-effectiveness will be greatest when all the personnel dedicated to insertion is adequately trained, according to the criteria set out by the WoCoVA Consensus published in 2012.

Cost-effectiveness of PICCs in a hospital setting

In a hospital setting, the choice of central venous access falls inevitably on a short-term device as a CICC or on a short/medium-term device as a PICC. Comparing CICCs and PICCs in terms of costs: (1) PICCs cost less at insertion (as long as the insertion is performed by a nurse at the bedside), notwithstanding the higher cost of the kit; (2) PICCs cost less in terms of insertion complications, that are virtually absent for PICCs, while can be severe and expensive for CICCs (for example, the average cost for treating a single episode of pneumothorax stands at around 5,000 euros); (3) PICCs cost less in terms of infective complications, considering that the incidence of CRBSI is approximately 0.3 – 1 episodes for 1,000 catheter days for PICCs and around 2-3 episodes for 1,000 catheter days for CICCs (each individual episode of CRBSI costs around 7,000 – 14,000 euros).

The latter point is one of the factors underlying the greater cost-effectiveness of PICCs compared to CICCs. Although the topic is still controversial, data from literature show a consistently lower incidence of CRBSI for PICCs (and especially for ultrasound-placed PICCs), probably due to a series of different reasons: the distance of the exit site from nasal/oral/tracheal secretions, the low degree of local microbial contamination and the physical characteristics of the skin of the arm, as well as the great ease in keeping the dressing stable and clean. A crucial fact could be that most PICCs are inserted following quite strict protocols, usually including the main recommendations on infection prevention (skin antisepsis with 2% chlorhexidine, maximum barrier precautions, etc.), whereas most CICCs are still inserted in a less rigorous manner in terms of precautions against infections. It is no coincidence that the recent EPIC guidelines – focused on infection prevention – recommend the preferential use of PICCs rather than CICCs, in the absence of local contraindications.

Apart from the advantage in terms of infections (that is not, however, associated with an advantage in terms of thrombosis, as mentioned above), the use of PICCs is associated with other "added" values: PICC insertion is virtually risk-free even patients in poor cardiorespiratory or coagulative condition (for example, according to the BCSH guidelines, PICCs are the only central access allowed in patients with severe thrombocytopenia); as medium-term central access, PICCs are expected to last longer than CICCs and are also appropriate for extra-hospital use (unlike CICCs).

In short, where a "PICC Team" is operating or where, in any event, there is an adequate hospital project for inserting PICCs, the first option for central access in hospital should be a PICC. As previously mentioned, the use of CICCs should be taken into consideration (a) in the case of local bilateral contraindications to the insertion of a brachial access (calibre of veins too small, fractures, burns, chronic paralysis, axillary lymph node resection, etc.), (b) in patients on chronic dialysis or candidates for dialysis, (c) in emergency situations in the operating theatre or in the intensive care unit, when a rapid-insertion central access is required for rapid blood volume repletion, (d) when the need for multiple lumina (>3) is expected, or (e) when a femoral access is indicated (mediastinal syndromes).

Hospital strategies aiming at cost-effectiveness

As mentioned, in the field of PICC-type short-term central venous access devices and, more generally, in the field of venous access for in-hospital infusion treatments, it has been shown that a limited number of general strategies that can be implemented relatively simply allow not only to significantly reduce the risk of complications suffered by patients, but also to significantly decrease the costs (and, in any event, an improvement in the cost-effectiveness ratio) and improve hospital efficiency.

Definition of a hospital strategy for the correct indication of vascular access (proactive vascular planning) This can be achieved using an algorithm that considers the characteristics of each device for venous access (central or peripheral, short-, medium- or long-term) and the complications potentially associated with it, and then chooses the venous access associated with the lowest risk of complications and the best clinical performance for any clinical situation, ensuring it is inserted at the right time in the most appropriate clinical phase. Examples:

- the timely insertion of a medium-term access (brachial PICC or Midline) in a patient who requires one or more weeks of in-hospital intravenous treatment enables the reduction of complications linked to the progressive depletion of the peripheral veins and avoids the forced recourse to a short-term central venous access (associated with more significant complications than a brachial access).
- in a patient who must be discharged with a venous access because he/she is a candidate for palliative care at home or in hospice for a period of a few weeks or months, the insertion of a PICC will imply significant savings in terms of costs and complications compared to a long-term access;
- in a patient with a tracheostomy or with a high risk of infection, the insertion of a brachial catheter will reduce the risk of septic complications compared to a catheter inserted in the cervical region.

Definition of the prerequisites for the insertion of venous access devices A series of structural and technical choices designed to minimise the incidence of mechanical and infective complications related to the device placement should be implemented. Obviously, insertion should be performed (especially in the field of medium and long-term accesses and, in particular, in the field of PICCs) by physicians and nurses specifically trained by means of appropriate courses (theoretical lessons, lab practice) and an adequate period of clinical training. The insertion by expert personnel significantly reduces not only the immediate complications linked to the insertion, but also a significant rate of complications that may appear later but are nevertheless linked to an incorrect insertion technique. Examples:

- the systematic adoption of ultrasound-guided venipuncture has been shown to be effective in reducing most of the complications linked to the insertion of any central venous access, leading to a significant improvement in the cost-effectiveness ratio;
- it has been shown that when the procedure is performed by specifically trained personnel is associated with a significant increase in procedural success, as well as a reduction in complications and costs.

Definition of the recommendations for the management of venous access devices

This can be implemented by defining and diffusely implementing hospital policies for venous access management. Such policies should be developed by a multidisciplinary group of local experts, based on specific national and international guidelines in the literature. Following these hospital policies, every clinical unit will be invited to define local protocols, tailored to the specific clinical needs of each unit and the specific devices used. In more recent times, it has been shown that an equally effective result can be obtained by defining one or more bundles of recommendations designed to minimise the risk of mechanical, thrombotic and infective complications (the latter being the most significant from an economical standpoint). These bundles collect a limited number of clinical recommendations, each one individually effective in reaching a specific goal – for example, the reduction of a certain complication – that, if implemented simultaneously and systematically, allow to reach an increasingly significant synergistic effect. For example, many international studies have shown that a systematic and continuous adoption of a simple bundle of few recommendations for preventing catheter-related infections led to a drastic reduction and sometimes even the elimination of the incidence of this complication, with significant clinical and economical benefits (reduction of mortality, complications, length of hospital stay and relative and absolute costs).

Many international studies in the last decade have also shown that the introduction in a hospital of a specific, dedicated venous access team leads to significant advantages in terms of safety, cost-effectiveness and efficiency.

The presence of a team (doctors and nurses or only nurses, depending on the type of venous access), such as, for example, a "PICC Team", enables:

- the complete and systematic implementation of a hospital-wide program of rational selection of devices *(proactive vascular planning)*, that includes the hospital pharmacy, so to purchase those devices with a better cost-effectiveness margin;
- the reduction of complications and costs related to insertion, thanks to the adoption of a standardised, shared technique, performed by experienced personnel with specific training;
- the implementation of a continuous service of counseling for venous access routine management (through identifying and implementing bundles or adequate operating protocols) and for extra-routine management of any infective, thrombotic, or mechanical complications;
- venous access cultural activities and educational training inside the hospital, with ongoing update of all procedures and protocols concerning the insertion and management of the devices.

In conclusion, the introduction of a "PICC Team" or a venous access-dedicated team not only increases patient safety by reducing many complications, but is also a crucial factor in reducing costs for managing hospital infusion treatments, through the following mechanisms:

- Reduction of the expense for purchasing devices and materials used:
  - increasing the rate of successful insertions reduces material waste;
  - preventing or effectively treating mechanical (obstructive) or infective complications that would usually lead to device loss reduces unscheduled procedures for removing devices;
  - implementing *proactive vascular planning* by careful selection of devices with better cost-effectiveness ratio.
- Reduction of the average duration of hospital stay:
  - reduction of the risk of catheter-related infections (which are constantly associated with a prolongation of the hospital stay);
  - systematic insertion of medium- or long-term devices that enable the patient to prolong certain intravenous treatments at home or on a day-hospital basis, plus the timely insertion of devices suitable for palliative treatments, allow to rapidly discharge patients and direct them to home care or hospice treatments;
  - reduction of the costs related to the working time of physicians and nurses inserting the devices.
- Reduction of the working time wasted by the nurses for repeated insertion of short-term peripheral access (needle cannulas).
- Reduction of the expenses related to the insertion of long-term devices by physicians, thanks to an appropriate implementation of brachial access (the insertion of which is mainly under the responsibility of nurses).
- Increase in efficiency:
  - minimisation of the waiting list for the insertion of medium- and long-term access;
  - possibility of implementing specific activities such as those connected to the management of oncological or haematological day-hospitals, centres for home artificial nutrition, optimisation of the perioperative care, and implementation of programmes of palliative care at home.

It is important to underline how the strategies listed above are simultaneously effective at several levels, in terms of safety, cost-effectiveness and efficiency.

Cost-effectiveness of PICCs outside the hospital setting

As mentioned above, PICCs are unparalleled as extra-hospital medium-term central access, as the Hohn catheter – usually classified as medium-term – shows a very low cost-effectiveness (it has a high cost but also a high incidence of complications, especially mechanical, such as ruptures and displacements).

In particular, in the field of palliative care (which typically requires a medium-term device), the adoption of a PICC-type central access also has clear cost-effectiveness compared to the use of peripheral venous or hypodermic access. In fact, the home use of needle cannula-type peripheral venous access, is not only inappropriate according to

most of the guidelines, but imposes strong limitations in terms of potential use, need for monitoring and periodic replacements, as well as a quite high incidence of several minor complications, such as thrombophlebitis, displacements and occlusions (estimated at around 150-200 events every 1,000 catheter days overall). On the other hand, hypodermoclysis involves the use of an uncomfortable and sometimes painful device for patients, with many limitations on usage and a high incidence of local complications and malfunctions (in 30-50% of cases), in addition to the obvious need for periodic replacements.
A recent cost-effectiveness simulation has demonstrated that PICCs, if compared to needle cannulas and hypodermoclysis, have indisputable benefits in patient management in palliative care, since they are associated with lower insertion and management costs, less working time for healthcare personnel and low costs connected to the treatment of expected complications. In this field, in fact, PICCs are a stable and reliable device that can be safely inserted – even at home – in the most fragile patients; PICCs do not need periodic replacement or close monitoring, require, on average, only a weekly dressing change and remain in the patient, in most cases, for the entire duration of palliative care. The economic advantage is also linked to the fact that device insertion, management and removal entirely depend on nurses working in the palliative care unit.
Long-term access (more than 4-6 months) is more complex. By definition, a long-term access device should be either cuffed (TCC) or equipped with a reservoir that can be implanted subcutaneously (chest port and brachial port, or PICC-port, which will be discussed in Chapter 5). Totally implantable ports should be limited to situations with long-term but infrequent access (less than once a week). For more frequent long term access, the choice is between silicone TCCs (for example, Hickman, Broviac, Leonard, cuffed Groshong) or power injectable polyurethane TCCs (for example, Pro-Line). In this regard, it should be noted that cuffed catheters in power injectable polyurethane completely revolutionised the world of TCCs, as they not only have great advantages compared to old silicone TCCs (greater resistance to mechanical complications, lower cost) but are highly versatile since they can be inserted either in central veins, in deep veins of the arm, or in the femoral vein (as CICCs, PICCs or FICCs, respectively, all cuffed and tunneled), depending on the clinical situation.
Recent data have shown that uncuffed PICCs can be used at home for long-term access as well, with remarkable advantages in terms of safety and cost-effectiveness. Recent retrospective and prospective studies have confirmed the possibility of the long duration of uncuffed PICCs, even for years, and comparison with TCCs has shown that the latter results in higher costs for insertion and complications. In this latter regard, PICCs have obvious benefits in terms of management in the event of mechanical or infective complications (they can be removed and replaced at home, unlike TCCs). Moreover, PICC stability can be increased by securing them with subcutaneously anchored sutureless devices (SecuraCath). In other words, an appropriately tunneled PICC secured with this device could potentially have the same advantages as a TCC, in terms of protection from infections and stability.
In conclusion, thanks to their cost-effectiveness, PICCs can today be regarded as the first choice for hospitalised patients who require central venous access and for patients treated

in home care settings or on a day-hospital basis - especially if they require a central venous access for extended but not indefinite periods - but also a possible and convenient option for selected patients who require venous access for frequent (more than once a week), long term or indefinite use.

PICC insertion to all patients, including those without palpable or visible veins, thereby overcoming a problem that until then had been an insuperable limit to the indication for PICCs.
In this form (which we named "ultrasound-PICC"), PICCs progressively spread not only in Anglo-Saxon countries, with North America at the forefront (currently, almost three millions of PICCs are sold every year in the United States, compared to around 100,000 ports, around 200,000 TCC and around 2,500,000 CICC) – but, in more recent times, also in continental Europe, particularly in Italy.
The **use of ultrasound** therefore underpins the advantages that now characterise PICCs as compared to CICCs. Indeed, ultrasound enables venipuncture of the deep veins of the middle third of the arm and no longer the antecubital superficial veins: this strategy not only allows the positioning of PICCs in patients whose superficial veins of the upper limb are neither visible nor palpable, but also allows the preparation of an exit site in an optimal position in terms of stability and ease of management (undoubtedly better than the one obtained with a non-tunneled CICC positioned in a supraclavicular site). Ultrasound-guided puncture also increases the possibility of the manoeuvremanoeuvre success to almost 100%, by minimising or eliminating failures and accidental injuries to arterial structures (brachial artery) or nerves (median nerve) that can now be identified and avoided through ultrasound examination.
The lower risk of severe bleeding complications also makes PICCs suitable for severely anticoagulated patients in whom CICC or FICC positioning would be dangerous. Finally, ultrasound visualisation allow to assess vein calibre and, as a consequence, to choose the most adequate catheter calibre.
This strategy is crucial for reducing thrombotic risk. It is important to underline that the use of ultrasound makes sense only if it includes (1) pre-insertion ultrasound examination of the arm, and (2) real-time ultrasound-guided venipuncture (that is, insertion of the needle in the vein under ultrasound control).
Unless an assessment of the anatomical conditions of the arm is made (position and size of the vascular and nerve structures), only a tiny part of the advantages of using ultrasound will be gained.
On the other hand, the use of ultrasound to localise the vein for "blind" puncture (so-called "ultrasound-assisted" venipuncture, as opposed to true "ultrasound-guided" venipuncture) is clearly an unintelligent and ineffective practice.
As a matter of fact, the benefits of ultrasound-guided insertion using modified Seldinger technique and micro-introduction kits are so high that ultrasound-free placing is contraindicated in almost all patients.
The historic switch from placing PICCs without ultrasound at the elbow to ultrasound-guided placing in the middle third of the arm not only increased patient comfort, but also brought about two specific benefits, in reducing both thrombotic complications and infective complications. In the pre-ultrasound era, it was already known that thrombotic risk was proportional to the PICC calibre; given the impossibility of measuring or assessing the internal vein diameter, the only way to reduce the incidence of thrombosis was to use very small catheters (3 Fr, for example), which, however, were associated with

flow problems. After the introduction of ultrasound-guided puncture, the catheter calibre could be properly matched to the vein calibre, following internationally accepted rules that do not recommend catheter placement if the internal vein diameter is not at least three times the external catheter diameter. Further progress in this direction was made in more recent times through the PICC tunneling technique, which will be discussed below: the tunneling rationale is based on the ability to select a vein that has sufficient calibre to be punctured in the proximal third of the arm, close to the axilla, thus enabling to prepare the exit site in the most appropriate location for good management (that is, in the middle third of the arm).

Another specific advantage of PICCs placed under ultrasound guidance is the great ease of exit site management and the consequent reduction of infective risks. The flat surface of the middle third of the upper arm enables the nurses – who are also the main inserters of PICCs throughout the world - to apply a stable and safe dressing. The infection risk of ultrasound-PICCs is significantly lower if compared to PICCs inserted in the antecubital fussa, or to CICCs; indeed, an exit site in the middle third of the upper arm is more preferable in terms of infective risk as compared to the elbow (typical of 20th century PICCs) or the supra- or infraclavicular region (typical of CICCs placed under ultrasound guidance in accordance with the most up-to-date techniques).

Needless to say, the worst exit sites for reducing the infective risk are placed at the mid neck (typical of CICCs inserted with the "blind" technique in the internal jugular vein) and in the inguinal region (typical of non-tunneled FICCs). As already mentioned when discussing the indications, the low infective risk of ultrasound-guided PICCs makes them especially appropriate in immunosuppressed patients, in patients with tracheostomies or digestive ostomies, and in oncoheamatology patients who are candidates for treatment lasting no longer than 3-6 months.

The exit site in the middle third of the arm is characterised, in fact, by low bacterial colonisation, due to particularly thin, dry skin (which discourages bacterial growth and favours antiseptic procedures), to the distance from "traditional" sources of contamination, such as the mouth, nose and tracheostomy, as well as to the possibility of maintaining a stable and easy to manage dressing.

All these factors contribute to reducing the risk of catheter contamination by the extraluminal route. Obviously, the advantages of ultrasound-PICCs in terms of infective risk do not depend exclusively on the exit site: other factors such as ultrasound-guided venipuncture (ultrasound lowers the risk of infection by increasing the success rate on first attempt and reducing repeated venipunctures, with the consequent extravasation and haematomas) as well as the consistent use of antisepsis recommended by the international guidelines and typical of PICC insertions are to be considered.

All these considerations have already been officially incorporated in various guidelines on the prevention of catheter-related infections. The CDC 2011 guidelines recommend considering a PICC insertion whenever infusion treatment is expected to last more than six days. The EPIC 2014 guidelines indicate PICCs as a preferable alternative option to CICCs whenever a non-tunneled catheter is indicated, in the absence, of course, of specific contraindications to the cannulation of the veins of the arm.

Principles of ultrasound anatomy of the arm and ultrasound-guided venipuncture technique

The skills required for ultrasound-guided insertion of PICCs and Midlines are: (1) being able to identify the main vascular and nerve structures of the arm using ultrasound and (2) knowing the most effective technique of ultrasound-guided venipuncture of the veins of the upper limb. These basic skills are fundamental for ultrasound-guided placement of any type of peripherally inserted venous access device (short peripheral cannulas, long peripheral cannulas or "mini-Midlines", traditional Midlines, PICCs), even if there are some relevant differences, depending on the technique chosen for venous cannulation (for example, the simple Seldinger technique *versus* the modified Seldinger technique). In the case of PICCs as central catheters, it is necessary to combine venous cannulation with some methods for the correct central placing of the tip (the so-called *tip location*) and some methods for controlling catheter progression inside the venous system (the so-called *tip navigation*).

Ultrasound anatomy of the veins of the upper limb

The superficial and deep veins of the forearm and the arm are usually visualised with ultrasound devices equipped with 26-38 mm large linear probes acting at a frequency higher than 7 MHz and therefore suitable for analysing structures located 2-3 mm below the skin surface. The probe must be oriented transversally to the axis of the limb and perpendicular to the skin, in such a way that the operator's left side corresponds to the left of the image on the screen but to the right side of the patient. The probe must be held in a solid, stable manner without exerting excessive pressure on the surface of the skin. Since most veins of the arm are oriented longitudinally, the transversal orientation of the probe leads to the visualisation of the veins in short axis, enabling a panoramic vision of the way veins relate to each other and other longitudinal structures, such as arteries and nerves (Figure 2.1).

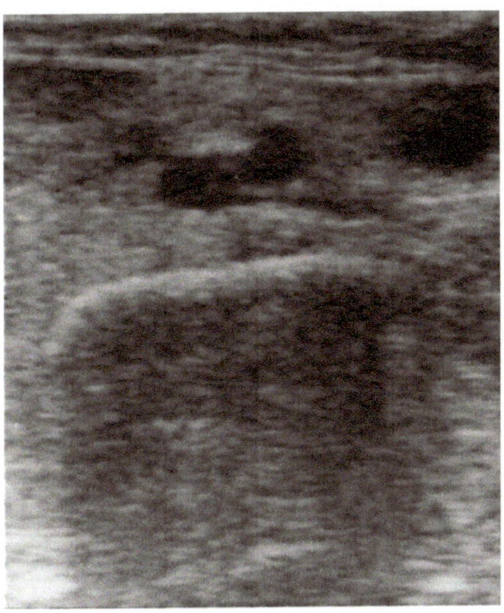

Figure **2.1**

Under ultrasound, the vein appears as a round, anechoic (dark) image in short axis, that can be easily compressed by the pressure applied by the ultrasound probe; a non-compressible image of this type should be interpreted as an artery (if pulsating) or as a thrombosed vein or a non-vascular structure (if not pulsating). In short axis, the arteries appear as round anechoic images, the pulsation of which can be shown by the compression of the probe against a bone surface. The nerves appear, on the other hand, as complex, multiloculated structures (a "beehive" image), mainly hyperechoic and not compressible.

There are very few veins of the upper limb that are potentially relevant for the purposes of puncture and cannulation. The longest is the **cephalic vein**, which starts near the so-called "anatomical snuff box" (on the radial edge of the wrist) and runs quite superficially along the entire forearm: in this tract, ultrasound-guided insertion of needle cannulas or long peripheral cannulas in the cephalic vein is allowed. An important collateral vein, called the antecubital, branches off from the cephalic vein and joins the basilic vein short before the antecubital fussa. At the elbow, the cephalic vein calibre increases significantly (it is the vein most used for blood samples) but then becomes thin once again and follows a rather irregular and superficial trajectory along the upper arm over the biceps, until it reaches the shoulder and crosses the deltoid-pectoral groove, finally joining the axillary vein short before the latter passes under the clavicle and over the first rib. At the elbow, the cephalic vein is large, superficial and easy to cannulate (often without the need for ultrasound) but insertion of peripheral venous access in this site is not considered appropriate, except in an emergency, since this is an area of flexion. As already mentioned, the cephalic vein very superficial in the arm and may be appropriate for the ultrasound-guided insertion of a short cannula or a "mini-Midline", but much less so for the insertion of a PICC. Notwithstanding this, PICC placement in obese patients may also take place in the cephalic vein in this area (Figure 2.2), as will be mentioned below.

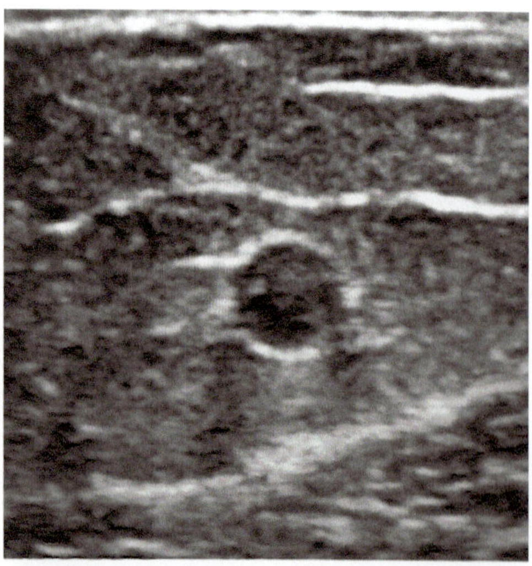

Figure **2.2**

The **basilic vein** runs along the ulnar border of the forearm and is usually thinner than the cephalic vein, even if equally superficial; cannulation is feasible in this tract with ultrasound-guidance for the positioning of needle cannulas or long cannulas. Close to the bend of the elbow, the basilic vein receives several tributaries (including the antecubital vein, described above, and a retro-olecranic vein) and becomes quite large (4-5 mm) in its passage along the upper arm in the bicipital-humeral groove. At this level, the basilic vein, which typically lies at a depth of 1-2 cm, has the perfect characteristics to be punctured and cannulated using ultrasound. Its size, depth and distance from arterial and nerve structures (with the possible exception of the medial cutaneous nerve of the arm, which is often very thin and negligible) make the vein ideal – or certainly the first choice – for placing a PICC or a Midline. In its passage to the upper part of the arm, the basilic vein tends to become closer to the neurovascular bundle of the upper arm (consisting of brachial artery, brachial veins and median nerve) (Figure 2.3), which runs just below the medial border of the biceps. After receiving all the brachial veins as tributaries, the basilic vein finally becomes the axillary vein and, as such, enters the axillary cavity.
The number of **brachial veins** varies from two to five and they appear as satellite veins of the brachial artery, also called humeral artery. This is the main and only artery of the upper arm, that divides into radial artery and ulnar artery in the forearm, usually 6-8 cm below the elbow. In most cases, the brachial veins are easily identified with ultrasound only above the elbow, and they appear as small round anechoic images, easily compressed, at the two sides of the brachial artery: the resulting image is often described as similar to the silhouette of "Mickey Mouse", with the artery forming the head and the two brachial veins the ears (Figure 2.4). In the upper arm, brachial veins run close to the median nerves and to the artery, from which they separate in extremely variable ways at extremely variable levels of the arm, to finally merge into the basilic vein. Usually, the venous system of the ulnar side of the arm (brachial-basilic-axillary) drains around 75% of the refluent blood of the upper limb, while the cephalic vein and its collaterals on the radial side drain the remaining 25%. The brachial veins are a second choice for positioning of PICCs and Midlines: although appropriate in depth, their calibre is very

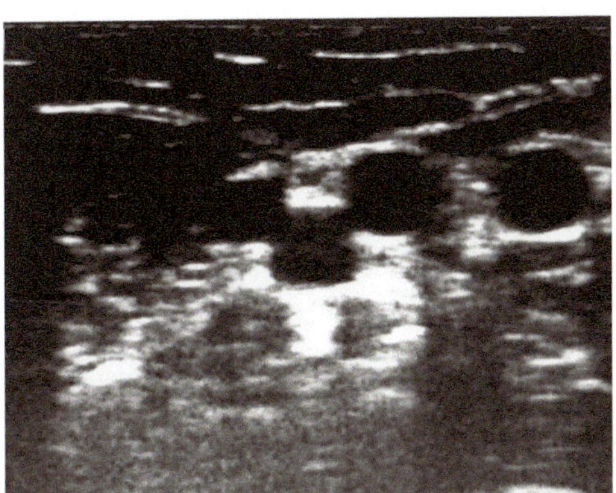

Figure **2.3**

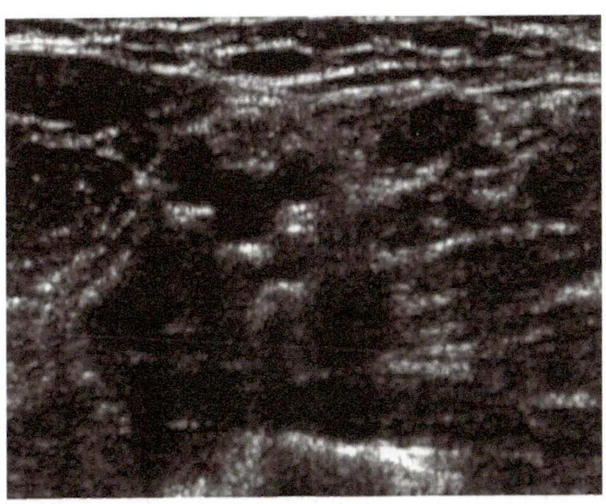

Figure **2.4**

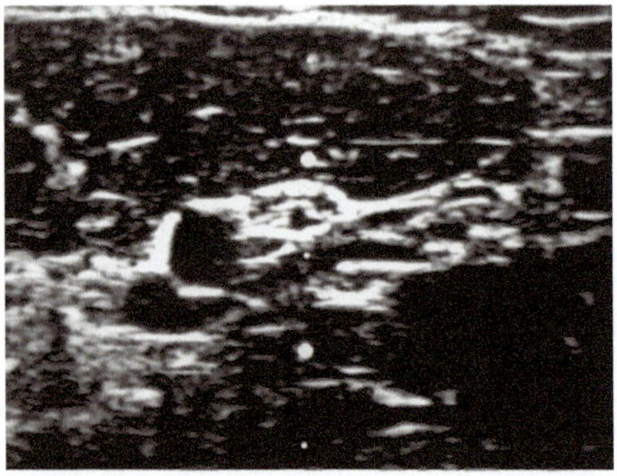

Figure **2.5**

variable (depending on the number, which is also variable) and ultrasound-guided puncture may be more complex due to their close relationship with the brachial artery and the median nerve. Furthermore, while the median nerve usually lies above the artery, brachial veins tend to run deeper than the artery (Figure 2.5).

In summary, several superficial veins (lying less than 8 mm under skin level) can be identified in the upper limb and can be cannulated with or without ultrasound for needle cannula or short peripheral cannula placement: the cephalic vein throughout its length along the forearm and arm, the antecubital vein near the bend of the elbow, and the basilic vein in the forearm. As with all peripheral cannulas placed in visible or palpable superficial veins without ultrasound, cannulation of veins close to areas of flexion (the wrist and the elbow) should be avoided. Deep veins (more than 8 mm from skin level) that are appropriate for ultrasound-guided insertion of PICCs and Midlines are all located in the upper arm and include (in order of preference): (a) the basilic vein in its passage in the bicipital-humeral groove, (b) the brachial veins inside the bundle of nerves and vessels in the arm, and (c) the cephalic vein (restricted to obese patients in whom it becomes a deeper, more stable vein).

PICCs and Midlines should be inserted in these veins in such a way that allows to obtain an exit site at a sufficient distance from the elbow (a flexion area) but also from the axillary cavity (a flexion area, whose skin has significant moisture and high bacterial contamination). It is recommended therefore to plan for the exit site to lie in the middle third of the upper arm, either by performing venipuncture directly in this area or by tunneling the catheter in order to obtain an exit site more distally from the puncture site, should venipuncture be performed in the proximal third of the arm (where a greater calibre of the basilic vein is generally expected) for practical reasons. The choice of the ideal location for the exit site was systematised by Rob Dawson with his Zone Insertion Method (ZIM): this method involves measuring the length of the arm (distance between the acromion and olecranon) and subsequently dividing the arm in three areas, a yellow zone (proximal third), a green zone (middle third) and a red zone (distal third). The exit site must be located within the green zone; this means that every time the ideal puncture

Table 2.2 RaCeVA Protocol
Visualisation of the following veins, in succession: 1. Internal jugular, at mid-neck (short axis) 2. Internal jugular, at the base of the neck (short axis) 3. Innominate, at the level of the upper mediastinum (long axis) 4. Subclavian and external jugular, in the supraclavicular area (long axis) 5. Axillary, in the infraclavicular area (short axis) 6. Axillary, in the infraclavicular area (long axis)

Table 2.3 RaPeVA Protocol
Visualisation of the following vessels, in succession: 1. Cephalic vein, at the elbow 2. Brachial artery and veins, at the elbow 3. Basilic vein, bicipital-humeral groove 4. Neurovascular bundle (brachial vessels + median nerve), mid-arm 5. Cephalic vein, mid-arm 6. Axillary and cephalic veins, infraclavicular area 7. Subclavian, internal jugular and innominate veins, supraclavicular

site falls within the yellow zone, PICCs should be tunneled in order to move the exit site into the green zone.

Beside choosing the right "level" of the arm at which the vein should be punctured, another crucial information for selecting the most suitable vein for a PICC or a Midline concerns the internal diameter of the vein (measurable with ultrasound) and its depth. As we will see below, the vein calibre should be at least three times the catheter calibre and it must be less than 3 centimetres deep (preferably within 2 centimetres).

To facilitate the systematic exploration of the veins of the arm susceptible to cannulation, both for didactic and pre-insertion diagnostic purposes, GAVeCeLT recently developed a protocol called RaPeVA (Rapid Peripheral Venous Assessment) aimed at standardising and simplifying the ultrasound examination. RaPeVA is similar to the RaCeVA protocol (Rapid Central Venous Assessment), that was developed a few years ago to systematise the supra-infraclavicular vein examination before central venipuncture (Table 2.2). The RaPeVA protocol (Table 2.3) initially involves the identification of the main veins and arteries of the bend of the arm, then the examination of the basilic vein, followed by the neuro-vascular bundle made up of the median nerve, brachial artery and brachial veins and, finally, the cephalic vein. The last step in the examination is the visualisation of the main veins in the infraclavicular and then the supraclavicular site, in order to identify potential anomalies or pathological alterations that could obstruct the PICC progression. In brief, the RaPeVA protocol involves the following sequence: visualisation of the cephalic vein at the bend of the elbow (1), sliding the probe from the radial side to the ulnar side in order to identify the artery and brachial veins and the confluence between the antecubital vein and basilic vein (2), identification of the basilic vein during its course along the bicipital-humeral groove sliding the probe upwards (3), lateral movement of the probe for an examination of the neuro-vascular bundle of the arm (4) and

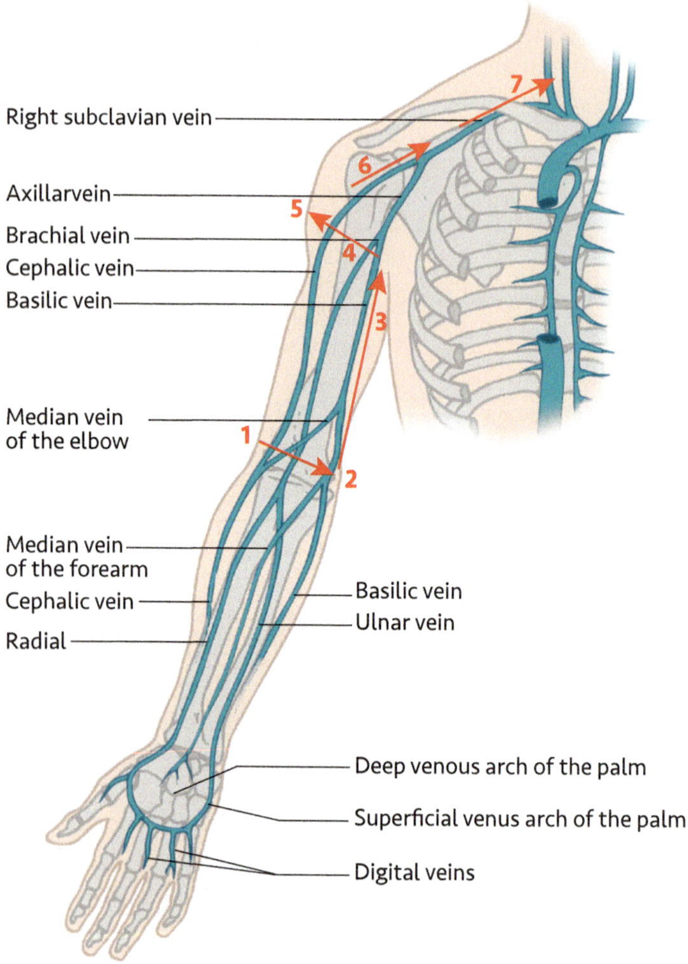

Figure **2.6**

still further laterally in order to visualise the cephalic vein at this level (5) and, finally, a rapid examination of the cephalic and axillary veins in the infraclavicular site (6) and the internal jugular, subclavian and innominate veins in the supraclavicular site (7) (Figure 2.6). The systematic adoption of the RaPeVA protocol enables to systematically analyse the characteristics of all the veins of the arm that are potentially suitable for adequately inserting a PICC or a Midline. This GAVeCeLT protocol has proved to be especially useful in teaching how to insert different brachial devices (long cannulas, Midlines, PICCs, tunneled PICCs, brachial CCTs, PICC-ports).

Ultrasound-guided venipuncture technique

The technique of ultrasound-guided venipuncture may potentially be applied to any vein that can be identified with ultrasound. Besides being used for the veins of the upper limb, it is typically performed for the veins of the lower limb (femoral and saphenous) and the veins in the supra-infraclavicular zone (axillary, subclavian, internal jugular, innominate, etc.). A description of any venipuncture technique under ultrasound control (or "echoscopy" as it is known) needs the definition of the spatial relations between vein, probe and needle used for puncture.

As far as the relationship between vein and ultrasound probe is concerned, there can be visualisation in short axis (when the main axis of the vein is perpendicular to the plane of the probe) or in long axis (when the axis of the vein is parallel to the plane of the probe). The obvious advantage of visualisation in short axis is that it provides a "panoramic" view of the various structures adjacent to the vein, which is particularly desirable with the limbs, where veins run alongside other longitudinal structures such as arteries and nerves (Figure 2.7). In terms of spatial relationship between needle and ultrasound probe, we identify an *out-of-plane* puncture when the needle trajectory is not contained in the plane of the probe and an *in-plane* puncture when the needle trajectory is entirely contained in this plane. The obvious advantage of *in-plane* puncture is that it enables the visualisation of the needle at any time, reducing the risk of accidental damage to neighbouring structures that could be caused, for example, by inadvertently puncturing the rear wall of the vein.

Although any combination between "long axis" or "short axis", and *out-of-plane* or *in-plane* is virtually feasible, clinical experience has substantially identified two main ultrasound-guided approaches: *in-plane* venipuncture in long axis (used mainly for central veins adjacent to the pleura, in which it is vitally important to avoid "going through" the vein: typically, ultrasound-guided venipuncture of the innominate vein or subclavian vein by the supraclavicular route) or *out-of-plane* venipuncture in short axis (typically used for the veins of the limbs) (Figure 2.8). *In-plane* venipuncture in short axis is an exception, and it is used exclusively for the internal jugular vein (the ultrasound-guided equivalent of the Jernigan technique – that is, the "lower-lateral" puncture of the internal jugular) (Table 2.4).

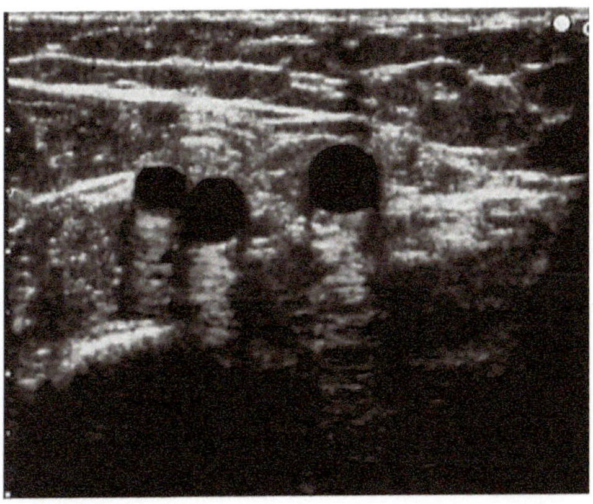

Figure **2.7**

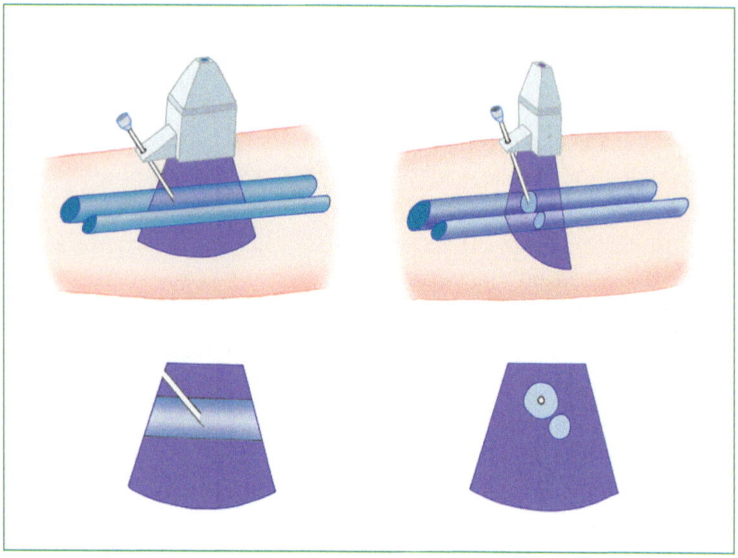

Figure **2.8**

Table 2.4 Ultrasound-guided venipuncture techniques		
	Out-of-plane puncture	**In-plane puncture**
Visualisation in short axis	• Veins of the arm (basilic, brachial, cephalic, axillary) • Femoral vein and saphenous vein • Axillary vein and cephalic vein in the infraclavicular area	• Internal jugular vein
Visualisation in long axis		• Innominate vein and subclavian vein in the supraclavicular area • External jugular vein in its last tract • Axillary vein and cephalic vein in the infraclavicular area

For the infraclavicular approach to the axillary vein, there is no clear indication of preference between *out-of-plane* venipuncture in short axis and *in-plane* venipuncture in long axis: both are feasible and have different advantages and disadvantages (the first reduces the risk of accidental arterial puncture, while the second reduces the risk of accidental pleural puncture).

As for ultrasound-guided venipuncture of the veins of the upper limb, experience and practice have established the prevalence of the *out-of-plane* venipuncture in short axis (Figure 2.9) beyond any doubt. Indeed, this approach allows for the accurate panoramic

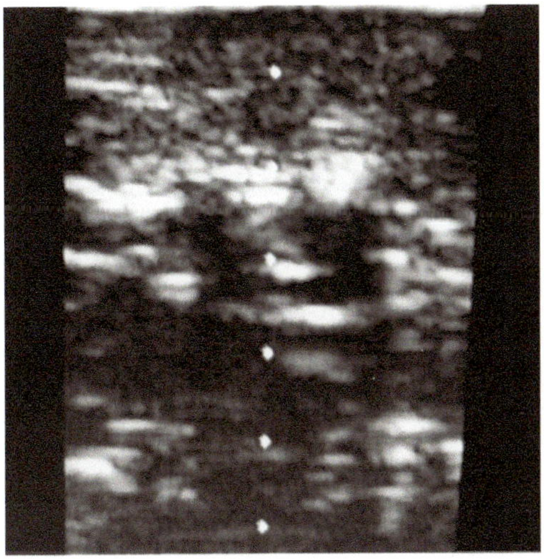

Figure **2.9**

display of the relations between the vein and other adjacent structures, thus minimising the risk of potential accidental puncture of the median nerve or the brachial artery. The lack of "complete" control of the needle trajectory does not lead to serious problems, considering the anatomical features of the arm.

Obviously, an accurate venipuncture of the basilic vein or the brachial vein, for example, requires adequate training (where possible, on appropriate simulators, such as the one used in GAVeCeLT courses), based on the following principles:

- appropriate technique for holding the probe, which must be held firmly by the operator (the non-dominant hand is used, leaving the dominant hand to manoeuvre the needle);
- visualisation of the chosen vein in short axis, exactly at the centre of the ultrasound display;
- positioning of the needle at an angle that is variously described as between 30° and 45° exactly at the centre of the probe and very close to the probe itself whenever possible; the closer the needle is inserted to the probe, the more acute the angle must be between the needle and the major axis of the probe;
- introduction and progression of the needle at an angle of inclination that depends on the depth of the vein; the needle trajectory can also be followed satisfactorily with the *out-of-plane* technique, as long as the probe is slightly inclined during the progression of the needle, so as to follow the tip.

Preparation for insertion

Once the appropriate venous site has been chosen, it is of the utmost importance that the insertion procedure is carried out correctly (following the recommendations of the international guidelines) and by specifically trained personnel. Indeed, it has been shown that an adequate insertion manoeuvre plays a crucial role in reducing the risk of mechanical, infective and thrombotic complications. While it was once believed that the only risks associated with the insertion procedure were those linked to any immediate mechanical damage from the venipuncture and from the catheter progress in the venous system, it is now known that many late complications (infective and non-infective) are caused or favoured by inappropriate actions at the time of insertion.

One example is the risk of bacterial contamination during insertion, which can translate into an infective complication that could be mild, severe or potentially lethal and may even arise after many days. One of the most important recommendations for inserting any type of venous access therefore concerns hand hygiene and the use of gloves.

Correct aseptic technique

Hand hygiene is the most effective and economical way of preventing infections related to healthcare. Effective healthcare operator hand decontamination reduces colonisation of the skin of the hands, with a consequent significant reduction in the transmission of microorganisms from one patient to another and, therefore, a reduction of healthcare-related infections.

Hand hygiene is recommended immediately before every contact with the patient, including the execution of clean/sterile procedures; immediately after every contact with the patient; immediately after contact with biological fluids, mucosa or not-intact skin; immediately after activity or contact with objects and instruments close to the patient, that could cause contamination of the hands; immediately after the removal of gloves. When inserting venous access devices, international guidelines recommend (1) "pre-surgery" hand hygiene before insertion of any short, medium or long-term central venous access devices or in-dwelling peripheral devices (Midlines or mini-Midlines) and (2) "routine" hand hygiene before and after insertion of peripheral needle cannulas (short cannulas). Both "pre-surgery" and "routine" hand hygiene, according to guidelines, must be preferably performed using an alcoholic gel rub; alternatively, soap and water can be used.

Gloves are the cornerstone of PPE (Personal Protective Equipment) and an essential part of daily compliance with of universal precaution rules. Generally, the two main indications for glove use to prevent infections related to healthcare are: (1) protection of the operator's hands from contamination with organic material and microorganisms; (2) reduction of the risk of cross-transmission of microorganisms to healthcare operators and patients. It is important to underline that the use of gloves does not replace hand hygiene in any way. The choice between sterile or non-sterile gloves is based on the assessment of various factors: who is at risk (patient or operator); whether the procedure specifically requires the use of sterile gloves; whether there is potential exposure to blood, body fluids or secretions; whether there is potential contact with non-intact skin or mucosa during the preparation or during the procedure. As a rule, gloves must be worn for:(1) invasive procedures; (2) contact with sterile sites and non-intact skin or mucosa; (3) all activities at risk of exposure to blood or body fluids; (4) when handling sharp or contaminated devices. Gloves must be: (a) disposable, (b) worn immediately before any contact with the patient, (3) removed as soon as possible once the activity on the patient has ended, (4) changed between patients (after appropriate hand hygiene), and (5) disposed of in accordance with local policies.

International guidelines for venous access device insertion recommend: (1) wearing non-sterile gloves during insertion of short peripheral venous catheters (needle cannulas), as long as the insertion site is not palpated after the application of skin antiseptic, and (2) wearing sterile gloves during insertion of any central venous catheter (short, medium and long term) and in-dwelling peripheral catheters (Midlines and "long" peripheral cannulas).

Bedside insertion versus *insertion in a dedicated setting*

For in-dwelling peripheral venous devices (Midlines and mini-Midlines) and short and medium term central venous access devices (CICCs and PICCs), the insertion can also be performed at the patient's bedside as long as the asepsis measures described below are observed.

Indeed, the current international guidelines confirm that the insertion of medium term venous access devices (PICC and Midline catheters) can also be performed at the patient's bedside, subject to basic aseptic technique principles and adequate barrier precautions (sterile gloves, etc.) and an appropriate insertion technique performed by specifically trained personnel.

Long-term venous access devices, including tunneled-cuffed catheters or TCCs (Pro-Line, Groshong, Hickman, Broviac or similar, including cuffed-tunneled PICCs) or totally implantable devices (ports and PICC-ports) manoeuvreimplantation setting must necessarily have the following characteristics:

- possibility of performing procedures with a guarantee of obtaining the necessary asepsis (for example: the environment must not be used for other procedures that carry a potential risk of bacterial contamination of the room; a facility for pre-procedural hand-washing must be provided);
- possibility of cleaning the environment completely (sanitised room; natural lighting; adequate room ventilation; absence of furniture, cupboards or surplus furnishings, that are beyond the scope of safe manoeuvre performancemanoeuvre; at least an additional bed for a pre-procedural visit and at least one cupboard dedicated to storing the materials strictly required for the manoeuvre);
- availability of adequate equipment (1) for patient monitoring during the procedure (for example: ECG monitor, oximeter), (2) for performing the procedure under safe conditions (for example: ultrasound device for ultrasound-guided puncture, shadow-free operating lamp or another adequate artificial light source), and (3) for treating the patient in case of adverse events (for example: emergency trolley with appropriate drugs, oxygen wall source).

This room, moreover, must be within a structural context that can guarantee:

- adequate space for patient access and for any waiting patient, should the procedure be performed in outpatient clinics or day-hospital units;
- separate hygiene facilities for operators and patients;
- telephone line;
- dedicated rooms for storing used materials and clean materials.

In a hospital setting, such environment may be an operating room, an interventional radiology suite, or a room specifically arranged for this use in a day-hospital facility, a clinical department (fully-equipped medical centre) or an outpatient department.
It is important to underline that one of the essential points mentioned above is the adoption of a room specifically dedicated to this type of procedure. Regardless of the wealth of equipment and structural prerequisites, even operating rooms or radiology suites should be considered inadequate or not entirely safe in terms of infective risk if the insertion of long-term venous access takes place at the same time or immediately after performing procedures that may be contaminated or at risk of bacterial contamination.

Insertion of needle cannulas, long peripheral cannulas and Midlines

The insertion of peripheral venous access devices can be carried out through the direct puncture of a visible or palpable vein (in the case of needle cannulas), ultrasound-guided cannulation of a deep vein with the direct Seldinger technique (long peripheral cannulas or "mini-Midlines") or modified Seldinger technique (Midline catheters).
The positioning of a needle cannula-type peripheral venous access involves a fully codified procedure:

- a vein of sufficiently large calibre and a needle cannula whose calibre must be proportional to the clinical use, but not exceeding this purpose, must be selected;
- it is recommended to choose veins in stable (forearm, arm) rather than unstable (hand, wrist, bend of the elbow) areas; considering the opportunity of saving the veins of the arm for any positioning of PICCs or Midlines, it is usually preferable to insert needle cannulas at the level of the forearm;
- the needle cannula is positioned using clean (not sterile) gloves, following hand-hygiene by the operator and skin antisepsis with 2% chlorhexidine in 70% IPA, as recommended by the EPIC 2014 guidelines;
- the needle cannula must be secured with sterile devices (preferably, a semipermeable adhesive transparent membrane) and never with a non-sterile tape; some transparent dressings are equipped with an integrated securement that avoids recourse to additional sutureless devices.

As already mentioned, ultrasound-guided insertion of short cannulas has not been associated with successful outcomes in clinical practice, due to device design (system with internal needle and external cannula), the stiff material they are made of (mostly Teflon) and their limited length (less than 6 cm). Given these characteristics, ultrasound-guided insertion of a needle cannula in a deep vein is initially successful but associated with a high incidence of complications (displacement, thrombosis, extravasation), which limits its duration to 24-48 hours.
More promising and potentially more useful as an aid to cannulation of superficial veins with "short" needle cannulas is the use of systems with Near-InfraRed (NIR) technology, that visualises superficial veins (7-8 mm deep) by exploiting the characteristic of 760 nm wavelengths in the "near-infrared" spectrum of being selectively absorbed by desaturated

haemoglobin (and therefore by venous blood). Such systems (VeinVewer, AccuVein, VeinSite) were introduced a few years ago in clinical practice; although there is no strong scientific evidence for their efficacy and cost-effectiveness, their use appears still to be recommended, especially for the visualisation, puncture and/or cannulation of superficial veins in pediatric and neonatal patients. It is important to underline that NIR systems do not overlap or conflict with the use of ultrasound, as the former are indicated for superficial veins (up to 7-8 mm deep) and the second for deep veins (over 9 mm deep).
While it is true that short needle cannulas (14-26 G calibre, 25-52 mm length) are placed by direct cannulation of visible or palpable superficial veins with or without the aid of visualisation by NIR technology, long peripheral cannulas (3-4 Fr calibre, 6-15 cm length) can be inserted both in superficial veins (visible and/or palpable and/or visualised with NIR devices) and in deep veins (which must be visualised with ultrasound). The common characteristic of long cannulas (or "mini-Midlines") is that they are placed with the "direct" Seldinger technique: that is, venipuncture with a needle, introduction of a guidewire in the vein through the needle, removal of the needle and progression of the cannula in the vein over the guidewire. The insertion technique of a long cannula in a superficial vein does not differ from the technique above described for short cannulas, except for the adoption of the Seldinger technique after venipuncture.

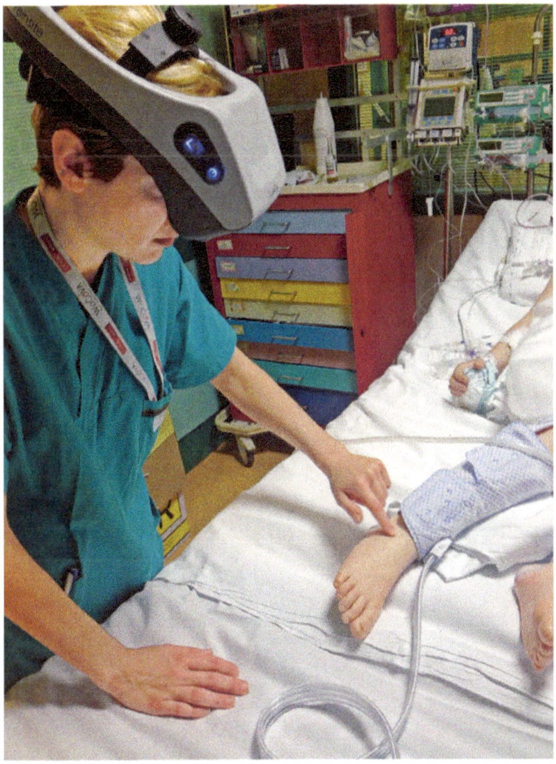

Figure **2.10**

Long peripheral cannula (mini-Midline) positioning with the ultrasound technique, on the other hand, is based on the following steps:

- Using ultrasound, selecting a vein whose calibre is at least three times the calibre of the chosen catheter, and preferably in a location that enables an exit site of the utmost stability (avoiding bending areas) (Figure 2.11).
- Appropriate asepsis and maximum barrier precautions, including: hand hygiene, sterile gloves, sterile gown, mask, cap, skin antisepsis with 2% chlorhexidine in 70% IPA, fenestrated sterile drape, and adequate sterile cover for the ultrasound probe.
- Out-of-plane ultrasound-guided venipuncture (vein visualised in short axis) (Figure 2.12), after infiltration with a local anaesthetic (for example: ropivacaine 0.75%).

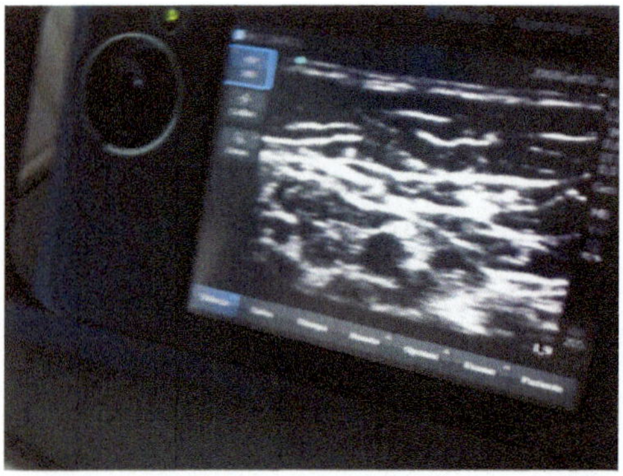

Figure **2.11**

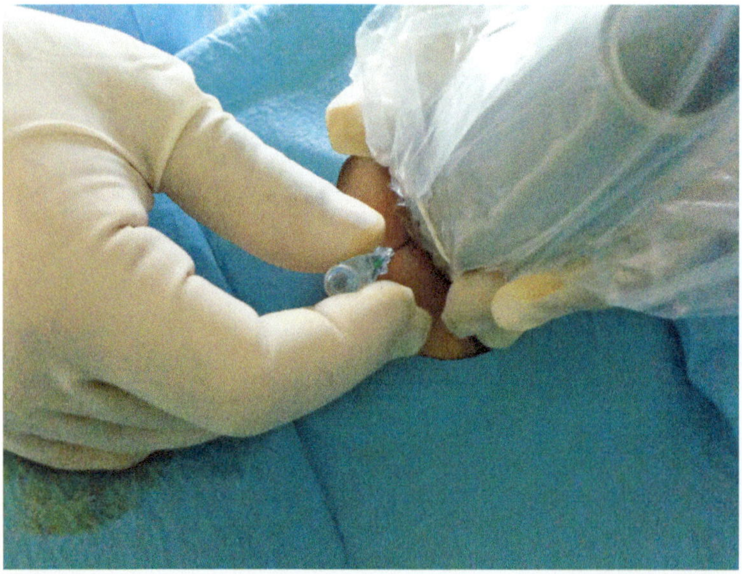

Figure **2.12**

- Catheter insertion using the direct Seldinger technique: the exact technique may slightly vary depending on the type of long cannula used; the most commonly used in Europe (LeaderCath and LeaderFlex) is a simple Seldinger technique with separate use of needle, thin straight-tip guidewire and cannula in succession (Figure 2.13 –Figure 2.15); some long cannulas are supplied as devices in which the needle, metal guide and cannula are integrated in a coaxial system (PowerWand, PowerGlide).

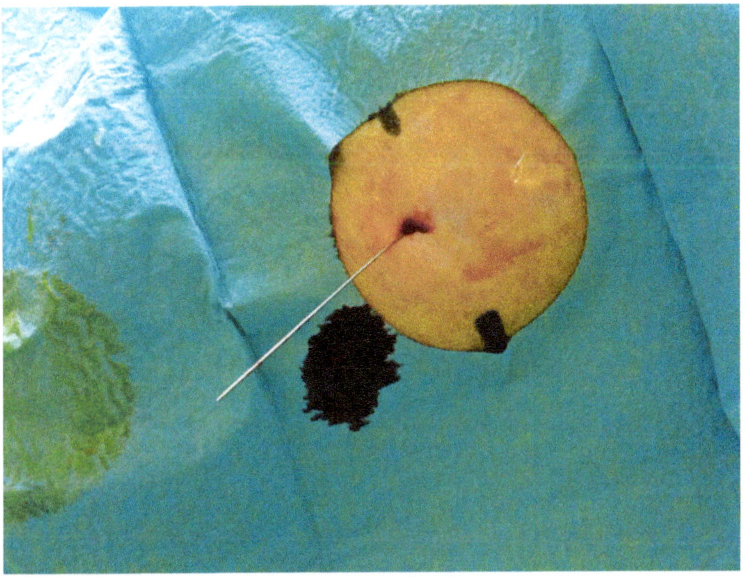

Figure **2.13**

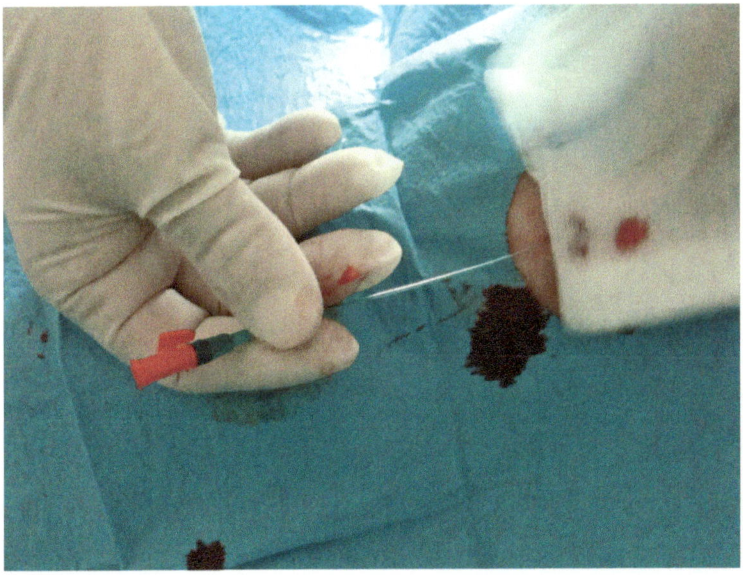

Figure **2.14**

- Catheter flushing and system closure with a Needle Free Connector (NFC) cap, preferably with neutral displacement (Figure 2.16).
- Appropriate catheter securement with sterile devices: semipermeable adhesive transparent dressing (Figure 2.17), with or without a sutureless device for additional securement (Figure 2.18).

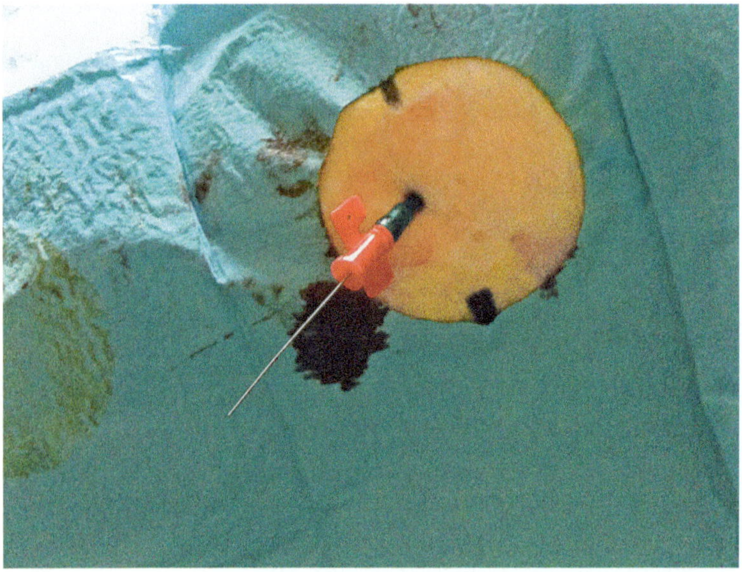

Figure **2.15**

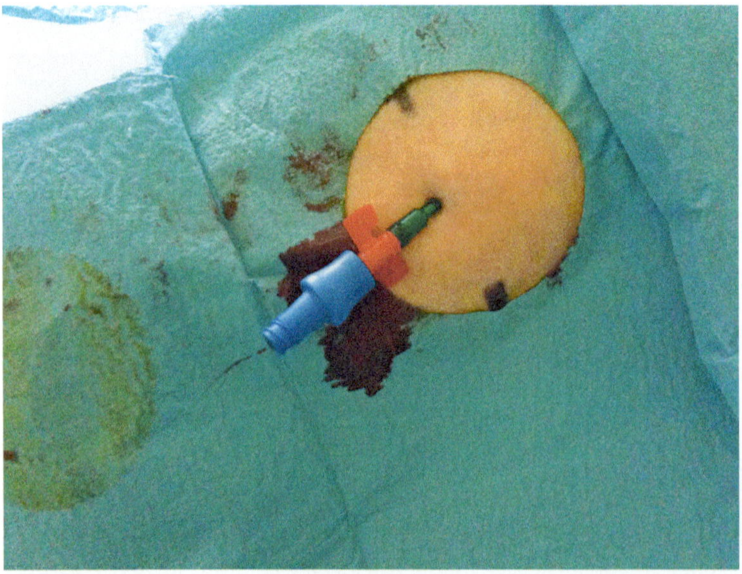

Figure **2.16**

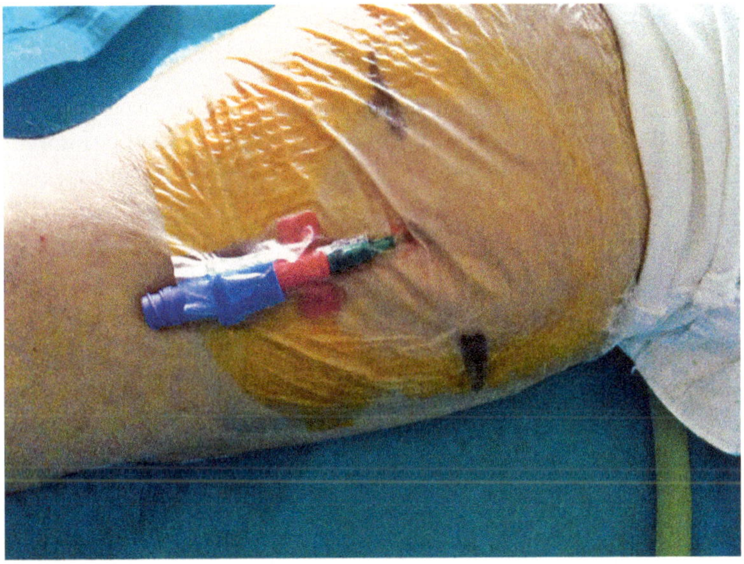

Figure **2.17**

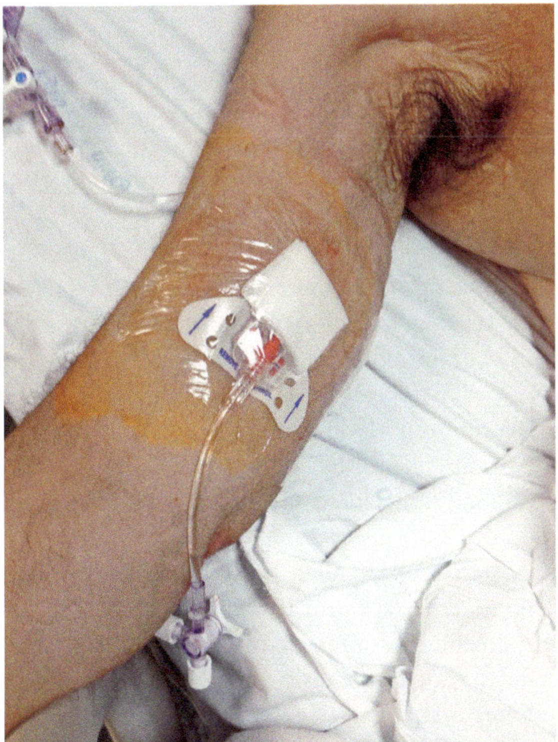

Figure **2.18**

The insertion of a "classic" Midline (4 or 5 Fr, single lumen, 20-25 cm) involves the adoption of the "modified" or "indirect" Seldinger technique, involving the following steps:

- Using ultrasound, selecting a vein whose calibre is at least three times the calibre of the chosen catheter, preferably located in the middle third of the arm (in Dawson's "green zone"); the first choice is the basilic vein (for the reasons given above), while the second choice would be one of the brachial veins; the cephalic vein (in its tract in the middle third of the arm) is cannulated only in special situations (in obese patients, for example, or when the basilic vein is being "saved" for a possible future insertion of a PICC).
- Appropriate asepsis and maximum barrier precautions, that is: hand hygiene, sterile gloves, sterile gown, non-sterile mask, non-sterile cap, skin antisepsis with 2% chlorhexidine in 70% IPA, fenestrated sterile drape, and adequate sterile cover for the ultrasound probe.
- Out-of-plane ultrasound-guided venipuncture (vein visualised in short axis), after infiltration with a local anaesthetic (for example: ropivacaine 0.75%).
- Insertion of a catheter using the "modified" or "indirect" Seldinger technique, that is: venipuncture with 21 G needle (preferably with echogenic tip) (Figure 2.19); insertion of a thin guidewire with a straight tip (0.018" calibre, soft straight tip, preferably in nitinol) (Figure 2.20); removal of the needle; introduction of a peel-away micro-introducer-dilator of an adequate calibre for the catheter (4.5 Fr for 4 Fr Midlines; 3.5 Fr for 3 Fr Midlines) with or without prior enlargement of the skin breach; guide and dilator removal; Midline catheter insertion in the introducer; peeling away the introducer to remove it. In many cases, it is possible to insert the introducer-dilator over the guidewire through the skin perforated by the needle without enlarging the breach, by separating the dilator from the introducer and inserting only the dilator, then reassembling the two pieces and reinserting them over the guidewire as a complete introducer-dilator system.
- The progression of a Midline catheter does not usually present relevant difficulties, especially if the insertion was preceded by a careful examination of the veins of the arm and the infraclavicular region by means of the RaPeVA protocol; contrary to what will be described below for PICCs, in most cases it is not necessary to use ultrasound to control the trajectory of the Midline, the entire length of which is inserted.
- Once the catheter has been placed, aspirating blood and infusing saline solution confirm the successful cannulation.
- The system is locked with normal saline and closed by a neutral displacement Needle Free Connector (NFC).
- The Midline must be adequately secured: in particular, only sterile devices must be used for Midlines. The use of non-sterile tapes must be avoided at all times. Semipermeable adhesive transparent dressings are preferred to dressings with gauze and sterile tapes (see EPIC 2014 guidelines). Depending on the clinical situation, it is possible to use them as the only securement strategy or combine them with a sutureless device.

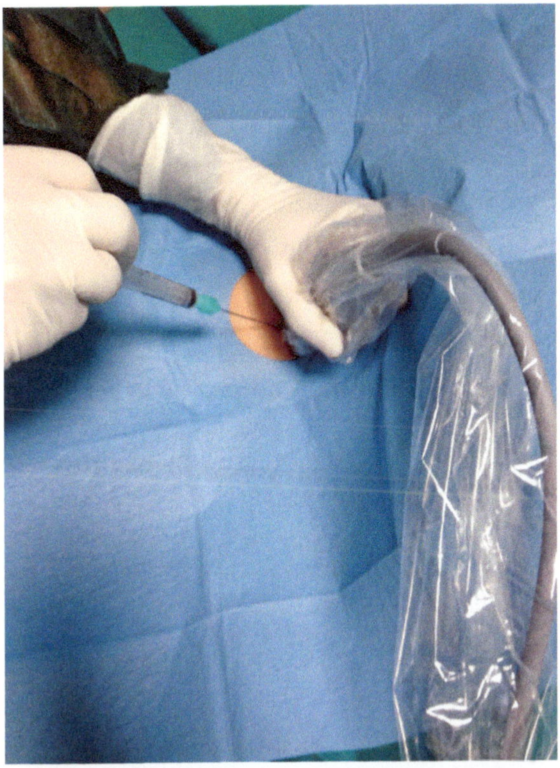

Figure **2.19**

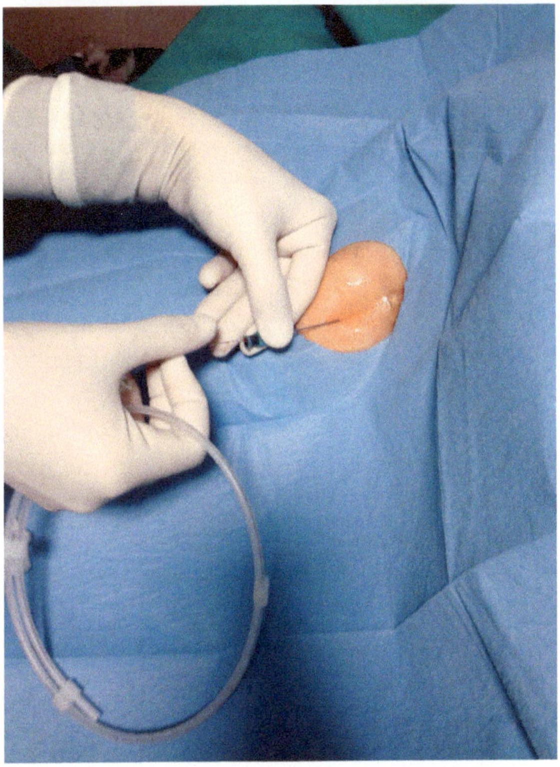

Figure **2.20**

PICC insertion

Several different skills are needed to correctly insert PICCs:

- appropriate examination of the venous system of the upper limb before insertion;
- manoeuvre performance according to a rigorous asepsis method;
- technique of ultrasound-guided venipuncture of deep veins;
- modified Seldinger technique;
- some method of controlling the catheter progression in the venous system;
- a method for verification of the central position of the tip;
- an appropriate securement of the catheter to the skin.

In addition to these skills, which are always necessary, in some cases the technique of tunneling the catheter is required (and is very useful, as already mentioned, in specific clinical situations). All these techniques must be integrated in an insertion protocol, such as the one already mentioned, called "SIP protocol" and developed by GAVeCeLT in recent years (see Table 1.2). The examination of the venous system, the ultrasound-guided venipuncture and the modified Seldinger technique do not differ from what was described above for Midlines. Before describing the SIP protocol in detail, it is appropriate to specifically discuss the methods used for progressing the catheter in the veins (*tip navigation*) and for verifying the central position of the tip (*tip location*), which are particular requirements of PICC insertion.

Tip navigation

Since the PICC is inserted in the arm but its tip is placed in a central venous site, this catheter has a particularly long intravascular course, varying from 25 to 50 cm depending on patient's age and physical constitution, the level of the arm in which the vein is cannulated and the side chosen. Along this course, catheter progression may encounter obstacles, due, for example, to kinking or stenosis of the vein, or it may not follow the centripetal direction (i.e., it may go in the wrong direction, such as towards the ipsilateral internal jugular or the contralateral innominate vein). Whereas stenosis can partially be predicted by carefully examinating the veins of the basilic-axillary-subclavian axis employing the RaPeVA protocol before insertion, or by the clinical examination of the patient (for example: presence of a pacemaker and its wires in the left subclavian region), the two crucial challenges for the progression are constituted, in most cases, by the junction between the subclavian, jugular and innominate veins and the point of confluence of the two innominate veins in the superior vena cava. In particular, one of the most frequent difficulties to catheter progression is encountered at the confluence between jugular and subclavian, especially when the catheter is coming from the right axillary, due to the narrower angle between the right subclavian axis and the right innominate vein axis (the left subclavian and the left innominate veins are almost coaxial). More rarely, limited to the left approach and more typically in patients of pediatric age, difficulties may occur in the passage through the confluence of the innominate veins.
In order to bypassing and minimising these challenges, the below techniques and recommendations are available.

- First, the linear progression of the catheter in the expected direction (axillary-subclavian-innominate-superior vena cava) will be aided by selecting sufficiently rigid catheters, such as polyurethane catheters, especially those in third-generation polyurethanes, used for power injectable PICCs; soft catheters (such as silicone ones) will encounter greater difficulties in their correct guidance in the right direction and may stop against obstacles or create catheter loops inside the vessel.
- It is important to remember that the catheter, like all intravascular devices, should be inserted slowly as needed, as inserting it too rapidly often leads to the risk of it taking a wrong direction.
- When possible the catheter passage from the right subclavian to the right innominate vein may be facilitated by tilting the patient's head towards the operator, lowering the right ear towards the right shoulder and the chin towards the clavicle; a preferable method would be compressing the internal jugular vein with the ultrasound probe, obtaining and visualizing its complete or semi-complete collapse (this manoeuvre will prevent the catheter from taking the wrong direction towards the jugular vein or at least reduce this probability).
- If catheter passage is difficult, the partial or total removal of the stylet usually does not have any significant effects (on the contrary, making the catheter softer increases the likelihood of it getting stuck or taking a wrong direction); it may, however, be useful to replace the stylet with a guidewire or, if using a double lumen PICC, insert the guidewire in the lumen not occupied by the stylet; if the guidewire is longer than the catheter, its protrusion outside the catheter into the lumen of the vein will not imply any risk, since the guidewire has a floppy tip. In general, the greater rigidity bestowed by the guidewire to the catheter will aid insertion.
- Difficulty in passing through the subclavian-innominate vein confluence can also be overcome by using the simplest and most economical system of *tip navigation,* or catheter progression under ultrasound control, positioning the same linear probe used for venipuncture above the clavicle in order to visualise the junction between the internal jugular, subclavian and innominate vein. If such manoeuvre has already been performed, the ultrasound view will confirm the absence of the catheter in the internal jugular vein ("negative" criterion) and/or the presence of the catheter in the first tract of the innominate vein ("positive" criterion). If the catheter gets stuck at the confluence, it will be possible to advance it slowly under ultrasound monitoring, rotating it if necessary in order to facilitate its course towards the innominate vein.
- Under normal conditions, a standard linear probe only enables the visualisation of the innominate vein (more precisely, the first tract of the innominate vein) but not the confluence of the innominate veins or the superior vena cava. In recent times, however, an ultrasound technique has been developed to enable the visualisation of the guidewire (or the catheter occupied by the guidewire) inside the superior vena cava, using a micro-convex ultrasound probe placed on the right supraclavicular fossa. Such economical and non-invasive technique could be increasingly useful in the future for positioning PICCs, especially considering the possibility of preventing the catheter from taking the wrong direction towards the contralateral innominate vein.

- Another option for having complete control over the catheter progression is positioning the PICC under fluoroscopy. However, this method is not recommended in clinical routine since it is not harmless (due to the x-ray exposure of both the patient and the operator) but primarily because it is extremely expensive and not logistically feasible in clinical practice. As mentioned elsewhere, the insertion of PICCs under fluoroscopy (1) conflicts with *bedside* positioning, which is a strongpoint of the cost-effectiveness of PICCs, (2) increases insertion costs (depending primarily on the costs of using operating rooms or radiological suites, or any other setting where the use of fluoroscopy is allowed) and (3) inevitably leads to a drastic reduction in the number of PICC insertions. When considering the main challenge of reaching the jugular-right subclavian confluence, actively steering the catheter or the guidewire coming from the subclavian vein towards the innominate vein is easier under ultrasound than radiological monitoring, since ultrasound enables the visualisation of both the intravascular device and the vascular structures, while fluoroscopy visualises the device but not the vasculature, unless contrast medium is used (with a further increase of costs and risks for the patient).

Alongside these general recommendations aimed at avoiding errors in directing the catheter and/or at correcting those errors, it is necessary to mention devices specifically designed and marketed for *tip navigation* purposes, which are available for clinical practice (Table 2.5).

Generally, we can distinguish between methods that enable the direct identification of the catheter course (direct visual methods), methods that project its course on a virtual screen (indirect visual methods) and, finally, non-visual methods.

Visual methods, including ultrasound and fluoroscopy that have already been mentioned, visualise the catheter inside the venous system (ultrasound) or in a space in which the venous system and the catheter position inside it are inferred from radiological landmarks (fluoroscopy).

Alongside these methods, a device (Navigator) based on a system for identifying electromagnetic impulses allows the direct identification of the catheter tip position below the cutaneous and subcutaneous planes. This system consists of a stylet with an electromagnetic tip that replaces the normal PICC stylet and the position of which inside the body

Table 2.5 Tip navigation methods

Visual methods	Non-visual methods
Direct vision • Ultrasound • Fluoroscopy • Electromagnetic systems - Navigator **Indirect vision** • Electromagnetic systems - Sherlock	**Based on Doppler** - Vasonova **Based on blood pressure detection** - Catfinder **Based on intracavitary ECG** - Delta

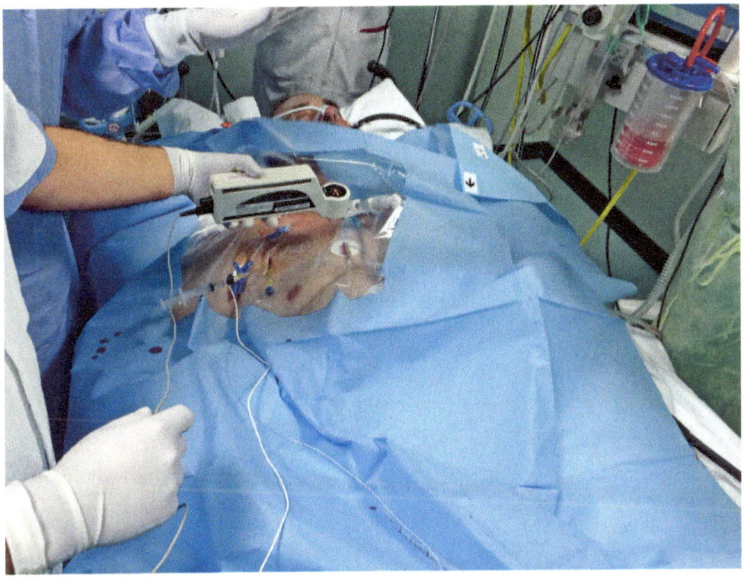

Figure **2.21**

is identified by an external detection device (Figure 2.21) with remarkable precision. The system allows to check whether the catheter is moving in the right direction, as well as identify anomalous tip positions, such as in the internal jugular vein or in the contralateral innominate vein. It also allows to monitor the tip position and whether the catheter tip is pointing in the right direction (Figure 2.22). Even though it has the ability to check whether the catheter tip is lying under the third intercostal space on the parasternal line and is pointing downwards, this system is not however adequate for proper *tip location* and should therefore be used together with an appropriate method for monitoring the tip position, such as the intracavitary ECG method. The benefits of the Navigator are its

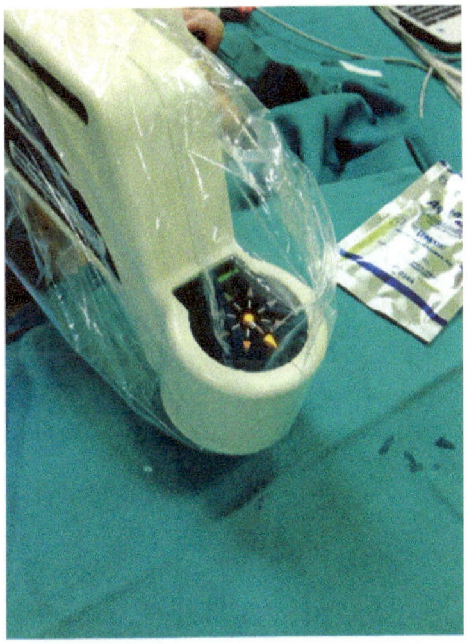

Figure **2.22**

limited cost, its adaptability to any type of PICC and the option of adopting it halfway through the manoeuvre whenever progression difficulties are encountered.
One example of an "indirect" visual method for *tip navigation* is Sherlock. This system is based on electromagnetic detection of the tip, like the Navigator, but instead of being detected in the patient, it is projected on a screen. Unlike the Navigator, this system does not allow for any detection, even an approximate on, of the actual position of the tip at any moment, but only checks whether the catheter is directed towards the superior vena cava or not. Although based on a similar system as the stylet with electromagnetic tip, Sherlock has numerous disadvantages compared to the Navigator, such as the high cost, its limited use to PICCs of a single brand and the need to use the system since the very beginning of the manoeuvre (from the catheter selection, in fact) and not only when required.
There are also "non-visual" methods of *tip navigation*. Their salient feature is that they only confirm that the catheter tip is "navigating" in the right direction and do not localize the position of the tip during its course, even approximately. An example is the Vasonova, based on a Doppler signal sent from a micro-probe inserted in the catheter in place of the stylet: the device connected to the micro-probe detects the Doppler signal to confirm that the catheter is navigating in the direction of the blood flow and not against it. The system is obviously very expensive, cannot be used with all PICCs and must be combined with an appropriate *tip location* system: indeed, the complete device, called Vasonova VPS, is the result of combining the Doppler method for navigation and the intracavitary ECG method for the exact verification of the position of the tip.
Another example of a non-visual method is Catfinder, based on the return pressure wave from the right atrium, the delay of which is compared to the moment of cardiac contraction (identified by ventricular depolarisation, inferred from the superficial ECG) to inform the device to whether the catheter is navigating in the right direction; the same method can also identify when the catheter reaches the heart, or, more precisely, the cavoatrial junction, with a certain precision. The Catfinder can be used with any catheter and has limited costs, but unlike the Navigator, the Sherlock and the Vasonova, it has yet to receive convincing validation based on clinical trials and has not been marketed in Europe.
Finally, one of the most promising methods in terms of accuracy, low cost and non-invasivity is the Nautilus Delta, a more recent version of the Nautilus, the first ECG monitor specifically dedicated to the intracavitary ECG method for *tip location.*
The system consists of a small ECG device connected to a traditional electrode, which uses tablet or smartphone screens as a display, via Bluetooth connection. The *tip location* is obtained through the ECG method that will be more fully described below and detects changes in the P wave on the intracavitary ECG trace, while *tip navigation* is based on changes in the R wave detected on a trace obtained by subtracting a stable reference trace (a vector between a surface electrode positioned at the jugular level and the surface electrode on the left side) from the intracavitary trace (a vector between the intracavitary electrode and the surface electrode on the left side). It is a simple, accurate and inexpensive system, that can be applied to any PICC (or any other central venous access device).

Table 2.6 Integrated methods (tip navigation + tip location)		
	Tip navigation	**Tip location**
Sherlock 3CG	Electromagnetic method	Intracavitary ECG
Vasonova VPS	Doppler Method	Intracavitary ECG
Catfinder	Both based on pressure measurement	
Delta	Both based on intracavitary ECG	

Table 2.6 shows a summary of the integrated *tip navigation* + *tip location* systems described above. To avoid any misunderstandings, it is important to stress that, while intraprocedural *tip location* systems, such as intracavitary ECG, have a well proven cost-effectiveness, there has been no convincing clinical demonstration of the actual cost-effectiveness of many *tip navigation* devices. Given the current state of knowledge, good sense would probably suggest two possible options: (1) routinely using a versatile and non-invasive integrated *tip location* + *tip navigation* system, such as the Delta, or (2) using a *tip location* system with the maximum cost-effectiveness, such as intracavitary ECG conducted with a non-dedicated ECG monitor, but resorting to navigation by ultrasound (scanning supraclavicular region) or to a low cost navigation system with the maximum versatility, such as the Navigator, in case of objective difficulties.

Tip location

PICC positioning cannot be performed without adopting adequate methods for verifying the central position of the tip. The optimal position of the tip of a central venous catheter, be it a traditional centrally inserted (CICC) or peripherally inserted (PICC), is of the utmost importance, since the wrong positioning of the tip is associated with a high risk of malfunctions, venous thrombosis, arrhythmia, vascular damage and other problems. The name "central venous catheter" is closely related to the position of the catheter tip, irrespective of its insertion point. There is currently a broad consensus, at least in Europe, that the optimal position of the tip lies at the level of the cavoatrial junction and, more generally, in the zone between the lower third of the superior vena cava and the first portion of the right atrium, in accordance with the guidelines of the European Society of Parenteral Nutrition (ESPEN) and the Royal College of Nurses (RCN) (see Appendix IV). The recommendations of the National Association of Vascular Access Networks (NAVAN, now AVA – Association for Vascular Access) are slightly different and suggest the lower third potion of the superior vena cava as the correct position. The overall incidence of primary malpositioning varies from 2 to 30%, depending on the various techniques of insertion used, and is more frequent during PICC insertion than CICC insertion. It is estimated that the incidence of malpositioned PICCs, in the absence of intraprocedural techniques for tip monitoring, may oscillate between 15 and 20%, with greater risk for catheters inserted in the left arm. A typical malposition is observed when the PICC tip lies in the upper third of the superior vena cava or even in the innominate vein; a PICC whose tip is wrongly positioned in this site will encounter various complications, such as malfunctions, high risk of venous thrombosis near the tip, increased risk of the formation of so-called *fibrin sleeves* (actually, a fibroblastic sheath), as well as an increased risk of tip migration (after a sudden increase of intrathoracic pressure, for example, as in the case of strong cough or vomiting).

Until a few years ago, the most commonly used method for verifying the position of central venous access (PICCs, CICCs, etc.) was performing chest X-ray after the insertion, with the strong limitation of being a post-procedural method. The catheter length was estimated on the basis of various surface landmarks, the direction was monitored (in the case of PICCs and CICCs positioned by the infracalvicular route) by placing the ultrasound probe on the internal jugular, as described above, and the correct direction of the catheter and the position of the tip at the cavo-atrial junction were visualised by a chest x-ray in anteroposterior view. If a malposition was diagnosed, as it was the case with PICCs more often than with CICCs, a new procedure had to be performed to reposition the tip. Currently, it is believed that the positioning of any central venous access should preferably be performed with an intraprocedural technique for the immediate verification of the central position of the tip. This recommendation is even more crucial for central venous access by brachial insertion (PICCs, PICC-ports) and, in general, for all medium and long-term access.

The intraprocedural assessment of the tip position may be performed with various techniques, such as fluoroscopy, transthoracic echocardiogram (TTE), transesophageal echocardiography (TEE), or intracavitary electrocardiography (see Table 2.7).

Fluoroscopy has already been discussed: the routine use of the fluoroscopy while positioning PICCs would undermine their cost-effectiveness and represent a major limitation on the number of PICCs that could actually be inserted in hospitalised and extra-hospital patients.

On the other hand, the use of echocardiography is more interesting. TEE is undoubtedly the most accurate method for the central positioning of the tip, but in most cases it is not practicable from the clinical point of view due to its invasive nature and cost; during TEE, it is possible to place the catheter tip exactly at the level of the *crista terminalis*, which is the anatomical equivalent of the cavoatrial junction and can be easily visualised by ultrasound. This method, however, is used exclusively for investigation purpose or,

Table 2.7 Tip location methods

Intraprocedural	Post-procedural
• Intracavitary ECG • Fluoroscopy • Echocardiography - transthoracic (TTE) - transeosophageal (TEE)	• Chest X-ray • Echocardiography (TTE) • CT, MRI, angiography, etc.

more rarely, for CICC positioning during heart surgery, when an esophageal ultrasound probe is also needed for interoperative haemodynamic monitoring.

TTE is a possible option for accurately assessing tip position. Although successful in performing many different tasks, TTE has never been integrated in the clinical practice of positioning PICCs in adult patients for various reasons, including: (a) technical difficulties of TTE in obese patients or with air in the stomach or colon; (b) difficult direct visualisation of the superior vena cava (though sometimes the infusion of echogenic contrast medium made of saline with air bubbles through the catheter may help to identify the tip position in the superior vena cava indirectly); (c) the need to use a different type of probe (sectorial, convex or micro-convex) than the one used for venipuncture (linear); finally, (d) the need for substantial training before being able to successfully interpret the echocardiographic images. TTE may be integrated more rapidly in tip position verification in pediatric patients, where the anatomic difficulties are fewer.

In the field of PICCs, therefore, the electrocardiographic method inevitably represents the most cost-effective option for the intraprocedural verification of the catheter tip position, even though it is not as accurate as the echocardiography.

The intracavitary ECG method was described for the first time in 1949 and, after the first experiences in 1960, it became widespread in clinical practice in Europe in the eighties and nineties, especially for CICCs and totally implantable central venous systems (ports). A few years later, following experiences in Italy and, specifically, at Università Cattolica del Sacro Cuore – Roma, the method was finally applied to PICC positioning.

The intracavitary ECG method is based on the observation that lead II (between the "red" electrode on the right shoulder and the "green" electrode on the left side) is more or less coaxial to the atrial depolarisation axis. In fact, the traditional "surface" lead II enables to clearly visualise the P wave, which corresponds to the atrial depolarisation. If the red electrode is removed from the right shoulder and appropriately connected to the venous catheter, an "intracavitary" lead II will result (as a matter of fact, semi-intracavitary) between the catheter tip and the "green" surface electrode placed on the left side, and the changes in the P wave will enable to identify the moment in which the catheter tip reaches the cavoatrial junction. The method is based on the fact that current catheters are made of electrically insulating material (polyurethane and silicone), while electrical impulses are easily transmitted by blood, tissue and saline solution contained in the catheter. In other words, when the "red" electrode is appropriately connected to the column of saline solution inside the catheter, the catheter becomes a sort of "travelling electrode", the position of which in relation to the heart can be inferred from the shape of the P wave. As the catheter tip gradually gets closer to the atrium, the P wave in the intracavitary ECG trace increases in height and reaches the maximum peak at the transition between the electrically-inactive tissue (superior vena cava) and the electrically active tissue (atrium), that is, at the cavoatrial junction (Figure 2.23); as soon as the catheter passes this point, directed towards the right atrium or towards the inferior vena cava, the P wave diminishes and/or becomes biphasic (negative-positive) and finally negative.

Given that the method has certain limits as to its applicability, as will be discussed below, we will now proceed with a description of how it can be applied to PICCs.

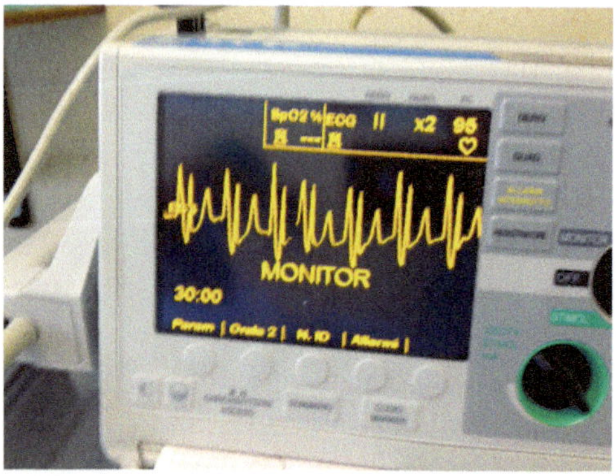

Figure **2.23**

First, the use of a method for tip location involves the assessment of the assumed length of the PICC on the basis of surface landmarks. The desired catheter length is estimated either by using the traditional method (distance in centimetres between the venipuncture site and the midclavicular point, plus the distance in centimetres between the midclavicular point and the third intercostal space on the right parasternal line) and/or with the Ocado method (distance in centimetres between the venipuncture site and the ipsilateral sterno-clavicle-costal joint, adding 10 cm, if on the right, or 15 cm, if on the left) in adult patients. If distal trimming is needed (see below), the catheter is cut by the equivalent or slightly superior length (1-2 cm) than the length estimated on the basis of the surface landmarks.
The intracavitary ECG method is performed using sterile cables that act as conductors between the catheter, filled with saline solution, and the red electrode connected to the ECG monitor (Figure 2.24-2.26). Given that the intracavitary ECG method uses the same travelling electrode in the intravascular tract, two different methods can theoretically be adopted: either connecting the electrode to the stylet inserted in the catheter (using a sterile wire with a clip at one end) (Figure 2.27) or connecting the electrode directly to the saline contained in the catheter (using an appropriate sterile cable-transducer)

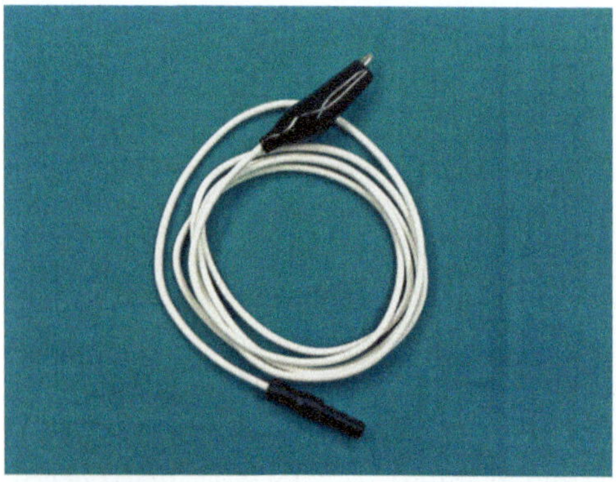

Figure **2.24**

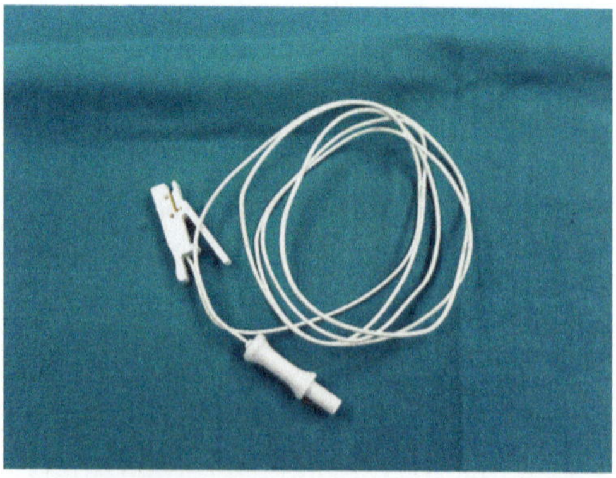

Figure **2.25**

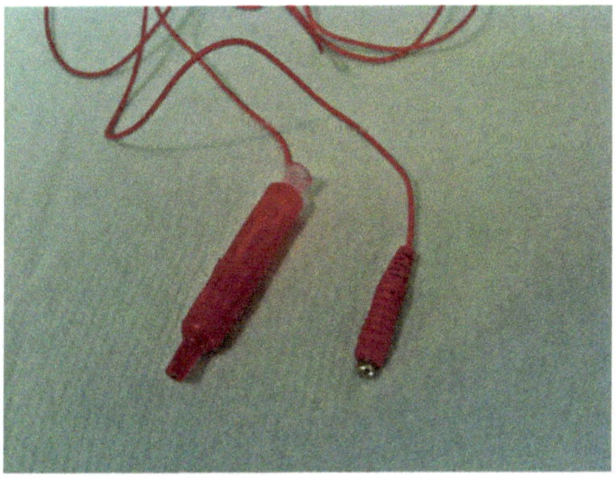

Figure **2.26**

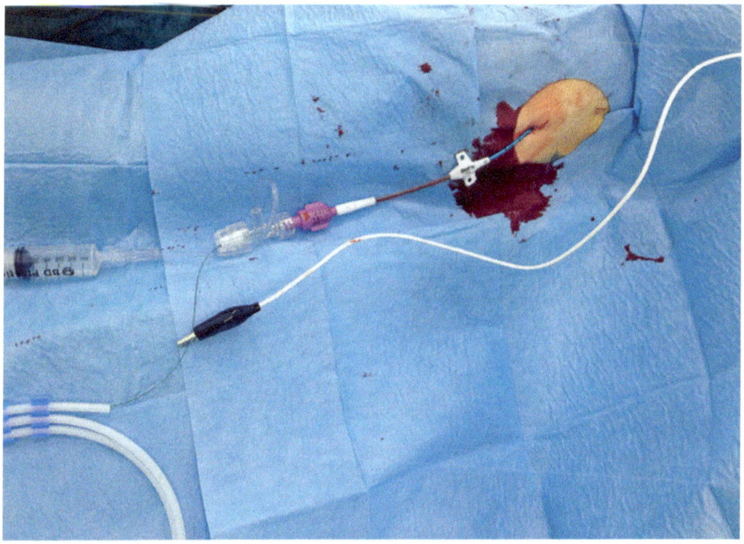

Figure **2.27**

(Figure 2.28). In both cases, the intracavitary ECG method is carried out according to the so-called "saline solution technique".
The method is performed using a normal ECG monitor, or an ECG monitor specifically designed for the intracavitary ECG method (such as the Nautilus, for example) (Figure 2.29).
The insertion of a PICC is performed in accordance with the SIP protocol (see below): careful ultrasound examination of the veins of the arm, selection of a vein whose calibre is proportionate to the catheter, ultrasound identification of the brachial artery and the median nerve, ultrasound-guided venipuncture in the middle third of the arm, cannulation of the vein with the modified Seldinger technique (that is, with micro-introducer-dilator). Following the SIP protocol recommendations, soon after the passage through the jugular/subclavian/innominate junction, the absence of the catheter in the ipsilateral internal jugular vein is confirmed by ultrasound. During the intrathoracic passage

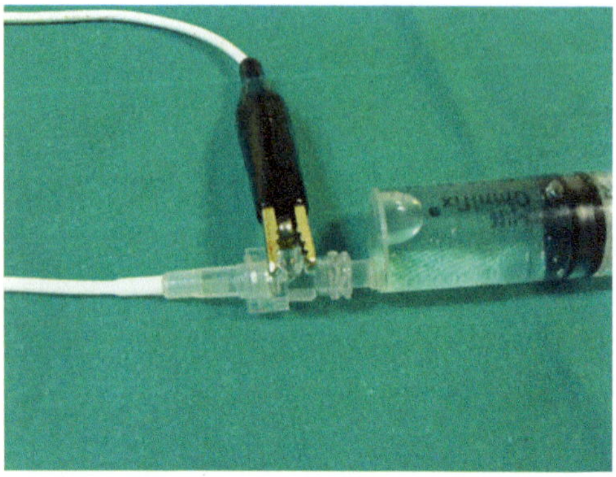

Figure **2.28**

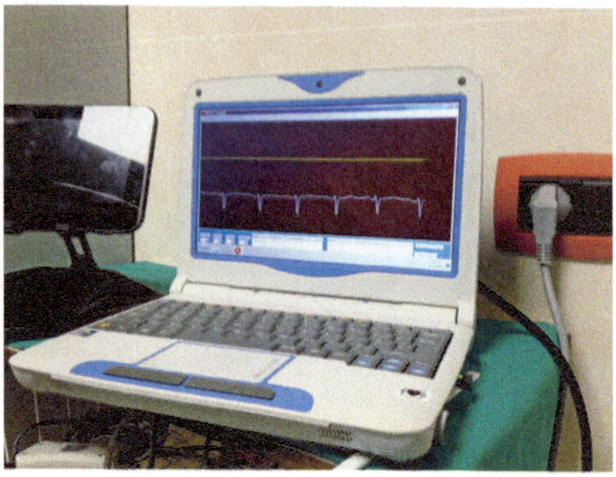

Figure **2.29**

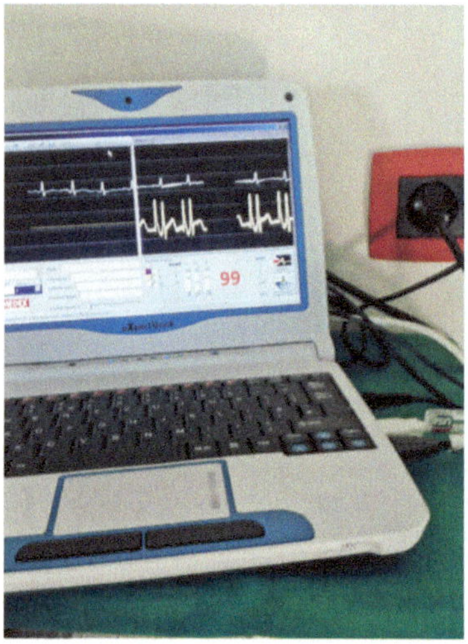

Figure **2.30**

of the catheter, typical variations of the intracavitary ECG lead II are observed. When the P wave reaches the maximum height, corresponding to the cavoatrial junction, the catheter is secured in this position. The best way of identifying the peak of the P wave is to push the catheter to the point in which a negative P component appears and then withdraw it until it returns to the maximum height. As mentioned, the most important benefit of the ECG method is that it enables to assess the tip position in real time, avoiding post-procedural repositioning procedures (complicated, costly and potentially risky). Intraprocedural verification may also be performed with other methods (fluoroscopy, etc.) that are, however, certainly costlier and logistically more difficult than the ECG method. As explained above, using fluoroscopy means renouncing to the cost-effectiveness of PICCs, at least partially. Furthermore, in most cases, the accuracy of the ECG method is greater that the accuracy of fluoroscopy and chest X-rays: in trials comparing ECG method and chest X-rays with the most accurate existing method,

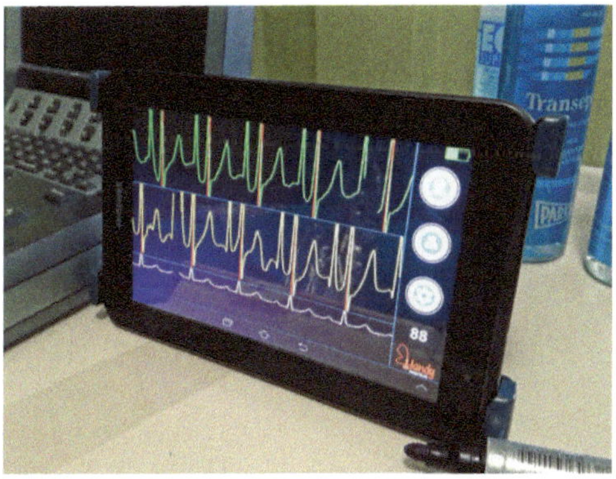

Figure **2.31**

TEE, the electrophysiological method was more accurate than radiological methods. This is not surprising, given the lack of objective radiological criteria for identifying the cavoatrial junction: the most reliable criterion, although relatively imprecise, is that of the tracheal carina, involving the algorithm according to which in adult the junction is positioned around 3 cm under the anteroposterior projection of the carina on the chest X-ray (or on a fluoroscopic image). The criterion is also applicable to pediatric patients, with some corrections (1 cm under the carina in newborns and infants; 2 cm under the carina in children up to 11 years old).
Another advantage of the ECG method is that it can be applied not only during insertion, but also days, weeks or months after insertion, to check that the tip has not migrated but is still in the correct position, among other things. The correct position of the tip can easily be documented in the medical records through a printout of the intracavitary ECG trace. This method has other advantages: it can be applied to clinical situations in which radiological verification is contraindicated (pregnancy) or logistically difficult (positioning of a PICC at home or in a hospice); it is safe and not expensive since it only requires a cable-transducer and the availability of an ECG monitor, and it can easily be performed by adequately trained nurses. More recent models of dedicated monitors, such as the Nautilus Delta mentioned above (Figure 2.31), also have the advantage of being smaller in size and easily portable. Two recent multicentre GAVeCeLT trials published in recent years have confirmed the great feasibility (98-100%) and utmost accuracy (95-100%) of the ECG method, both in adults and in pediatric patients.
The only significant limitation of this method is its limited applicability. In its traditional formulation, in fact, the method relies upon the interpretation of the P wave changes. The method is therefore not applicable in patients with cardiologic conditions that prevent the P wave from being visualised (especially atrial fibrillation).
Alternative options therefore apply to this category of patients:

- use of the traditional system (estimate the length by surface landmarks + control of the direction by ultrasound scan of the subclavian/internal jugular junction + final radiological verification of the tip position);

- use of the Navigator to position the tip below the third intercostal space, then checking the final position with a chest X-ray;
- use of alternative intraprocedural methods, such as TTE, with or without using ultrasound contrast medium;
- targeted use of fluoroscopy.

Specific electrocardiographic methods (based on the interpretation of the TQ tract, for example) that could be validated in the future for identifying the cavoatrial junction, even in fibrillating patients, are currently being investigated.

General principles for PICC insertion

No pre-/post-insertion antibiotic prophylaxis is indicated. Before carrying out the insertion, it is advisable to perform a careful, pre-procedural ultrasound examination to assess all the veins of the arm and the main veins of the supra-infraclavicular region, as described in the aforementioned RaPeVA (Figure 2.32-2.34). This will enable the selection of the most suitable vein in terms of calibre and position, in relation to the most desirable exit site.

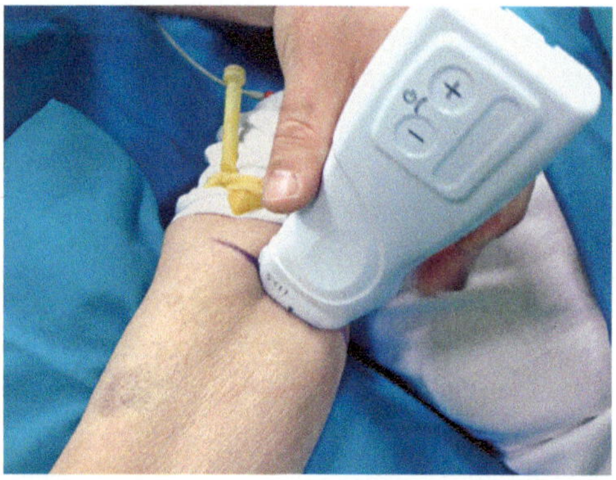

Figure **2.32**

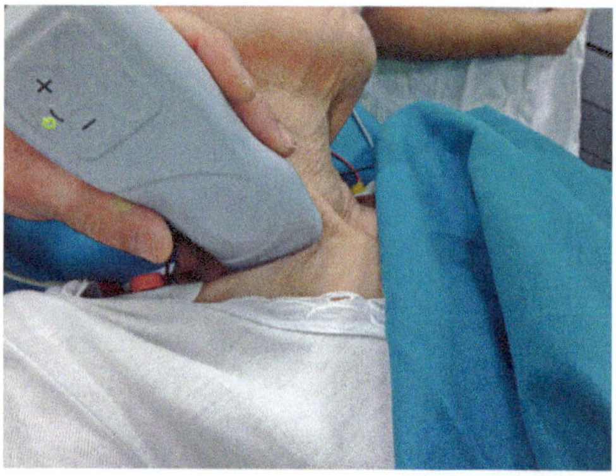

Figure **2.33**

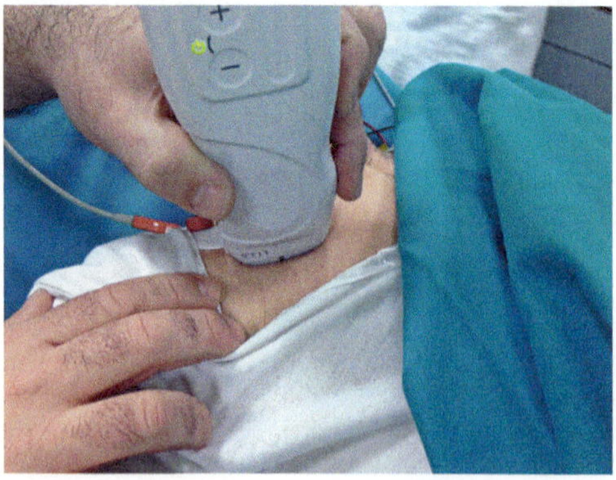

Figure **2.34**

As regards the preparation of the skin, trichotomy should only be carried out if indispensable and preferably using specific atraumatic trichotomy devices (clippers). Whenever possible, it is recommended to wash the patient's skin from the neck down with soapy solutions of 4% chlorhexidine before the start of the procedure.
As previously mentioned, the correct aseptic technique involves operator hand hygiene (Figure 2.35) but also the adoption of maximum barrier precautions (sterile gloves, sterile gown, non-sterile mask, non-sterile cap, ample patient cover, sterile cover for the probe) (Figure 2.36). Skin must be disinfected with 2% chlorhexidine in 70% IPA (Figure 2.37). The use of 10% povidone iodine should be restricted to patients with a known allergy to chlorhexidine.

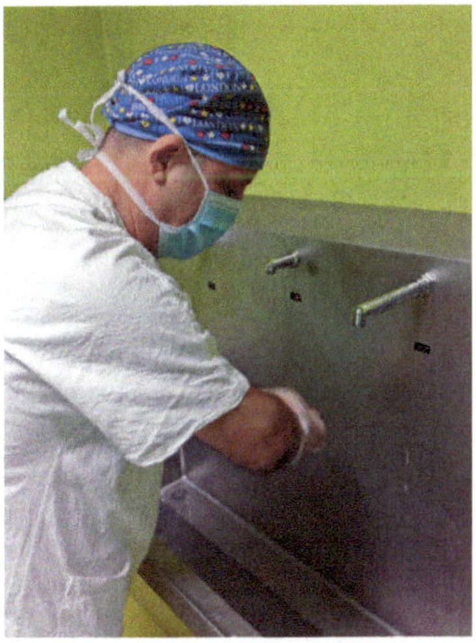

Figure **2.35**

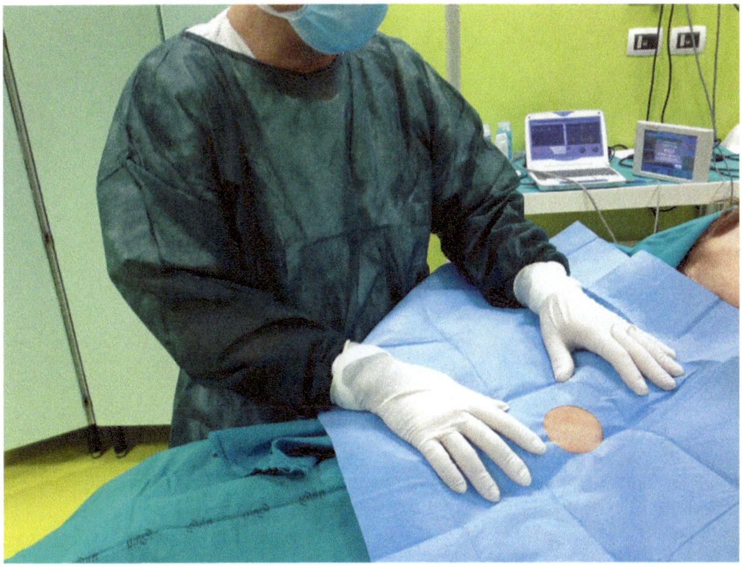

Figure **2.36**

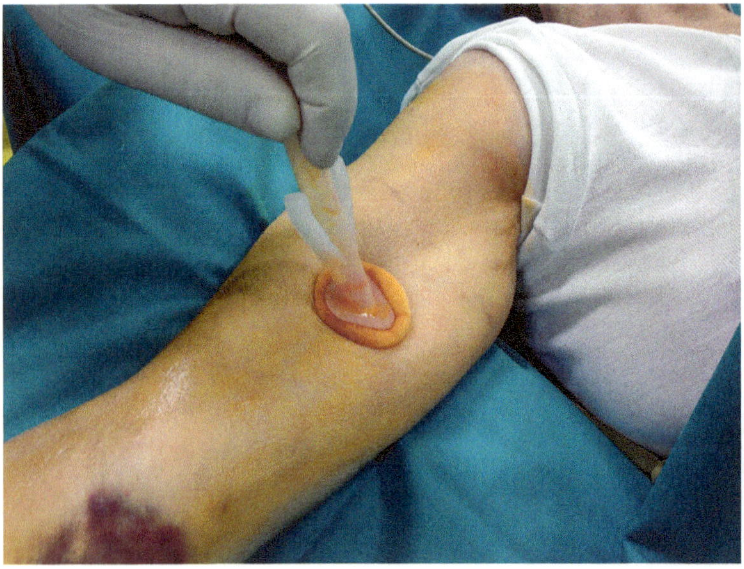

Figure **2.37**

Under local anaesthesia (a few millilitres of ropivacaine 0.75%, for example), the selected vein (brachial, basilic, axillary in the brachial tract, cephalic) is punctured in short axis employing *out-of-plane* ultrasound-guided technique (Figure 2.38-2.41).
After venipuncture, the cannulation manoeuvremanoeuvre is performed using the indirect (or "modified") Seldinger technique (Figure 2.42-2.45). The planning of the catheter exit site has particular importance for the PICC future. The ideal exit site is located in the middle third of the upper arm, halfway between the elbow and the axilla; should the

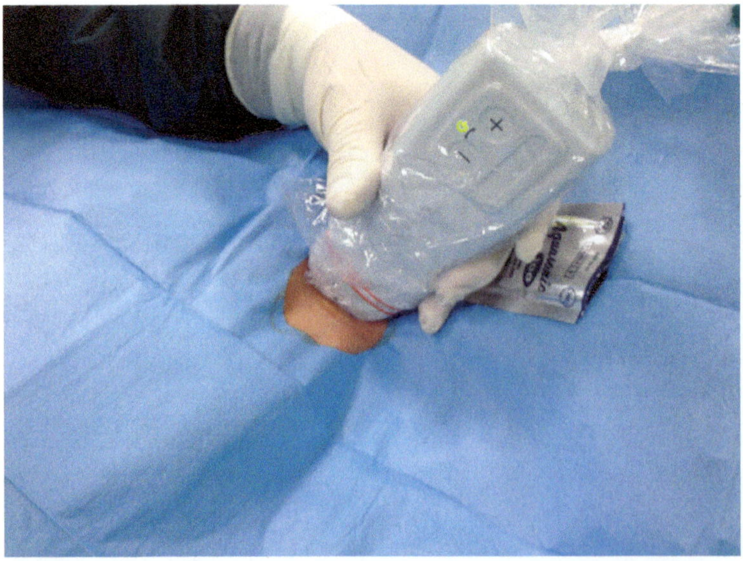

Figure **2.38**

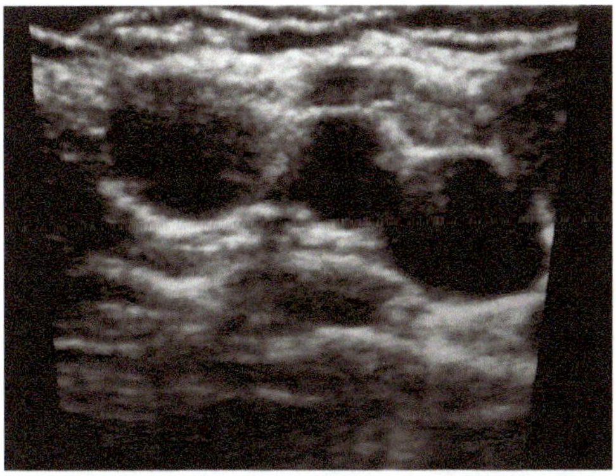

Figure **2.39**

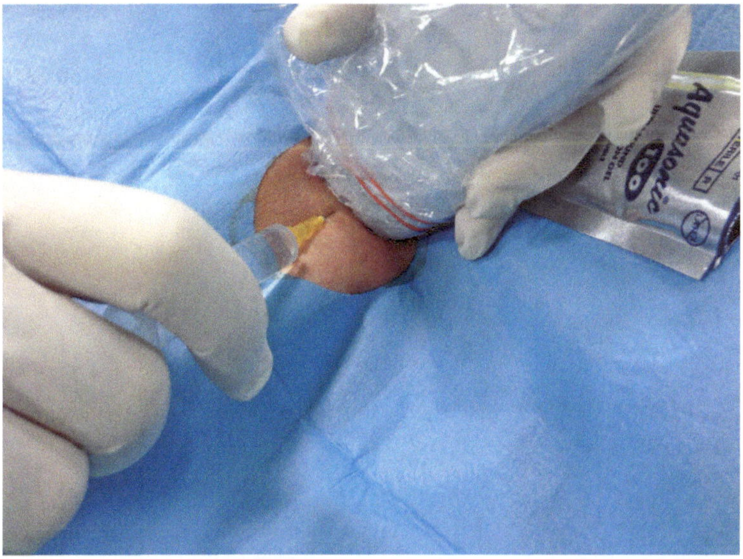

Figure **2.40**

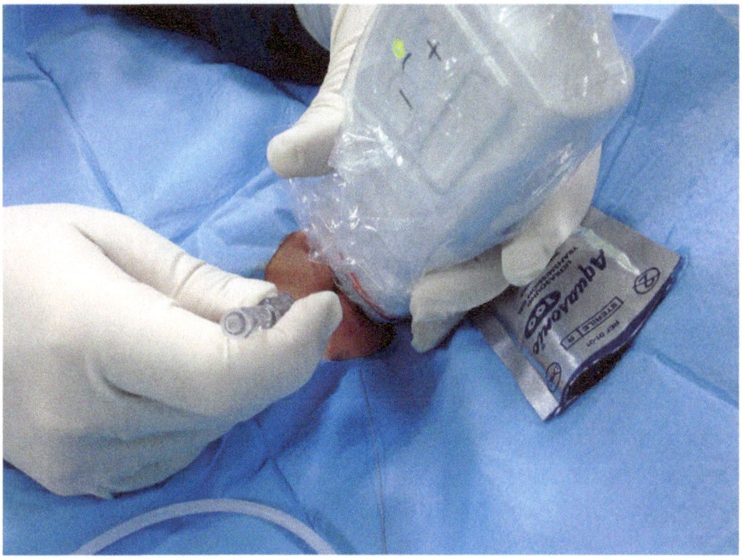

Figure **2.41**

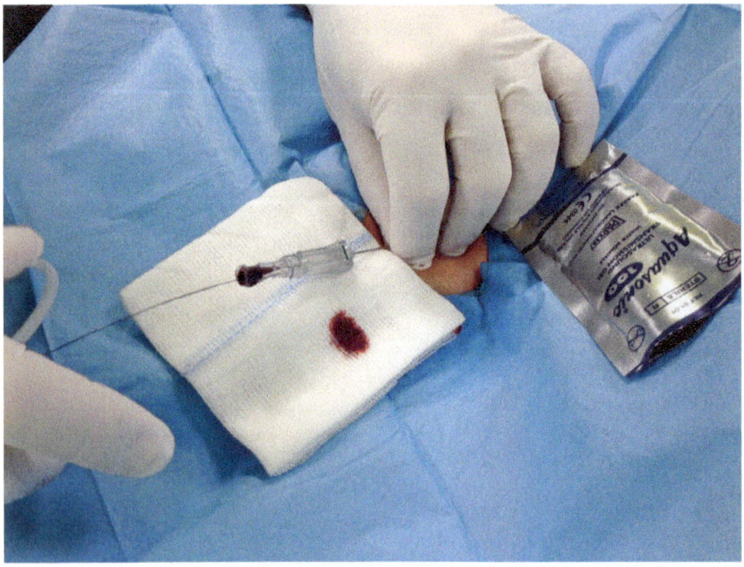

Figure **2.42**

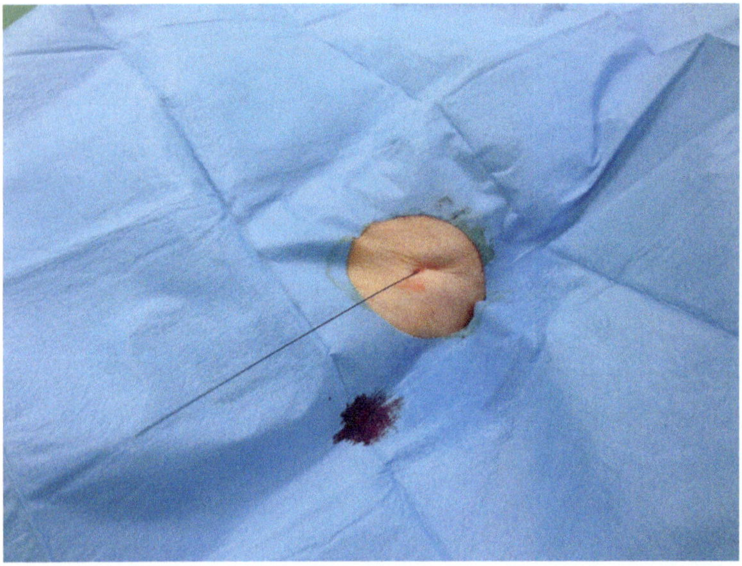

Figure **2.43**

venipuncture site be too high and fall within the proximal third of the arm, it is recommended to move the exit site down through appropriate tunneling (see below).

As with all central venous access devices (inserted in the superior caval district), during PICC insertion it is good standard practice to proceed directly to assessing the tip position, which should lie in proximity to the cavoatrial junction (immediately above or immediately below). As explained earlier, the safest, most accurate and most cost-effective technique for this purpose is the intracavitary ECG method.

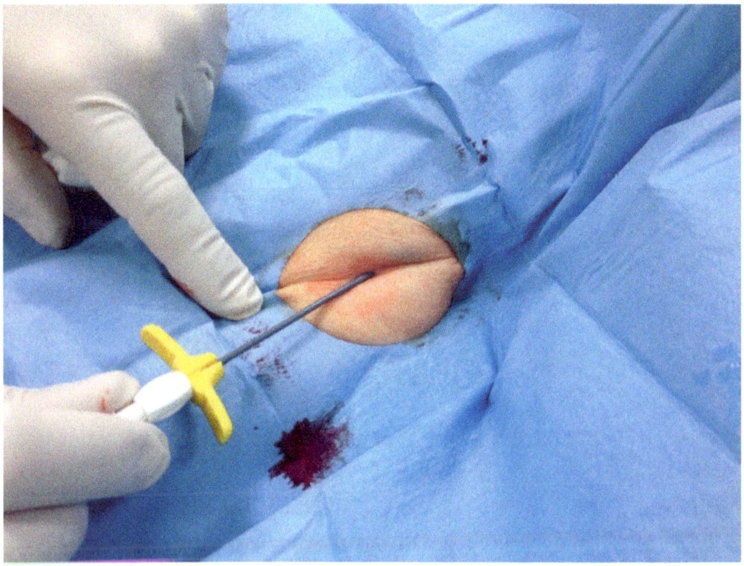

Figure **2.44**

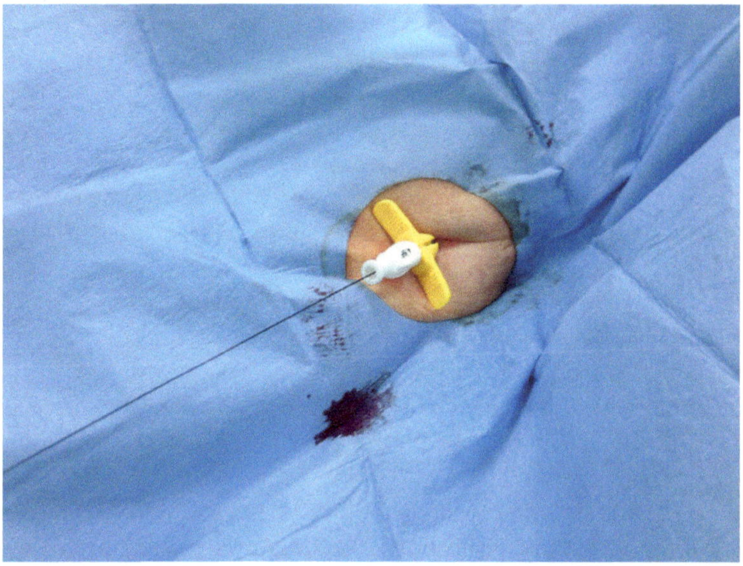

Figure **2.45**

The correct position (cavoatrial junction) corresponds to the visualisation of the P wave peak on the intracavitary ECG. Whenever this method is not applicable (in patients with atrial fibrillation, for example) or has not produced clear and unequivocal results, it is necessary to estimate the approximate catheter length with one of the methods based on skin markers described above, with or without the aid of a *tip navigation* system, and then perform a post-procedural chest X-ray. The correct tip position at the cavoatrial junction will be inferred from the presence of the catheter tip at around 3 cm under the

tracheal carina (in adult patients): any position between 1 and 5 cm under the carina are considered acceptable.
As recommended by the guidelines, securing the catheter with a stitch must be avoided whenever possible. The presence of a suture creates a chronic cutaneous granuloma, which inevitably favours the extraluminal contamination of the venous access device. The catheter should instead be secured with *"sutureless"* or skin adhesive systems (such as Statlock or GripLok or WingGuard), or subcutaneously anchored systems (SecuraCath). Should there be any risk of immediate or early bleeding from the puncture site and/or from the catheter exit site (typically in patients suffering from coagulopathy due to drugs, liver disease, nephropathy or other causes,; or following PICC insertion where the skin has parted too much), the best way of obtaining immediate and safe haemostasis is through cyanoacrylate glue application.
The exit site should be protected with semipermeable adhesive transparent dressing. If gauze is placed under the dressing to cover the exit site, the dressing should be replaced after 24 hours. In the absence of gauze, it can remain in place for 7 days.

SIP protocol for safe insertion of PICC

The concept of *zero targeting* based on the possibility/necessity of reducing predictable complications to zero has become very widespread in the prevention of bacteraemic infections from venous catheters. It is possible to minimise or reduce to zero all types of predictable complications, not only infective, but also mechanical and thrombotic. We can now adopt low-cost technologies and devices that can significantly reduce the risks connected to the insertion of venous access devices, and we have learned methods and strategies of conduct that, based on scientific evidence, are effective in reducing the incidence of complications without increasing the costs or times for insertion manoeuvres. Although no strategy or technology on its own is sufficient to minimise the complications of insertion, it is possible to identify a series of recommendations of particular significance and clinical efficacy, that are able to produce a positive synergistic effect on the clinical outcome of the procedure.
In other words, it is possible and even desirable to use an *insertion bundle*, that is, a series of recommendations to optimise the execution of the insertion, thereby minimising potential immediate, early or late complications.
Bundle refers to a few rules of clinical conduct that, if adopted simultaneously and consistently, can reduce or eliminate specific complications, thus significantly improving the clinical outcome. The *bundle* must contain a limited number of recommendations each based on scientific evidence and must be simple to apply, since its effectiveness is based on the ability to perform it on any patient.
A few years ago, GAVeCeLT developed a *bundle* for the safe insertion of PICCs (SIP protocol, SIP: Safe Insertion of PICCs).
The SIP protocol (see Table 1.2) consists of eight recommendations, explained in detail in the chart on page 87. It is advisable to underline that the SIP protocol is clearly only one of the possible *bundles* that are effective in reducing complications. Literature presents other similar *insertion bundles*, that often more complex, but all quite similar since they are based on the same *evidence-based* recommendations.

1. Hand hygiene, aseptic technique and maximum barrier precautions

The first point of the ISP protocol illustrates the aseptic technique. Contrary to what was thought in the past, many infections related to PICCs (and venous access devices in general) originate from incorrect conduct at the time of the insertion and may manifest on the third to fourth day, or even later.

Hand hygiene before performing the manoeuvre is one of the most effective behavioural strategies in reducing the infective risk, as is the adoption of maximum barrier precautions, such as sterile gloves and gowns, non-sterile mask and cap, as well as a large sterile field that covers the entire patient (Table 2.8). The adoption of a large sterile field is particular important for PICCs, where the risk of contamination during the manipulation of catheters, stylets and metal guidewires of a certain length is very high. Hand hygiene and maximum barrier precautions are considered to be manoeuvres with the utmost evidence of efficacy and the maximum force of recommendation in all the guidelines, such as Atlanta CDC guidelines in the USA and EPIC (evidence-based Practice and Infection Control) guidelines in the UK. In addition to "traditional" barrier precautions, an appropriate ultrasound probe cover is also required, as recommended by the GAVeCeLT-WoCoVA-WINFOCUS Consensus of 2012, which examined the evidence for all aspects connected to the ultrasound-guided insertion of vascular access.

Skin preparation should include a careful scrub of the area using 2% chlorhexidine in alcohol solution (best done twice). A solution of 2% chlorhexidine in 70% isopropyl alcohol (IPA) (ethanol is more aggressive both to the skin and to the polyurethane catheters) is preferable, with a disposable applicator if possible. Disposable sterile applicators are available with 2% coloured chlorhexidine in 70% IPA, which is the gold standard for skin antisepsis before inserting a venous access. Solutions of povidone-iodine at 10% are less effective and should only be adopted for patients with known allergies to chlorhexidine (a very rare occurrence).

Table 2.9 summarises the main recommendations included in the guidelines for the infection prevention during insertion of venous access: it will be noted that, with the sole exception of short peripheral cannulas, the use of sterile gloves and maximum barrier precautions is mandatory for positioning any device. Similarly, hand hygiene before the procedure and skin antisepsis with 2% chlorhexidine are recommended in the insertion of all venous access devices, including needle cannulas.

Table 2.8 Maximum barrier precautions
• Non-sterile, clean cap • Non-sterile, clean mask • Sterile gloves (after hand-washing) • Sterile gown • Large sterile field (coverage of 80% of the patient and more) • Sterile cover of the ultrasound probe and the cable connected to the ultrasonograph

Table 2.9 Recommendations for the prevention of infections during the insertion of venous access			
	Short cannulas	**Long cannulas Midline PICC CICC**	**TCC Port PICC-port Cuffed PICC**
Hand-washing	Yes	Yes	Yes
Gloves	Clean not sterile	Sterile	Sterile
Antiseptic	2% chlorhexidine	2% chlorhexidine	2% chlorhexidine
Maximum barrier protections	No	Yes	Yes
Environment	Bedside	Bedside	Dedicated room

2. Ultrasound exploration of the veins of the arm and the neck before the procedure

Before choosing the vein in which to insert a PICC, it is advisable to perform a bilateral ultrasound scan of all the deep veins of the arm (basilic, brachial), as well as the central veins of the region above the clavicle (axillary, subclavian, internal jugular, innominate) to exclude any anatomical anomalies or previous venous thrombosis and select the vein most probably associated with the successful outcome of the procedure. This manoeuvre is recommended by the aforementioned Consensus, in order to use ultrasound to its full potential. For a long time, indeed, ultrasound was only seen as a system for obtaining a safer and more precise venipuncture, therefore underestimating the impact it could have in examining the veins before the procedure (which it may be true not only for PICCs but also for traditional CICCs) so to select the most appropriate vein for a specific catheter in a specific patient. The deep veins of the arm should be evaluated with and without tourniquet applied.

3. Selection of the most appropriate vein

Selecting the optimal vein to cannulate is crucial for the procedure success and to reduce the risks related to it. The first important parameter is the calibre of the vein: it is advisable to choose veins having diameters at least three times the diameter of the catheter (that is: the diameter in millimetres is equal or greater than the catheter diameter according to the French scale) as evaluated without tourniquet, in order to reduce the risk of PICC-related peripheral venous thrombosis. Therefore, a 3 Fr catheter would require a 9 Fr (3 mm) or larger vein; a 4 Fr catheter a 12 Fr (4 mm) or larger vein; a 5 Fr catheter a 15 Fr (5 mm) or larger vein; a 6 Fr catheter a 18 Fr (6 mm) or larger vein.

Furthermore, to optimise the PICC exit site management, to prevent catheter malfunction due to repeated mechanical stress and to reduce the infective risk, the PICC should emerge from the skin at an appropriate distance both from the elbow and the axilla,

specifically at the level of the middle third of the upper arm. This concept was recently systematised by Rob Dawson in his ZIM (Zone Insertion Method). The tract of the upper arm between the bend of the elbow and the axillary cavity is divided into three zones of equal length: a middle third (*green zone*), a proximal third near the axilla (*yellow zone*) and a distal third close to the elbow (*red zone*). To obtain an ideal exit site, the venipuncture should always be performed in the *green zone*; however, in clinical practice, this is not always feasible due to the calibre of the veins being too small, or because of unfavourable anatomical relations (the anatomical position of the brachial artery and median nerve, for example, may impede the puncture of a brachial vein), etc. In these cases, it is possible to overcome the problem through the tunneling technique, that allows for the puncture site to be at an appropriate distance from the exit site. In practice, venipuncture can be performed at a higher level, in the proximal third of the arm up to the axillary cavity in the *yellow zone*, where the veins usually have a greater calibre, and a subcutaneous tunnel can be built so that the catheter exits lies in the *green zone*, further away from the area with high bacterial contamination. In this way, infective and mechanical risks related to the very "high" position of the catheter are limited and the potential discomfort for the patient during movements of the arm is avoided (Figure 2.46).
A third aspect to be considered is the depth of the vein. Although there are no insurmountable difficulties in placing venous catheters even in very deep veins, the excessive depth of the cannulated vein can give rise to malfunctions during the maintenance manoeuvres, due to the kinking of the catheter. Therefore, the veins to be selected for the insertion of PICCs should ideally be situated at a maximum of 2 cm from the skin surface (Figure 2.47). The puncture and cannulation of veins deeper than 3 cm must always be avoided.

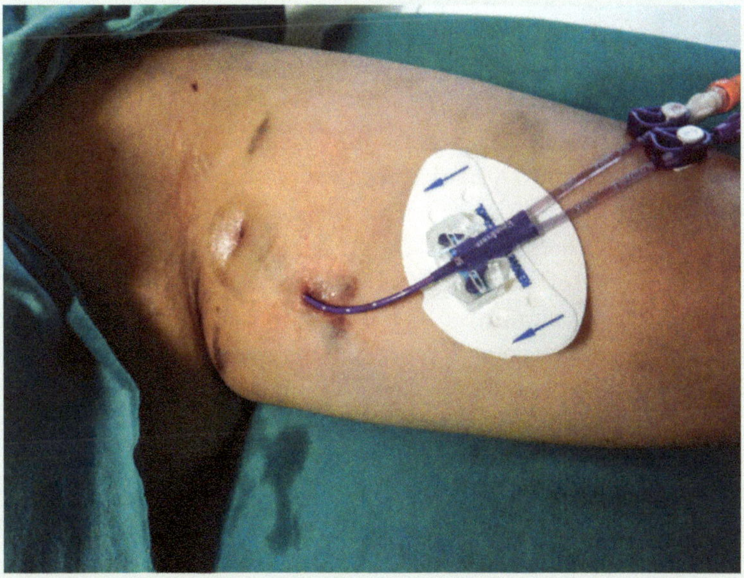

Figure **2.46**

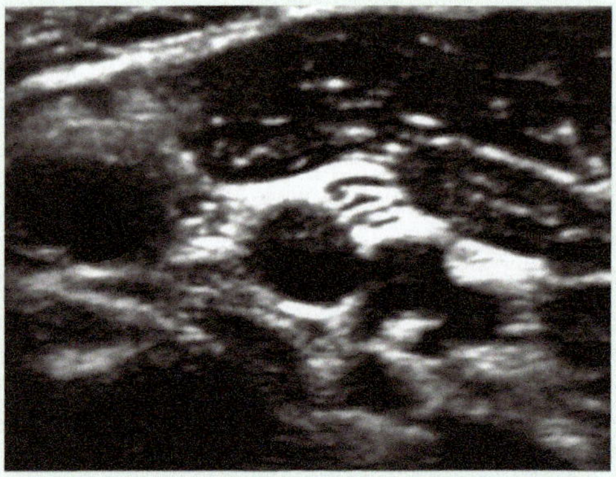

Figure **2.47**

Once the "ideal" venipuncture site has been found (that is, the site where the vein appears to be of an appropriate diameter and at an appropriate depth), the operator must verify the estimated distance between the future exit site and the cavoatrial junction with one of the two methods described above. In this phase, it will also be necessary to verify that the puncture site lies in Dawson's green area (middle third of the arm): if the puncture site is too high (in the proximal third of the arm, Dawson's yellow zone), a short tunneling of the PICC must be planned.
At this point, in the case of PICCs designed for distal trimming, the catheter must be shortened so to obtain a PICC with a length 1-2 cm greater than the length estimated by surface landmarks. In the case of PICCs designed for proximal trimming, the catheter is left intact, taking note of the desired length (this will be useful later).

4. Ultrasound identification of the median nerve and the brachial artery before venipuncture

In the arm, in addition to the deep veins, which are the target of the PICC inserter, there are other structures of fundamental importance that must be preserved during PICC insertion, such as the median nerve and the brachial artery. The most effective method for avoiding accidental damage to the median nerve is through direct ultrasound identification of the nerve, both before and during venipuncture. Normally, the median nerve is found close to the brachial artery (often immediately above) and appears as a hyperechoic not compressible structure, with an internal "beehive" pattern (Figure 2.48) under ultrasound. Close to the basilic vein (often immediately below), there is a much thinner, exclusively sensory nerve, the medial cutaneous nerve of the arm: its accidental puncture (rare) during basilic venipuncture may lead to some symptoms, but without the serious consequences of damaging the median nerve. The same warning is valid for reducing the risk of an accidental arterial puncture. While the latter may lead to local haematomas of varying extent, but always reversible, damage to the median nerve can be associated with a chain of consequences, that can be permanent. Ultrasound identification of these "dangerous" structures involves, on one hand, appropriate ultrasound instrumentation and, on the other, appropriate training.

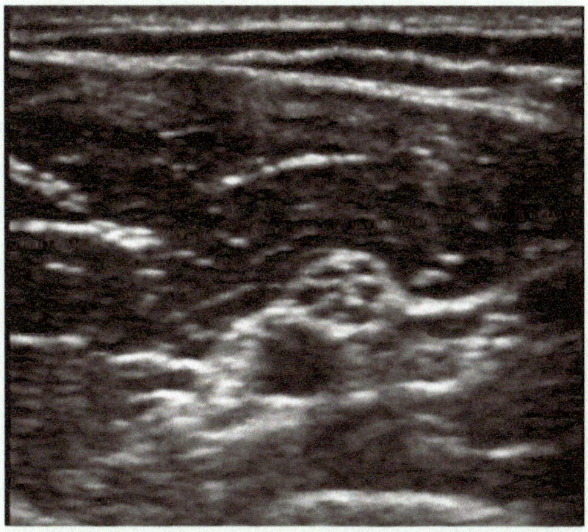

Figure **2.48**

5. Ultrasound-guided venipuncture

Ultrasound-guided venipuncture of a deep vein of the arm (basilic or brachial) is the standard technique for venous cannulation for PICC positioning, with enormous benefits in terms of safety, cost-effectiveness and efficiency. PICC positioning at the level of the elbow or the distal third of the arm using cannulation of a visible or palpable vein without ultrasound guidance is not currently recommended, since it is associated with a high risk of failure, malpositions, thrombosis and infective complications. Many studies in recent years have shown the importance of the ultrasound-guided technique for PICCs: see the recommendations of the ESPEN guidelines (European Society of Parenteral and Enteral Nutrition).

Along with the constant use of the ultrasound-guided technique, the micro-introducer technique (using the modified Seldinger technique) is also recommended. It consists of puncturing the vein with a thin 21 G needle with an echogenic tip and cannulating the vein with a thin metal guidewire (0.018"), with a straight but extremely soft tip *(floppy straight tip)* preferably in nitinol (nickel-titanium). Apart from the experience of the operator (and therefore the quality of the training received), the most important factors in determining a successful cannulation are the quality of the ultrasound device (the minimum prerequisite of which is the clear visualisation of the median nerve) and the quality of the micro-introduction kit. An inadequately stiff guidewire or a micro-introducer of mediocre quality can be associated with failures, even if used by expert hands.

6. Ultrasound scan of the internal jugular vein during the catheter progression

During the insertion of the catheter in the micro-introducer, it is useful to visualise the ipsilateral internal jugular vein by ultrasound and compress it with the ultrasound probe, in order to facilitate the passage of the catheter from the subclavian vein to the innominate vein (Figure 2.49). Alternatively, the patient can be asked, if cooperative, to turn her or his head towards the operator's side. After the manoeuvre, it is recommended use the ultrasound probe to verify the absence of the catheter in both jugular veins (Figure 2.50).

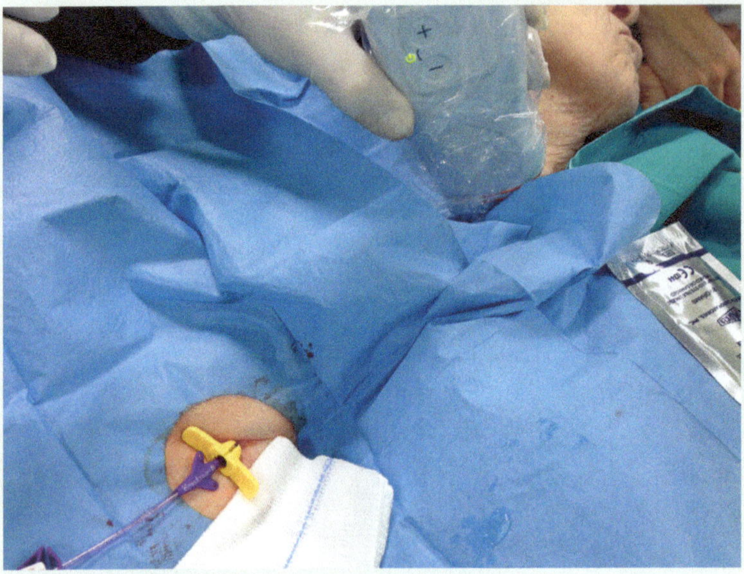

Figure **2.49**

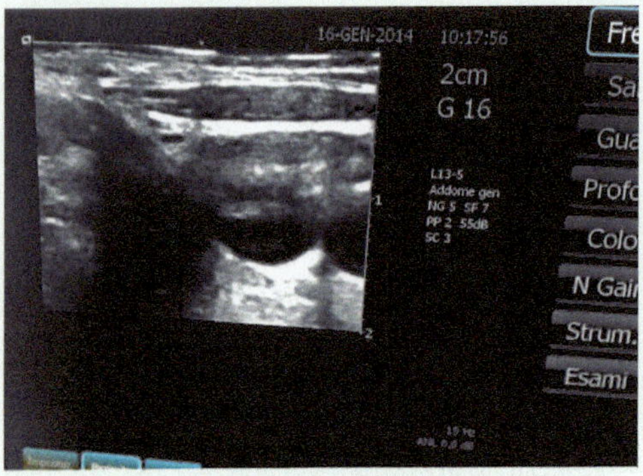

Figure **2.50**

This simple and easy procedure enables the immediate identification of the potential malpositioning of the catheter (failure to enter an innominate), without having to resort to fluoroscopy or costly electromagnetic-based *tip navigation* systems or any another type in most cases.

It is clear that this point also underlines the importance of the ultrasound instrument at various times during the positioning of venous access, beside venipuncture.

7. Use of the intracavitary ECG method to verify the tip position

The intracavitary ECG method is an economical, effective, simple and safe system for verifying the central position of the PICC tip during the procedure. This technique exploits the amplitude variations of the P wave in an intracavitary ECG lead II trace, in which the venous catheter takes the place of the red electrode: when the tip is in the

correct position, corresponding to the cavoatrial junction, the P wave at the intracavitary ECG reaches the maximum height whereas, in more proximal positions, the amplitude is reduced and, in more distal positions (entirely in the atrium), it becomes biphasic and negative if it reaches the inferior vena cava. The technique has been fully described above. As already explained, the only limitation is the applicability of the method since, being based on P wave variations, it cannot be employed in patients with atrial fibrillation (or other conditions that prevent the visualisation of the P wave on ECG).
Currently, other devices are also available for precisely locating the catheter tip in patients in whom the intracavitary ECG technique cannot be used (for example: patients suffering from atrial fibrillation). By replacing the stylet with a purpose-built one with an external navigation system that recognises the guide tip through electromagnetic signals (Navigator, Corpak), it is possible to identify the site and direction taken by the catheter. Transthoracic echocardiography can be of great help in children since it can also be applied during the procedure. In selected cases, it is possible to adopt fluoroscopy (which, however, must remain the exception, since it jeopardises PICC safety and cost-effectiveness) as well. The correct position of the tip significantly reduces the risk of arrhythmia, catheter malfunction, formation of a pericatheter fibroblastic sheath (so-called *fibrin sleeve*) and catheter-related central venous thrombosis. Verification during the procedure (rather than after the procedure, as it was done traditionally by chest X-ray) avoids the costs and risks associated with the need to reposition PICCs whenever the tip has not been positioned in the correct site.
As already mentioned, in the case of PICCs designed for distal *trimming*, the catheter is shortened so to obtain the desired length (slightly more than that calculated from the surface landmark methods) and then inserted into the introducer (Figure 2.51-2.53).

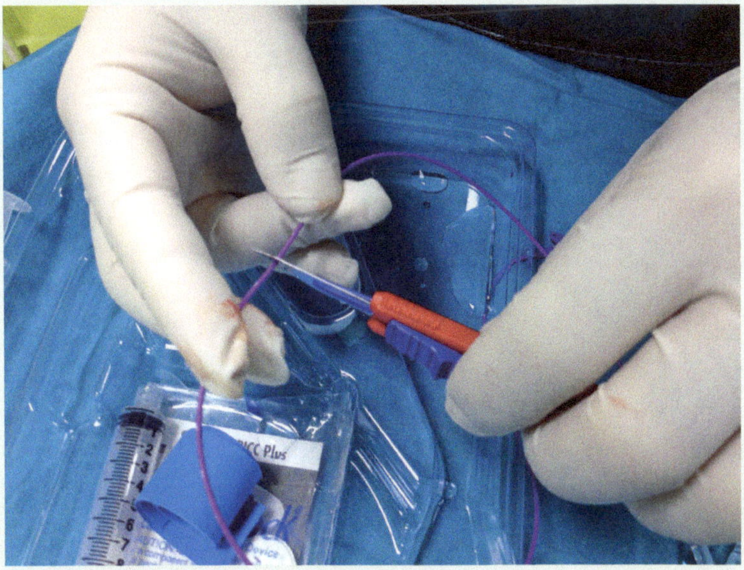

Figure **2.51**

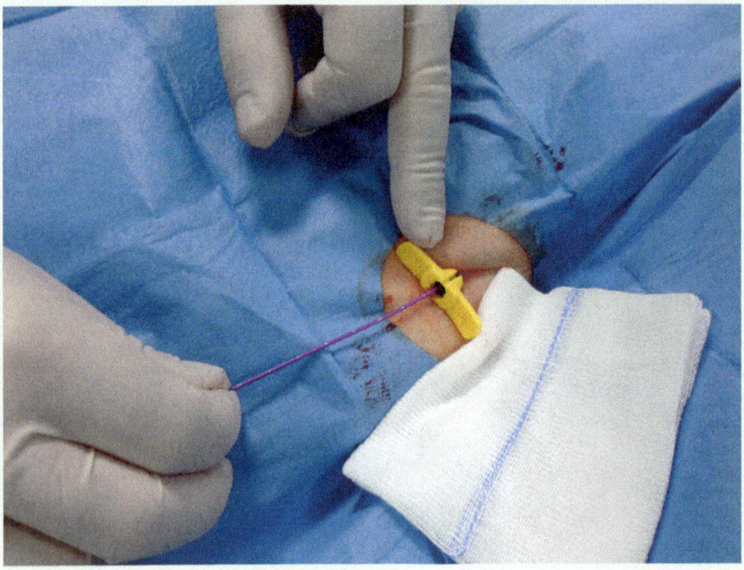

Figure **2.52**

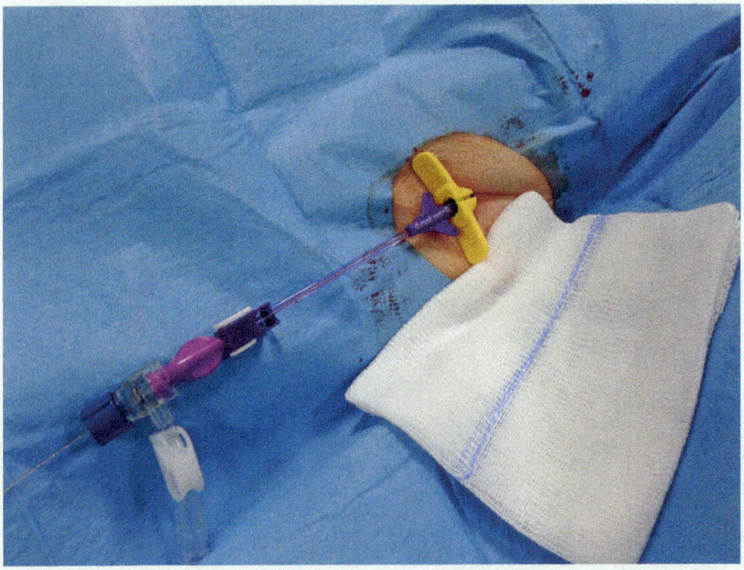

Figure **2.53**

After connecting the catheter to the ECG monitor using the sterile cables available on the market, the ECG technique can be performed and the catheter secured in the position that corresponds with the maximum height of the P wave (Figure 2.54-2.58). It should be noted that some of these cables cannot be connected directly to the electrode of the ECG monitor but need an intermediate switch-box (Figure 2.59-2.60).

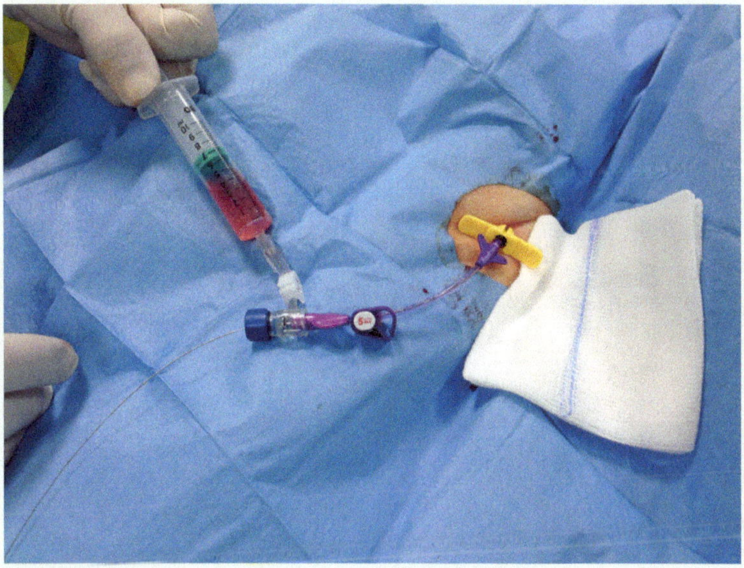

Figure **2.54**

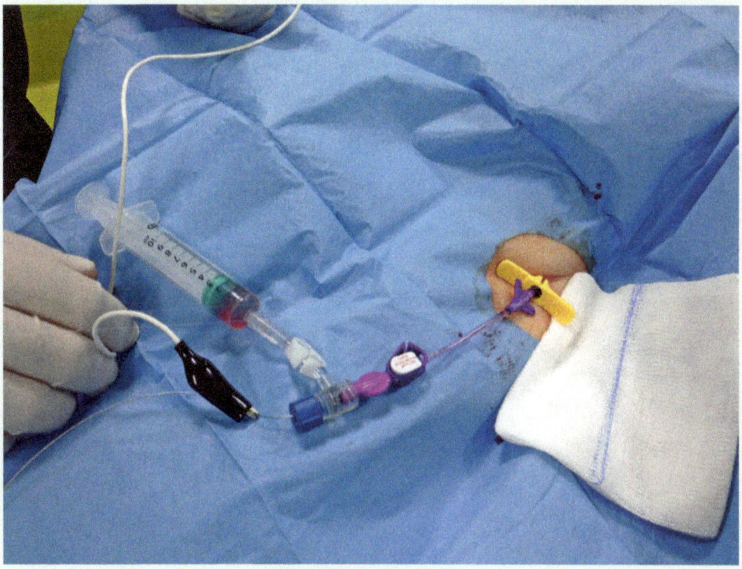

Figure **2.55**

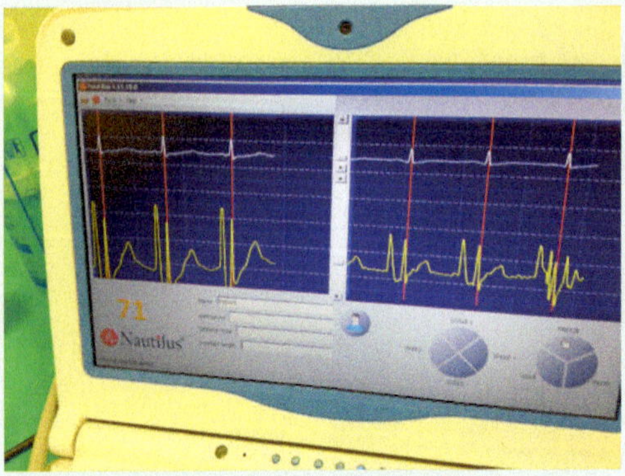

Figure **2.56**

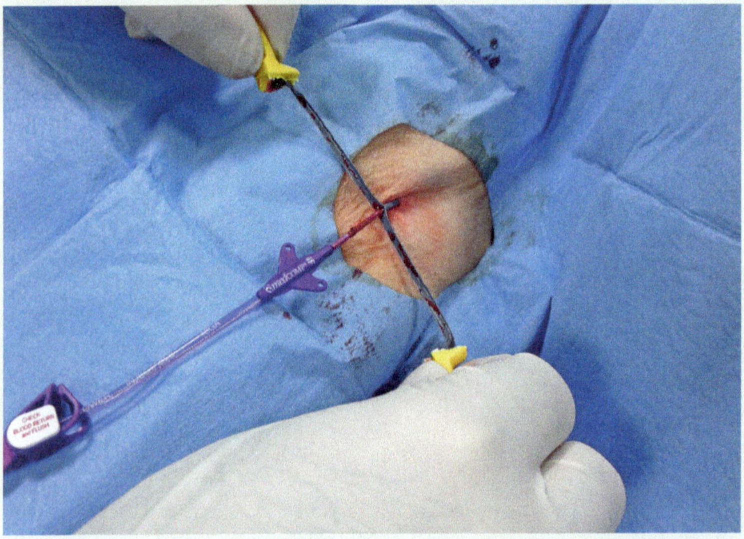

Figure **2.57**

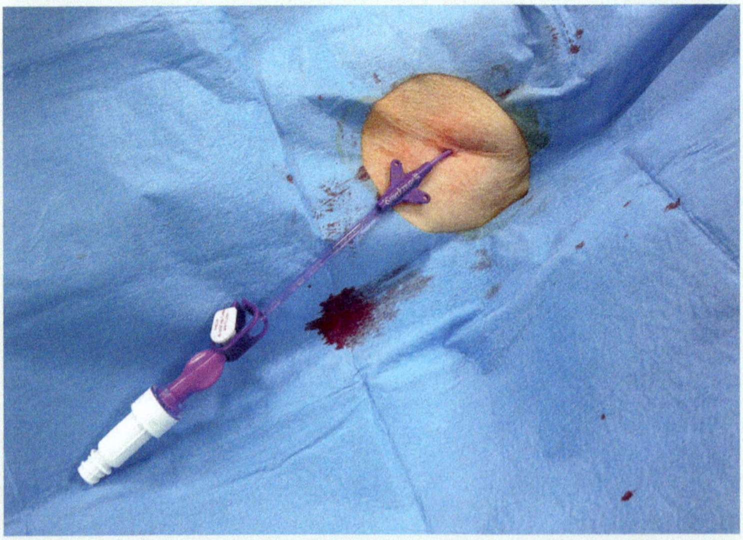

Figure **2.58**

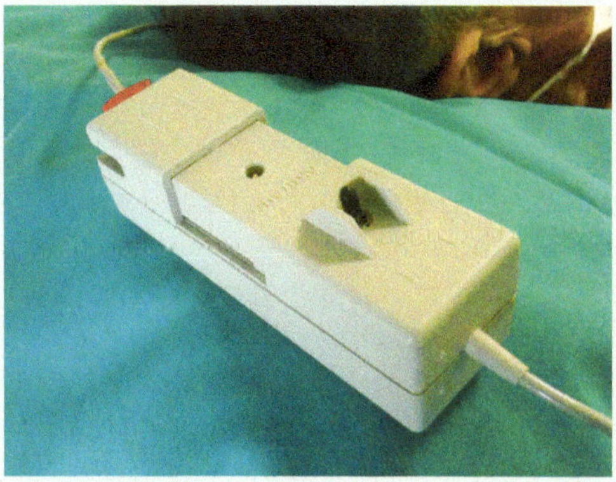

Figure **2.59**

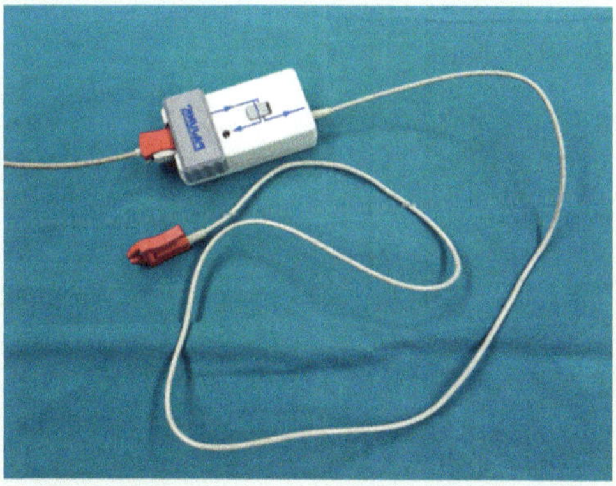

Figure **2.60**

In the case of PICCs designed for proximal rather that distal *trimming* (such as certain PICCs with "specialised" tips, for example), the intact PICC is inserted in the micro-introducer at the time of the ECG intracavitary manoeuvre and note is taken of the distance between the exit site and the maximum height of the P wave. Then, depending on the type of PICC, the catheter is proximally trimmed (with subsequent connection with a winged extension, then secured to the skin), or directly secured to the skin in this position using a moveable wing to be applied along the catheter, close to the exit site.
Groshong PICCs designed with closed-end tip and distal valve (still in use in some facilities even if greatly surpassed by open tip PICCs in terms of cost-effectiveness) display a peculiarity during the intracavitary ECG manoeuvre: in its neutral position, the Groshong valve closes and prevents communication between the catheter lumen and the venous lumen, so electrical conductivity between the saline contained in the catheter and the venous blood is created only applying a light infusion pressure with a manually operated syringe that is connected to the proximal end of the catheter. This allows to keep the valve open for as long as needed to create the electric connection and verify the signal of the intracavitary ECG.
In the case of PICCs designed with proximal valve and open-end tip, there are no major problems: it is sufficient to keep the stylet partially inserted in the catheter to create an electrical connection with the stylet: the existence of the latter is sufficient to keep the valve open and maintain the electrical connection between the column of saline solution proximal to the valve and the column distal to the valve.

8. Securement of the PICC to the skin using a sutureless device

At the end of the procedure, the PICC must be secured to the patient's skin avoiding sutures but employing an appropriate *sutureless device*, as recommended by the Atlanta CDC guidelines. The use of these devices is potentially effective in reducing the risk of infections, displacement and venous thrombosis. Ideally, the *sutureless device* should be used together with a semipermeable transparent dressing, which, however, in the case of blood secretion from a PICC exit site on the skin, could be contraindicated in the first

24 hours after insertion. In this case, it is advisable to cover with a gauze dressing, to be replaced as soon as possible with a transparent dressing, as recommended by the EPIC guidelines.

Currently, apart from skin adhesive securement devices (for example: StatLock or GripLok or WingGuard), there are some new devices that anchor the PICC by means of two small nitinol bars inserted under the skin at the catheter exit point at the time of attachment (SecuraCath). Compared to other *sutureless devices*, this type of securement device must not replaced periodically, but lasts as long as the catheter lasts and is specifically indicated for patients whose PICC had previously accidentally dislodged or, generally, whenever an increased risk of the catheter displacement is expected due to uncontrollable behaviour (children, or elderly patients with cognitive deterioration) or specific local cutaneous condition (erythroderma from medicines, burns, dermatitis, allergies or intolerance to dressings or to the adhesive of standard *sutureless devices*).

Moreover, patients in whom PICCs are inserted in outpatient clinics or those with a higher risk of bleeding (cirrhotic, under treatment with anticoagulants or suffering from oncohaematological diseases) may benefit from the application of a cyanoacrylate-based glue to reduce post-procedural bleeding from the exit site, thereby enabling optimisation of the device management.

The association of *sutureless device* + cyanoacrylate glue + semipermeable transparent membrane will guarantee the utmost stabilisation and protection of the catheter at the exit site (Figure 2.61-2.63).

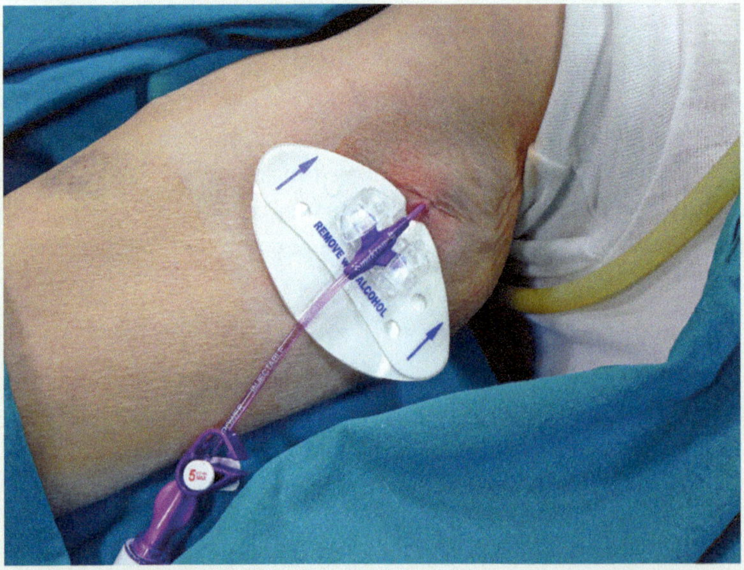

Figure **2.61**

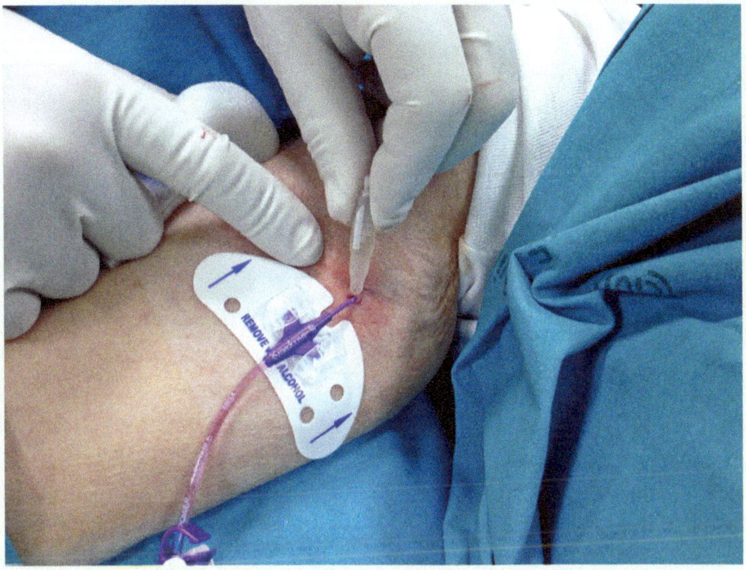

Figure **2.62**

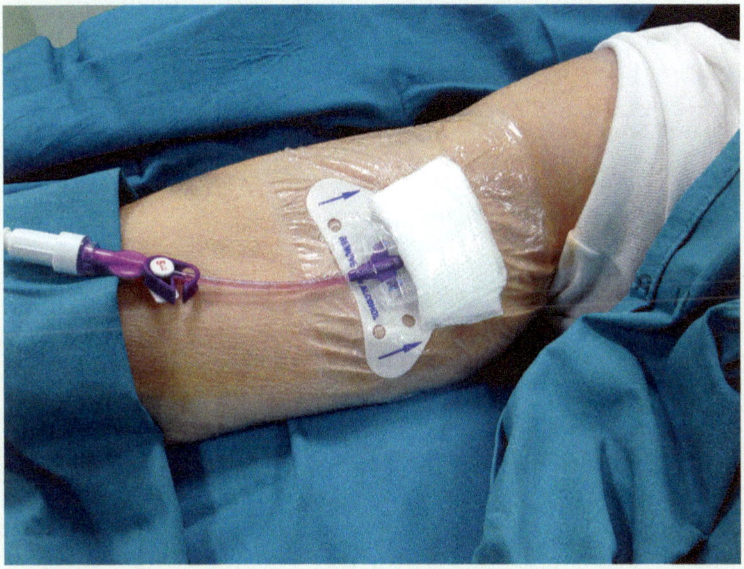

Figure **2.63**

Tunneled PICC insertion technique

As previously mentioned, in certain situations it is advisable that the PICC exit site is not too close to the venipuncture site (typically, when the only vein with a sufficient calibre for the catheter is in the proximal third of the arm or Dawson's so-called "yellow" area). Under these conditions, a short tract of the PICC can be tunneled subcutaneously with various, simple techniques, in order to simultaneously obtain both a venipuncture site in the yellow area and an exit site in the green area.
The tunneling instrument may be a proper metal tunneler or a needle cannula of adequate size. If a tunneler is used, it is advisable to select purpose-made instruments for PICC tunneling (there are various types available on the market), which have a blunt tip at one end to penetrate the subcutaneous tissue, and a connection system at the other end, of an appropriate size so as to guarantee the connection with 3-6 Fr calibre PICCs. If a needle cannula is used, a 14 G can be used for 4-5 Fr catheters or a 16 G for 3F catheters. The needle cannula passes through the subcutaneous tissue from the puncture site to the exit site (or vice versa) and then, after needle removal, the PICC is threaded inside the cannula.
The tunnel is usually created in an anterograde fashion: the PICC is first passed into the subcutaneous tissue (drawn by the tunneler or pushed into the cannula) from the exit site up to the puncture site, and then inserted into the vein through the introducer. Only for PICCs designed for proximal *trimming* is it possible to choose between anterograde tunneling (as described above) and retrograde tunneling (the catheter is first inserted in the vein and then tunneled, in a retrograde fashion, from the puncture site to the exit site).
When positioning cuffed PICCs (see below), tunneling is mandatory and must be performed so as to place the cuff inside the subcutaneous tunnel at least 2 cm away from the exit site.

PICC-port insertion technique

The term PICC-port refers to brachial ports inserted with the same principles as 20th century PICCs: ultrasound-guided venipuncture of the deep veins of the arm + micro-introducer technique (modified Seldinger technique) + positioning the tip with the intracavitary ECG method.
The venipuncture and the venous cannulation, as well as the placement of the tip at the cavoatrial junction, are performed as described for PICCs.
The only difference is that the punctiform incision of the venipuncture, used for introducing the metal guidewire first, then the micro-introducer/re-dilator and finally the catheter itself, is enlarged transversally through lateral broadening, in order to prepare the incision in which to insert the reservoir.
By means of an appropriate infusion of 10-15 mL of local anaesthetic (for example: 0.5-0.75% ropivacaine), a subcutaneous pocket is created by blunt dissection in which the reservoir is housed. The skin incision is then closed with a layer of absorbable intradermal stitches + adhesion of the skin with cyanoacrylate glue.

Prevention of immediate and early complications connected to PICC insertion

There are few immediate complications directly related to PICC positioning (Table 2.10) and they rarely occur. We can classify them as follows.

Venipuncture failure or success after repeated punctures

This usually depends on two reasons: insufficient operator training and/or use of inadequate materials. For example, metal guidewires which are too stiff or micro-introducers with inadequate tapering can make the manoeuvre difficult and may be associated with repeated attempts; obviously, repeated attempts are inevitably associated with greater local trauma, venous intramural haematomas and other local alterations that may lead to an increased risk of venous thrombosis.

Prevention strategies

- Adequate operator training (for example, on a simulator, as described above) before proceeding to the insertion in the patient.
- Selection of the appropriate material: high quality 21 G echogenic needles, microguidewire in nitinol with a sufficiently soft tip.
- Adequate vein selection (sufficient calibre and adequate depth of the vein).
- Appropriate *out-of-plane* venipuncture technique (vein visible at the centre of the screen, skin puncture at the centre of the probe, vertical progression of the needle, appropriate *tilting* movement of the probe to follow the needle tip up to its entry in the vein).

Accidental nerve injury

The most feared injury involves the median nerve, which is often found in close relations of contiguity with the brachial artery or with one or more of the brachial veins (Figure 2.64). Accidental damage to the median nerve leads to one of the potentially most serious complications following PICC positioning, that may cause permanent functional damage. Accidental damage to the medial cutaneous nerve of the arm, which often lies in direct contact with the basilic vein, has also been described but the actual possibility of this type of nerve damage leading to a significant clinical problem is, however, more theoretical than real.

Table 2.10 Immediate and early complications after PICC insertion
• Failure or repeated punctures • Accidental nerve lesion • Accidental arterial puncture/local haematomas • Pain during and after insertion • Difficulty in the progression of the guide and/or catheter • Primary malposition • Bleeding from the insertion site

Prevention strategies

- The best way of preventing this complication is using an ultrasound device of sufficient definition to identify the median nerve: the appropriate identification of the nerve is, in fact, the only effective way of preventing accidental damage to it.
- Alongside the use of an ultrasound device of sufficient quality, good clinical operator training is also essential and must include practicing ultrasound anatomy of the arm with recognition of the nerve structures.

Local haematomas

Local haematomas are often secondary to an accidental puncture of the brachial artery or to significant damage of the vein to be punctured (with intra- or extramural haematoma) (Figure 2.65); the cause in this case can also be found in insufficient training or in the use of an inadequate micro-introduction kit.

Prevention strategies

- Operator training, including practising ultrasound anatomy of the arm for the selective recognition of the arterial structures.
- Use of a metal guidewire and a good quality micro-introducer (if the guide is too rigid or the micro-introducer has insufficient tapering, an excessive trauma of the venous wall is more likely to occur).

Pain during insertion

This may be due to inadequate local anaesthesia of the zone, erroneous tourniquet positioning , accidental puncture of a sensitive nerve (median nerve; medial cutaneous nerve of the arm) or an excessive prolongation of the manoeuvre due to technical difficulties, sufficient to make the patient not tolerate the tourniquet anymore.

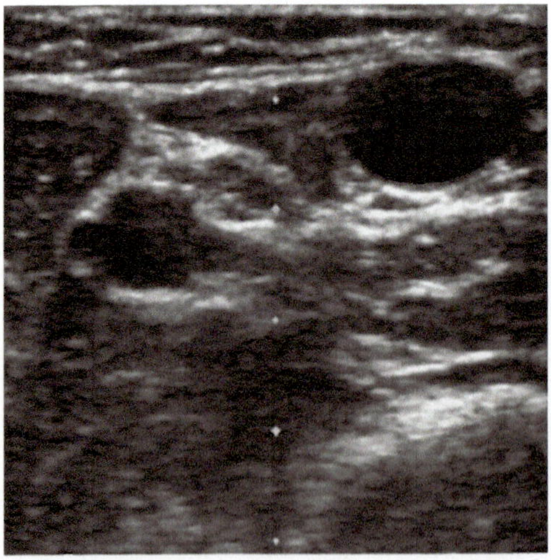

Figure **2.64**

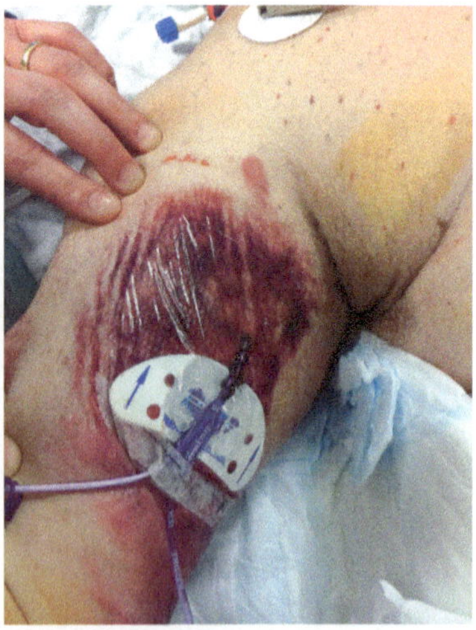

Figure **2.65**

Prevention strategies

- Before starting the manoeuvre, place the patient's arm in a comfortable, stable position.
- Place the tourniquet appropriately (very high, at the axillary level, and leaving clothing between the skin and the band, if possible).
- Avoid using the tourniquet for very high veins (in the proximal third of the arm) or for veins with a significant calibre (from 5 mm up) or that cannot easily be collapsed.
- Use local anaesthesia (a few millilitres of ropivacaine 0.75%, for example) before venipuncture, injecting it with a small needle (25 G, for example) and performing ultrasound-guided technique (that is, checking the antiseptic infusion with the ultrasound probe).
- Add a few millilitres of local anaesthetic after positioning the metal guidewire and removing the needle, before inserting the micro-introducer.

Difficulty in the progression of the metal guide or the micro-introducer

This may be the result of an erroneous venipuncture maneuver (typically, due to insufficient operator training) or the use of poor quality material (for example, a guide with an insufficiently soft tip or a micro-introducer/dilator with inadequate tapering).

Prevention strategies

- Adequate operator training (on a simulator).
- Appropriate venipuncture technique.
- Use of a good quality metal guide and micro-introducer (see above).

Difficulty in catheter progression

This may be the result of an objective difficulty connected to a partial or complete obstruction of the axillary-subclavian venous axis (post-thrombotic stenosis; pacemaker wires in the subclavian lumen) or a particularly acute angle between the subclavian and innominate axes (typically on the right side, rather than the left) or suboptimal material (for example, use of a catheter made of a material that is too soft: it is no coincidence that difficulties with progression and/or the unwanted progression of the catheter in the ipsilateral jugular occur more often if silicone PICCs are used).

Prevention strategies

- Choose the appropriate side for PICC insertion, considering the presence of a pacemaker as a relative contraindication and using the complete RaPeVA protocol (therefore also examining the patency of the central vessels – axillary, subclavian, innominate – and not only the vessels of the arm).
- As a preference, use power injectable PICCs in polyurethane, characterised by greater rigidity (note: to increase PICC rigidity, replace the stylet with the guidewire or, in case of double lumen PICCs, introduce a metal guidewire in the lumen not occupied by the stylet).
- After inserting the PICC in the introducer, turn the patient's head towards the insertion side, with the chin pointing towards the clavicle, if possible.

- If there are difficulties at the subclavian-innominate passage, place the ultrasound probe on the patient's neck: the compression of the jugular by the probe can assist the catheter in directing the right way towards the innominate vein. Moreover, by visualising the subclavian and innominate vein with the supraclavicular ultrasound approach, it is often possible to direct the catheter under direct vision under "echoscopy".
- In selected cases, it is virtually possible to carry out the manoeuvre under fluoroscopic control, although this is rarely indicated and certainly not cost-effective.

It is important to underline that many *tip navigation* systems among those described above (Navigator, Nautilus Delta, Sherlock 3CG, or Vasonova VPS) enable to assess whether the catheter tool a wrong turn towards the internal jugular, but they are of little use in helping the operator reposition the catheter and direct it towards the innominate vein. On the contrary, positioning under ultrasound or fluoroscopic control enables the operator to send the catheter in the right direction by applying appropriate manipulation (for example: rotation of the catheter or advancing the guidewire beyond the catheter tip). In this regard, ultrasound is undoubtedly more useful than fluoroscopy, since the former enables to visualise both the venous lumen and the catheter (or guide), while the second does not directly visualise the venous system.

Primary malpositioning

A catheter is considered malpositioned when its tip does not reach the lower third of the vein of the upper vena cava or is positioned deeper than the upper third of the right atrium. The term primary malposition, that is linked to the insertion manoeuvre, is used to distinguish it from secondary malposition, occurring after some time due to the spontaneous "migration" of the catheter tip (if, for example, intrathoracic pressure increases, as explained below) or to displacement of the tip following displacement of the catheter external tract. As mentioned above, the constant use of the intracavitary ECG method minimises the incidence of primary malpositioning. Malpositioning may also occur in patients in whom the ECG method is not applicable, such as, for example, patients with atrial fibrillation or, in any case, where there is no possibility of visualising the P wave in the surface ECG trace.

Prevention strategies

- Using the intracavitary ECG method for every PICC insertion, as long as the P wave can clearly be visualised on the surface ECG (that is, when the method is applicable).
- If the P wave cannot be visualised, as recommended above, the operator may adopt some alternative strategies: (1) the traditional method (assessment of the length of the catheter by surface landmarks + control of the direction by means of ultrasound scan of the subclavian/internal jugular junction + final verification of the tip position through chest X-ray); (2) using the Navigator to position the tip below the third intercostal space, then checking the final position by chest X-ray; (3) using alternative intraprocedural methods such as TTE, with or without 'echo-contrast medium'; (4) targeted use of fluoroscopy.

Bleeding from the insertion site

PICC insertion is often associated with bleeding at the exit site, mainly because the modified Seldinger technique necessarily involves an enlargement of the exit site to allow catheter insertion through a skin breach larger than the diameter of the catheter and at least equal to the PICC calibre plus an additional half Fr, which is the external diameter of the micro-introducer. Bleeding from the exit site is a frequent cause of logistical problems (the need to replace the dressing after a few minutes or a few hours) and patient anxiety. Because of the risk of early bleeding, it is usually recommended to place an initial temporary dressing with gauze, to be replaced after 24 hours with a definitive dressing consisting of adhesive transparent membrane. To this end, early placement of Biopatch-type sponge dressings is also feasible. In addition to releasing chlorhexidine, these dressings have excellent liquid absorption properties (in this case: haematic and sero-haematic secretions from the exit site). However, the cost-effectiveness of this strategy is uncertain.

Prevention strategies

- Avoid using a scalpel to make the incision before introducing the micro-introducer/re-dilator: rather than cutting the skin, the operator may disassemble the micro-introducer into two pieces (*peelaway* introducer and dilator), insert the dilator into the skin opening, withdraw it, reassemble the introducer and the dilator and insert them together.
- Use a *reverse tapering* PICC with the enlargement having the same size as the catheter calibre in its most proximal tract. The enlarged proximal tract has a greater diameter than both the catheter and the introducer, therefore can effectively reduce the bleeding from the skin cut by applying mechanical compression.
- The most effective system for preventing bleeding from the skin cut is, without any doubt, the application of cyanoacrylate glue around the catheter exit site. Cyanoacrylate seals the skin breach, thereby stopping the bleeding and reducing the risk of catheter displacement and of bacterial contamination by the extraluminal route. If glue is used, the definitive dressing with transparent membrane can be applied directly, without using a temporary dressing with gauze to be replaced after 24 hours. To date, no harmful effects from cyanoacrylate on the skin or on catheter materials, have been described. Glue sealing is highly recommended in the following situations: (1) evident bleeding at the end of the manoeuvre; (2) PICC insertion in patients with predictable coagulation problems (hepatopathy, use of anticoagulants, thrombocytopenia, etc.); or (3) in patients to be sent home immediately after insertion.
- Some preparations to prevent *exit site* bleeding are available on the market, as sponge dressing with anticoagulation properties (StatSeal, Guardiva), but they currently do not seem to have any benefits in terms of efficacy or cost-effectiveness compared to cyanoacrylate glue.

Finally, it must be remembered that, as the most recent guidelines recommend, the minimisation of any of the complications described above is connected to the presence of a well-trained PICC Team, the definition of a precise insertion procedure that is systematically adopted by all operators, as well as the adoption of a checklist to ensure that every insertion manoeuvre is performed in a consistent and controlled manner, according to the various steps laid down by the procedure.

CHAPTER 3

Management

General framework

The proper management of PICCs and Midlines plays a fundamental role in the prevention of most late complications or, rather, complications that occur 48 hours or later after insertion. Although an etiopathogenesis for many remote complications can be recognised in less than optimal conduct during the insertion, there is no doubt that surveillance during management and implementation of correct conduct in the exit site and infusion line maintenance plays a fundamental role in the prevention, or at least in the early diagnosis of infective (infection of the exit site, catheter-related blood stream infection) and noninfective complications (catheter-related venous thrombosis, fibroblast sheath, catheter lesions, displacements).

For PICCs in particular, the old classification of complications by time period (immediate, early, late complications) has lost clinical significance compared to the new classification, which distinguishes between complications directly or indirectly related to insertion and those related to management. The pathogenesis of many remote complications (traditionally classified as late) can originate from inappropriate choices and conduct during PICC and Midline insertion procedures. For example:

- an *infection* occurring a few days after the insertion could have been caused by the inadequate observance of antisepsis measures (hand hygiene, maximum barrier precautions, skin antisepsis with 2% chlorhexidine in alcohol solution), by the selecting an inadequate exit site, that lies, for example, too close to the axillary cavity, or from accidental contamination during guidewire or catheter manipulation;
- the pathogenesis of *catheter-related thrombosis* can originate, apart from patient's predisposing factors, from selecting a wrong catheter that is too large for the vein diameter, from a difficult venous cannulation procedure (repeated punctures with the formation of intramural venous hematomas, use of suboptimal micro-introduction kits with increased trauma of the endothelium, etc.), from the non-central positioning of the PICC tip, from the inadequate securement of the catheter to the skin, or from choosing to insert a Midline rather than a PICC, while knowing that the patient is

to be given intravenous treatments (vancomycin, chemotherapy, parenteral nutrition etc.), which notoriously require a central line;
- *mechanical lesions* of the catheter, even if they occur weeks or months after insertion, can be caused by a suboptimal exit site selection, or the decision to leave a long part of the catheter outside the skin or to insert a catheter made of particularly fragile material like silicone;
- *lumen occlusions* can be favoured by deciding to insert catheters with calibres that are too small for the intended use or to bend the catheter in the extravascular tract;
- PICC *displacement* (or Midlines) can be favoured by choosing an inappropriate exit site (in Dawson's "yellow zone" or in "red zone") or the wrong securement method (for example, by suturing);
- a *malfunctioning* catheter may be secondary to the selection of a suboptimal catheter (silicone valved catheter with Groshong-type tip, which is known to be associated with a higher risk of malfunctions) or a primary tip malposition, such as a PICC left with the tip too high in the innominate vein or in the upper third of the superior vena cava (positions associated with malfunction due to the high risk of fibroblast sheath formation or to contact of the tip with the venous wall).

It is true, moreover, that the role of management in preventing complications is also fundamental and can be separated into two different aspects:

- *exit site management* plays a fundamental role in preventing exit site infections, bacteraemic infections from contamination by the extraluminal route, catheter displacement and mechanical lesions in the external tract;
- *connection and infusion line management* plays an essential role in preventing bacteraemic infections from contamination by the interluminal route, as well as lumen occlusions.

An integrated prevention strategy covering all complications must therefore include not only an appropriate insertion procedure but also, and above all, a series of standardised procedures for managing the exit site and the infusion lines.
Complications must obviously minimised for the following reasons: venous access complications, especially infective, are a significant cause of morbidity and mortality, extend hospitalisation times and increase healthcare costs. It has been calculated, for example, that a single episode of catheter-related sepsis in Intensive Care costs around 13,000 euros and leads to an average hospitalisation time extension of around 12 days. A single episode of catheter-related venous thrombosis leads to an additional cost of around 1,000 euros (in the absence of major complications).
Fortunately, medical literature extensively describes and validates strategies that involve simple actions for proper venous catheter management and have led to a considerable reduction or complete elimination of complications, particularly infective ones. The application of *bundles* has been found to be particularly useful for preventing many of the complications related to the use of venous catheters, for example by assessing adherence through a dedicated checklist.

In brief, a structured strategy is crucial is essential to eliminate or minimise complication incidence and should cover the following points.

- Surveillance: in order to identify the need for complication prevention strategies and evaluate their effects, it is vital for every operating unit to record the incidence of the most significant complications (for example: catheter-related bacteraemic infections, symptomatic catheter-related venous thrombosis, catheter occlusions/malfunctions) expressing them in units of measurement so that it is possible to compare operating units to different policies and the literature (for example: number of complications every 1,000 days of catheter life or every 1,000 days of catheter use for devices used outside hospitals, with episodic frequency).
- Local adoption of clear, unambiguous definitions of each complication. For example, the diagnostic definition of catheter-related bacteraemic infection must correspond to the one indicated in the IDSA's 2009 guidelines: patients with central venous catheter with signs of SIRS, who do not have alternative sources of infection and present at least one of the following criteria: (1) isolation of the same microorganism (same species and same antibiogram) from a blood culture taken from a peripheral vein and from the culture of the catheter tip; or, (2) isolation of the same microorganism (same species and same antibiogram) from a blood culture taken from a peripheral vein and a blood culture taken from the central venous catheter with a positivisation time of two or more hours in favour of the blood culture taken from the venous catheter.
- Every clinical unit must take into consideration the possibility of identifying a physician or a nurse who will take care of recording catheter-related complications, according to established definitions, in order to be able to evaluate them within the unit and the whole hospital, involving the committees assigned to the surveillance of infections, risk management, etc.; regular audits should be carried out periodically involving the responsible physicians and nurses in each department, to discuss the reporting for the period and deal with any problems that may have occurred.
- Use of *bundles* and *checklists*: as previously mentioned, in accordance with the international guidelines, *bundles* and *checklists* are the main instruments available for healthcare operators to apply in daily clinical practice for preventing venous catheter-related infections.

  Bundles are a series of simple recommendations that have proven to effectively prevent specific complications (we have given a number of examples of the GAVeCeLT bundles for preventing infections, insertion complications, etc.), while checklists are detailed lists covering the salient points of each individual manoeuvre to check off the correct execution of each procedure in real time.
- Operator training: this is probably the most important point. Just as providing sufficient training (and education) for the operators executing the insertion drastically reduces the incidence of insertion-related complications, an adequate personnel training program for the operators in charge of the management is related to a reduction in late complications and the possibility of the PICC remaining *in situ* until the end of the planned intravenous treatment.

Management of PICC and Midline exit site

Protection of the exit site from bleeding

As already explained with insertion-related complications, it is not uncommon for the PICC or Midline exit site to present complications of persistent local bleeding that may last for several days unless treated appropriately. The phenomenon is more likely in patients with coagulation problems (thrombocytopenia, hepatopathy, treatment with antiplatelets or anticoagulants, fragile skin, etc.) and when the previously described preventive measures are not adopted during insertion (avoiding the use of scalpels to enlarge the cutaneous passage, using PICCs with *reverse tapering*, applying cyanoacrylate glue on the exit site at the end of the manoeuvre). Among these measures, the most effective and simple from the logistical point of view is definitely the application of glue to the exit site (Figure 3.1).

For bleeding control purposes, in centres where cyanoacrylate glue is not used, a gauze dressing is often applied over the exit site at the end of an insertion (Figure 3.2) (or a gauze plus a transparent dressing) (Figure 3.3) as a "temporary" dressing to be replaced after 24 hours. During the replacement procedure, if the risk of local bleeding persists, the

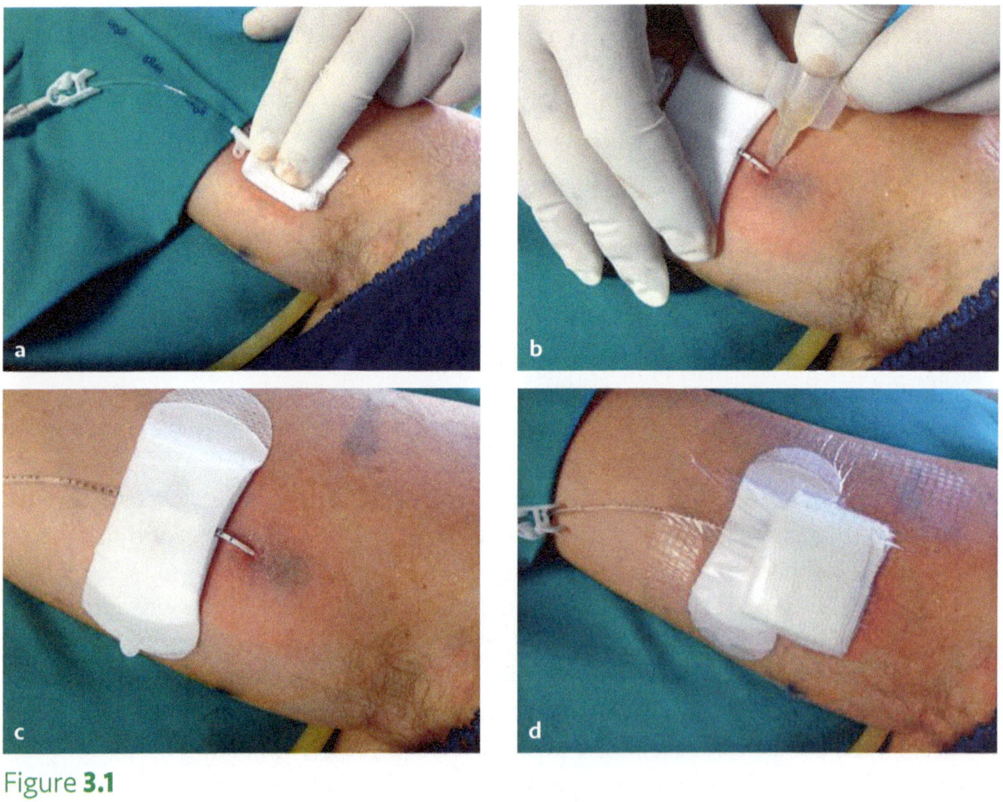

Figure **3.1**

option of first choice is to apply cyanoacrylate glue to the exit site; an alternative option (rather less cost-effective) is applying a new "temporary" dressing to be replaced after 24 hours. It is needless to underline that the local application of vasoactive or pro-coagulant drugs has no effect.
At other times, the operator performing the insertion may not foresee any risk of bleeding and place a "permanent" dressing directly on the exit site, or a transparent dressing with or without chlorhexidine releasing systems (dressing with chlorhexidine-releasing hydrogel or transparent dressing + chlorhexidine-releasing sponge in polyurethane). In this case,

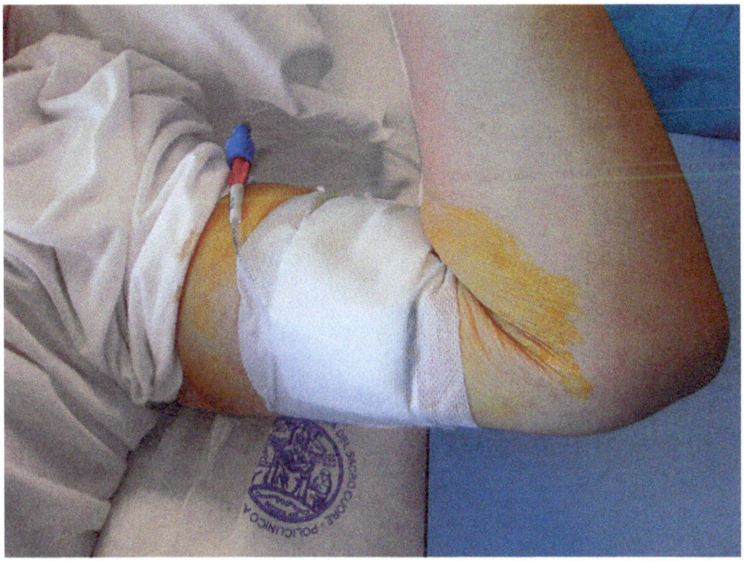

Figure **3.2**

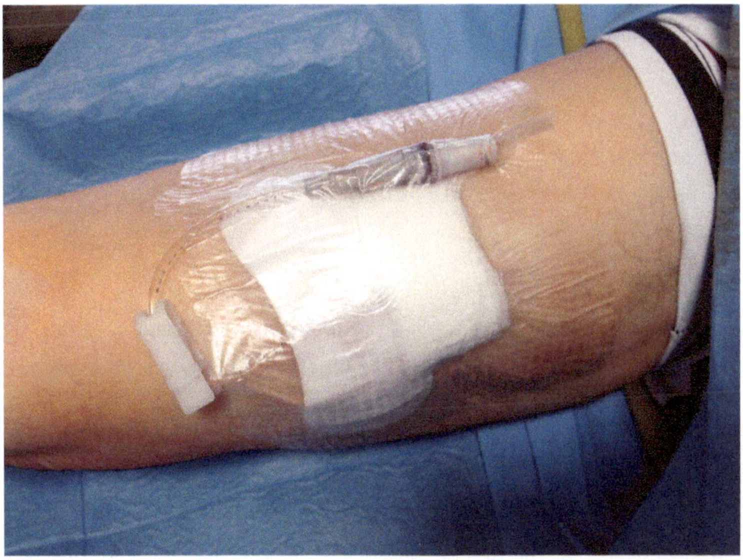

Figure **3.3**

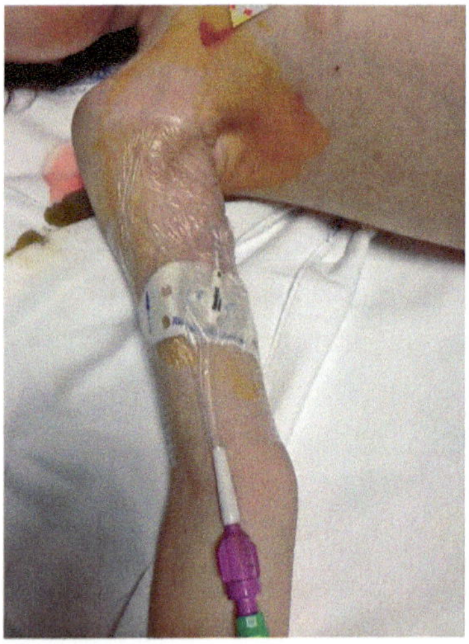

Figure **3.4**

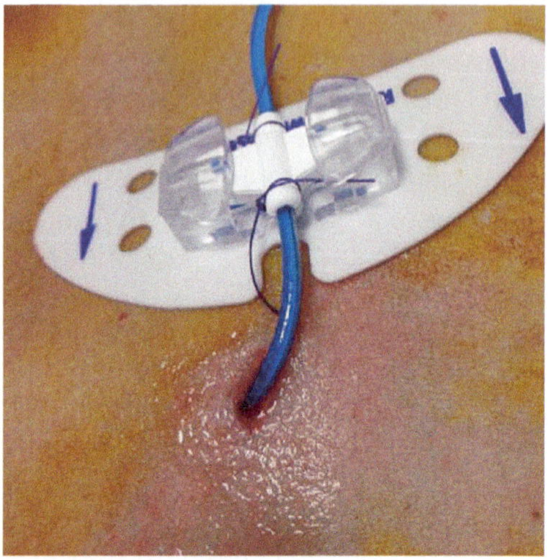

Figure **3.5**

a blood collection under the transparent dressing or soaking the sponge (Biopatch) is a clear indication to change the dressing.

Finally, the operator may apply cyanoacrylate glue placing the transparent dressing in direct contact with the exit site. In this case, local bleeding is an extremely unlikely occurrence; should this occur, the transparent dressing should be removed and cyanoacrylate glue re-applied; if, on the other hand, the exit site appears bloodless, the transparent dressing can be left *in situ* for a week without causing any problem, since it will allow exit site inspection. In special cases (especially in pediatric patients) (Figure 3.4), it is possible to leave the transparent dressing *in situ* in direct contact with the glue, even for periods longer than seven days, since the dressing removal entails a significant risk of device displacement. Currently, significant phenomena of skin intolerance to cyanoacrylate have not been described, nor damage by the glue to the catheter material: it is possible to use the glue not only on third-generation polyurethanes but also on potentially more fragile materials like silicone (Figure 3.5).

Obviously, as will be reiterated below, in all cases in which the transparent dressing appears loose or dirty or damp, its replacement is indicated at any time, irrespective of the presence of cyanoacrylate glue beneath.

Disinfection of the exit site

One of the fundamental objectives of an appropriate management of the exit site of PICCs or Midlines is to minimise the risk of local infections and catheter-related bacteraemic infections from extraluminal bacterial contamination (i.e., from bacteria from the patient's skin or operator's hands that could contaminate the external surface of the catheter, thus penetrating inside the organism through the it). The most effective prophylaxis of extraluminal bacterial contamination is based on appropriate skin antisepsis at and around the exit site, hence in all the areas covered by the dressing.

The purpose of the antisepsis is to reduce the "environmental" bacterial flora covering the host's skin to a critical level; it is, however, unlikely that an antisepsis – however meticulous – can significantly reduce the "residential" bacterial flora that typically accumulates in hair follicles. On the other hand, environmental flora is the only kind of flora that causes potential local or bacteraemic infections and is often represented by pathogenic germs lying on the operator's hands (if not adequately washed), on other contaminated areas of the patient's skin (for example: ostomies), or deriving from the hospital flora (in the case of hospitalised patients). A thorough skin antisepsis at a PICC or Midline exit site, as well as for any venous catheter, both peripheral and central, must be carried out with 2% chlorhexidine gluconate in 70% isopropyl alcohol (IPA) by means of single-dose, disposable, sterile applicators (Figure 3.6). This solution is currently considered to be the best antiseptic available. Please bear in mind that, while there are many varieties of "disinfectants", few have been shown to be effective as "antiseptics" or "disinfectants for the skin".

More than a decade of studies has led to the identification of three antiseptic solutions that are clinically effective on the skin: isopropyl or ethyl alcohol (at 70% concentration), chlorhexidine gluconate (at 2% concentration or, in any case, higher than 0.5%) and povidone-iodine (at 10% concentration). All the main international guidelines (see EPIC 2014 guidelines) agree on the recommendation to use a solution combining the first two disinfectants (alcohol and chlorhexidine), both in sufficient concentrations, as first choice antiseptic. The use of povidone-iodine is seen as a second choice, to be adopted in patients who have a known allergy to chlorhexidine. Note that many disinfectants that are sometimes mistakenly used for skin disinfection during venous access insertion or management (such as, for example, sodium hypochlorite) have no proven clinical efficacy in this regard in any kind of patients.

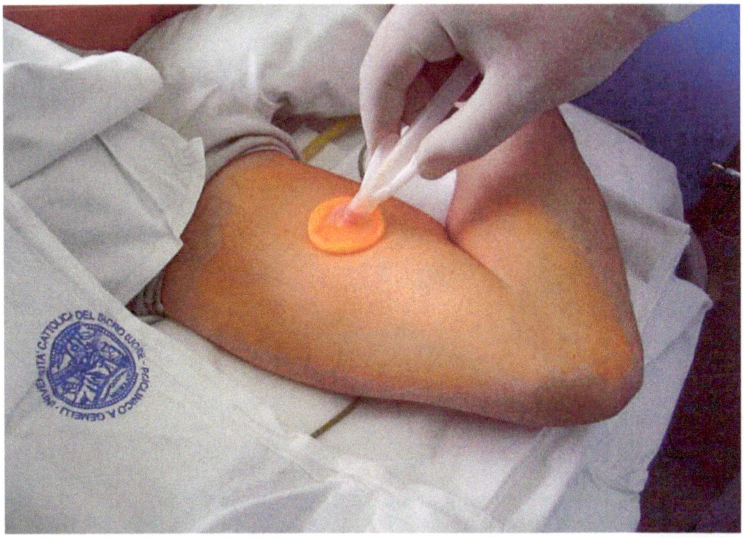

Figure **3.6**

Chlorhexidine in alcohol solution must be applied to the exit site, wiping vigorously with the *no touch* technique for 30 seconds and leaving it to dry for 30 seconds. The requirement to wipe vigorously derives from the chance to benefit from a double action of chlorhexidine in alcohol, both as a "detergent" (removal of skin debris, detached epithelial cells, bacterial biofilm, accumulations of secretions or blood cells, etc.), and as an "antiseptic" acting specifically for antibacterial purposes. The *no touch* technique can reach its best effect if a disposable sterile applicator is used, as recommended by the EPIC 2014 guidelines. It is necessary to wait 30 seconds to allow the alcohol to evaporate, thus fixing the chlorhexidine to the skin, where it can initiate its antibacterial action.

Alternatively, when 10% povidone-ionine is used in patients that are allergic to chlorhexidine, it will always be necessary to vigorously wipe with the *no touch* technique, leaving to dry for at least 120 seconds (the time required to allow the solution water to evaporate).

In addition to the lower latency time before the antibacterial action takes place, chlorhexidine has many other advantages over povidone-iodine, such as a broader spectrum of action and a greater duration of the antiseptic effect. Finally, the lower efficacy of povidone-iodine is also linked to inadequate use (for example, if the operator does not wait for the mandatory 120 seconds), ineffective detergent action and the risk of being inactivated in the presence of blood, serum and biological secretions in general.

After an appropriate disinfection of the exit site, an adequate level of antisepsis is assured for a few hours. During this period, the skin flora is reconstituted, starting with the residential flora remaining in the hair follicles and, in part, the surviving environmental flora. In patients at high risk of infection, it may be necessary to apply strategies to maintain a sufficient level of antisepsis for prolonged periods, or even several days, until the following dressing. To this end, local application of antiseptic or antibiotic ointments on the exit site has been proven ineffective and even counterproductive, at least as regards PICCs and Midlines, and is not recommended by the international guidelines.

The possibility of providing local chlorhexidine release 24 hours a day, for a whole week is more promising. To this end, the use of polyurethane sponge dressings that continuously release 2% chlorhexidine (Biopatch) (Figure 3.7) has been proven to be an effective strategy for protecting CICC or PICC central venous catheter exit sites and must be considered for preventing catheter-related infections, especially in specific situations (see SHEA 2014 guidelines):

- clinical units where standard prevention measures (hand hygiene, skin antisepsis with chlorhexidine, use of the maximum barrier precautions for the insertion, etc.) adoption and application are not successful in reducing the incidence of bacteraemic infections from central venous catheters;
- individual patients with repeated episodes of catheter-related infections and limited possibility of venous access repositioning;
- immunosuppressed patients;

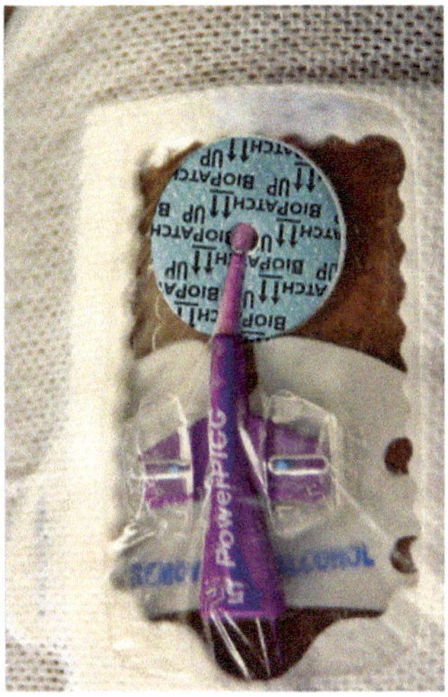

Figure **3.7**

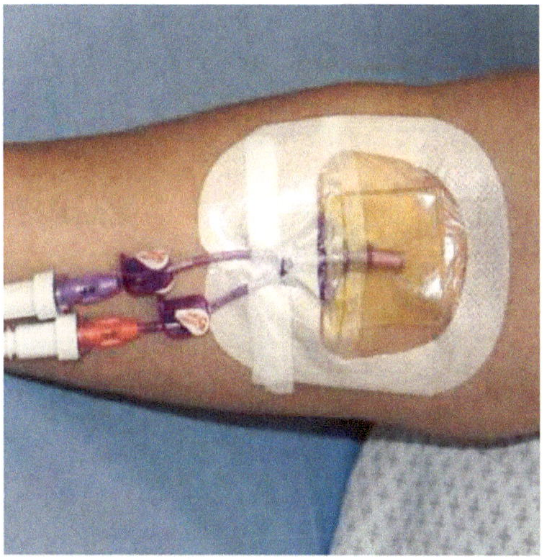

Figure **3.8**

- patients in whom a catheter-related infection could have quite serious consequences (for example, patients with heart valve or aortic prosthesis implants).

Besides polyurethane sponges, whose effectiveness has been proven by numerous randomized, controlled, clinical studies published in the last ten years, transparent dressing attached to a chlorhexidine releasing hydrogel pad (Tegaderm CHG) (Figure 3.8) have been recently marketed and proven to be effective in at least one multicentre clinical study. The main advantage of Tegaderm CHG is the visibility of the exit site; its greatest weakness is that the gel does not have absorbing properties (unlike the polyurethane sponge of the Biopatch), therefore rapidly decays and becomes ineffective in a humid environment.

Protection of the catheter from the risk of displacement

Apart from minimise bacterial contamination by the extraluminal route, the other main goal of exit site management is to minimise the risk of PICC or Midline displacement.

Considering that a safe intravenous infusion requires the tip of the PICC to be in a properly "central" position, close to the cavoatrial junction or a little above or below it, especially when infusing solutions that are potentially harmful to the endothelium. Catheter dislodgement even by a few centimetres can therefore be associated with an increased risk of central venous thrombosis and/or catheter malfunction, originating from a "secondary" tip malposition (whereas a wrong tip position at insertion is indicated as "primary" malposition). When using CICCs or PICCs, a dislodgement of 2 cm or less can still be associated with an "acceptable" position of the tip, while a dislodgement of more than 4 cm is always indicates to remove the PICC or to replace it over guidewire (see Chapter 4). If the catheter is dislodged by 2-4 cm, it is necessary to verify the tip position with a chest X-ray: to this end, the criterion of the carina will be useful, as illustrated elsewhere. If the PICC tip projects at or below the tracheal carina level, the PICC position is still acceptable. On the contrary, if the tip projects above the carina, it is likely to be in the upper third of the superior vena cava or in the innominate veins, or in another unacceptable positions, therefore the PICC should be removed or replaced with ultrasound guidance. An excessively dislodged PICC could be considered as a Midline. It is not, however, safe to leave it in place, due to the risk of inadequate use.

Midline and a long peripheral cannula (mini-Midline) displacement is less dangerous in terms of potential clinical consequences; it should be noted, however, that the closer the tip is to the exit site, the more likely is a catheter malfunction (for example, due to the fibroblast sheath), with leakage of the infused solutions from the breach of the skin at the exit site.

Catheter instability not only influences the displacement risk, but it also negatively impacts other potential complications. If the catheter mobility inside a vein of the arm is too high, it traumatises the endothelium, increasing the risk of local thrombotic complications at the entrance of the catheter in the vein, be it a short cannula, a mini-Midline, a Midline, or a PICC.

A poorly stabilised catheter showing a to-and-fro movement at the entrance to the skin, carries an infection risk, as its extraluminal contamination will be facilitated. Sometimes the operator may directly cause the contamination, should an improper attempt be made at reinserting a displaced catheter via the skin incision.

Displacement must clearly be prevented by applying a multimodal strategy that involves those who insert the PICC and those who manage it. Catheter displacement in the extravascular tract, in fact, typically occurs due to poor catheter securement or improper manoeuvres while applying the dressing to the exit site.

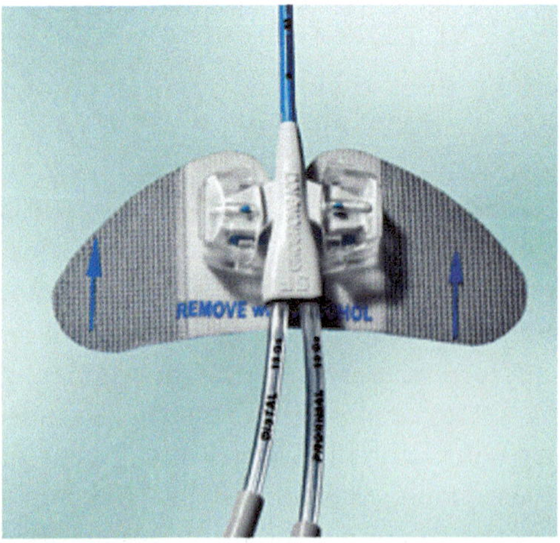

Figure **3.9**

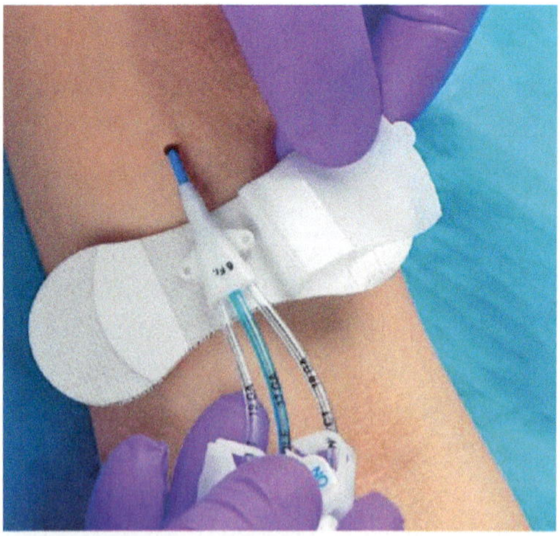

Figure **3.10**

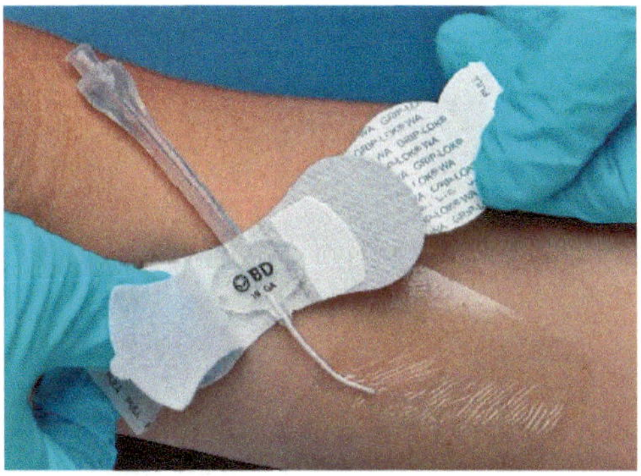

Figure **3.11**

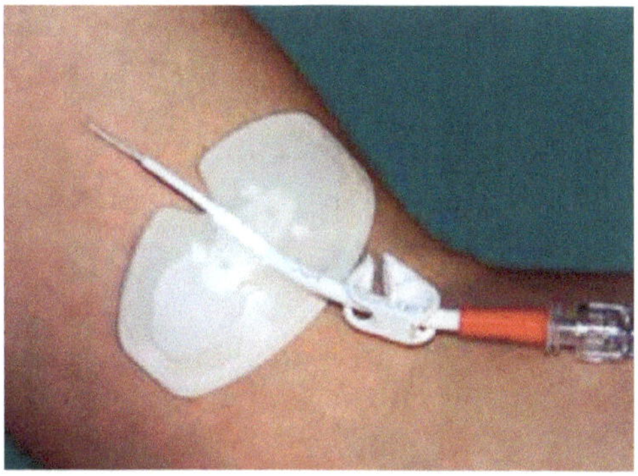

Figure **3.12**

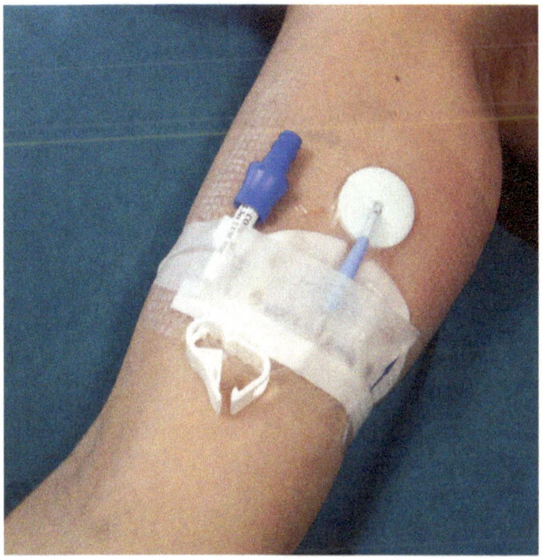

Figure **3.13**

PICC or Midline stabilisation strategy is based primarily on a few recommendations that must be thoroughly observed at the time of insertion (see Chapter 2, SIP Protocol).

- Selecting a suitable PICC/Midline exit site lying in Dawson's "green zone" (the middle third of the arm). Should the best vein for puncturing lie in the "yellow zone", it is always possible to tunnel the PICC so that the venipuncture site in the "yellow zone" corresponds to an exit site in the "green zone".
- Using a sutureless device, such as StatLock (Figure 3.9), Griplock (Figures 3.10 and 3.11) or WingGuard (Figure 3.12). Contrary to expectations, using suture to stabilise the catheter has more uncertain outcomes than employing a sutureless device, as with the latter the risk that stitches may become loose and compromise the wing stabilisation is avoided. Sutureless devices is perfectly compatible with the use of chlorhexidine sponge dressing (Figure 3.13).

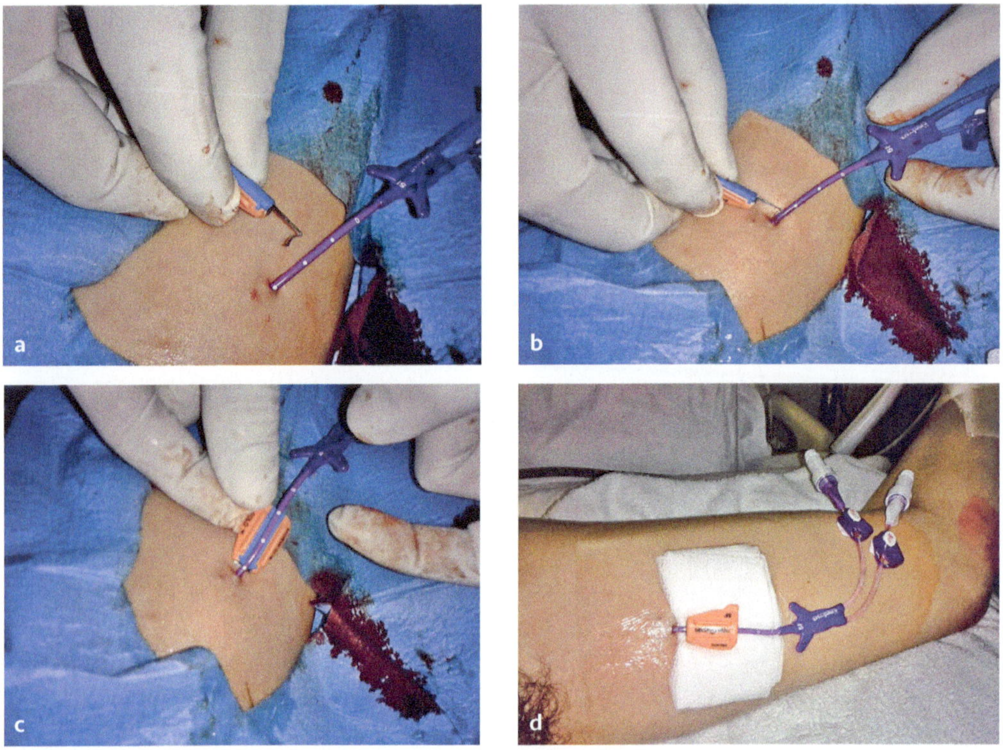

Figure **3.14**

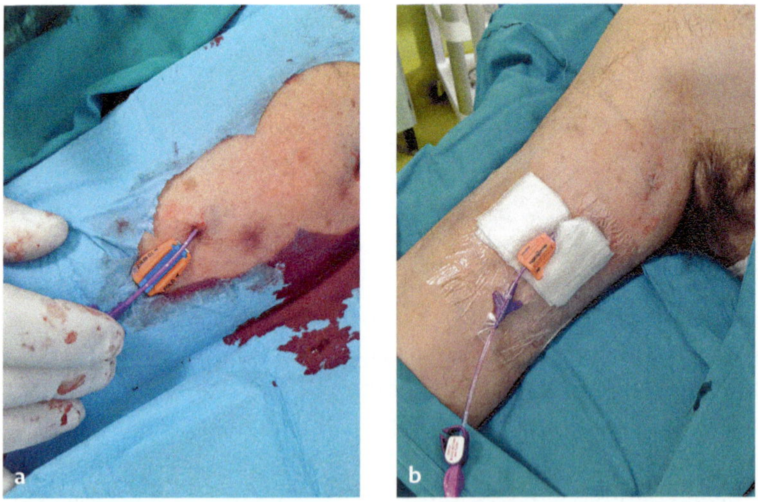

Figure **3.15**

- Using subcutaneously anchored sutureless devices (SecuraCath) in patients who are at higher risk of PICC dislodgement (uncooperative elderly people, restless children, patients with chronic skin lesions or local hyperhidrosis, etc.), where traditional sutureless devices adhesive to the skin (StatLock, GripLok, WingGuard) may be unreliable. One of the substantial differences between these new devices and traditional sutureless devices lies in the fact that SecuraCath is placed at the time of the insertion and removed at the time of the removal of the PICC, therefore accompanying the catheter for its entire life, whereas skin adherent sutureless devices are replaced weekly. Moreover, SecuraCath application requires a special technique that is easily learned (Figure 3.14) and it can be used on tunnelled PICCs (Figure 3.15).
- Using cyanoacrylate glue, especially in agitated patients or in children. In addition to stopping the bleeding from the exit site, glue are also used for better stabilising the catheter at the exit site, at least in the first week. The application of a SecuraCath is not incompatible with the application of cyanoacrylate glue (Figure 3.16).

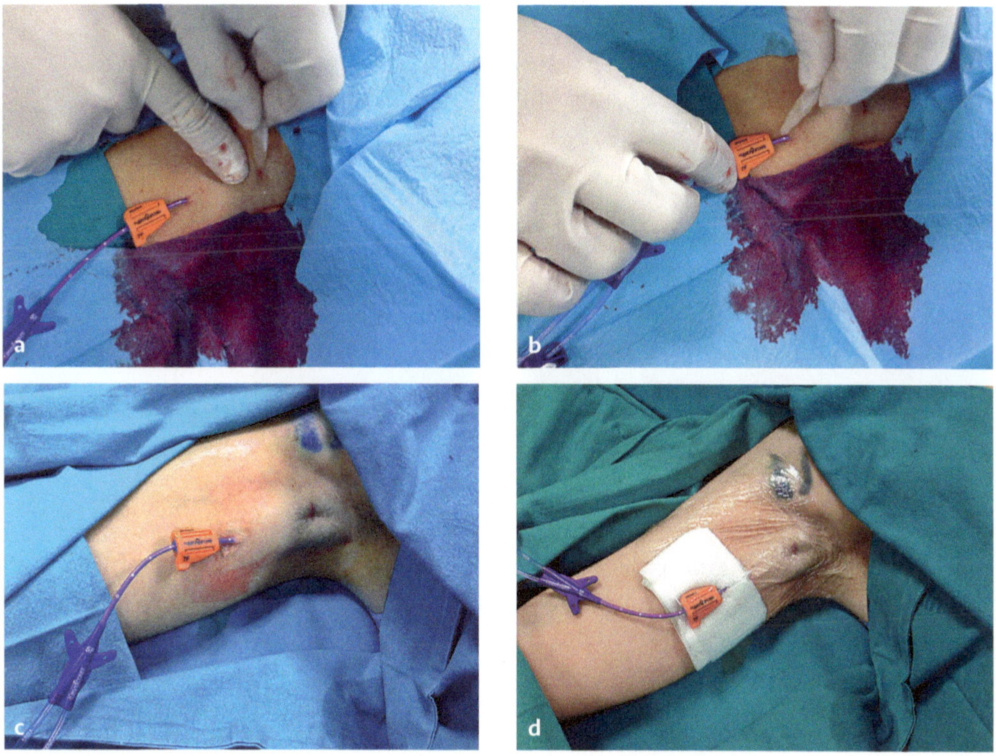

Figure **3.16**

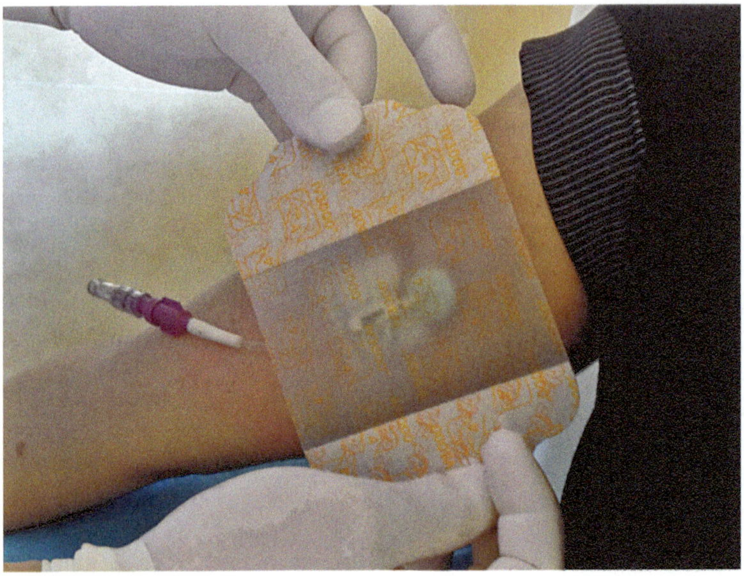

Figure **3.17**

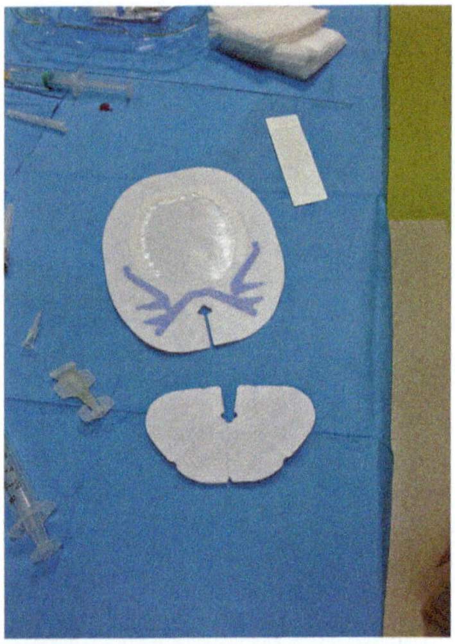

Figure **3.18**

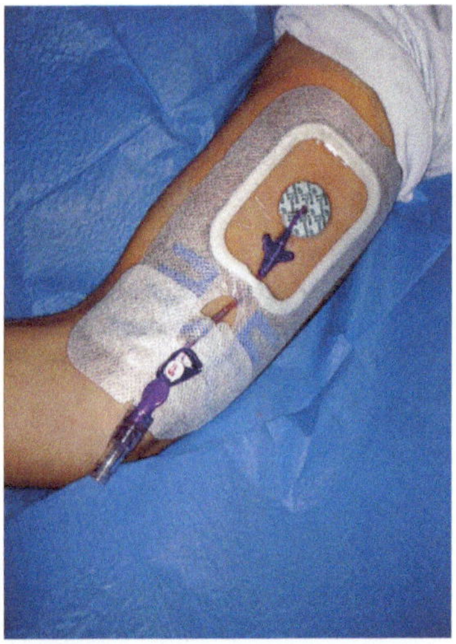

Figure **3.19**

- Using semipermeable adhesive transparent membrane (Figure 3.17) dressing. As will be further explained, transparent dressings are currently considered preferable to gauze dressings in terms of infection prevention (see EPIC 2014 guidelines); in addition to protecting from environmental bacterial contamination, these dressings also show superior catheter stabilisation, especially if used in association with sutureless devices. Recently, transparent dressing integrating sutureless device-type stabilisation systems (Figure 3.18) have become available, and they can also be used simultaneously with chlorhexidine releasing sponges (Figure 3.19). Their main advantage is combining

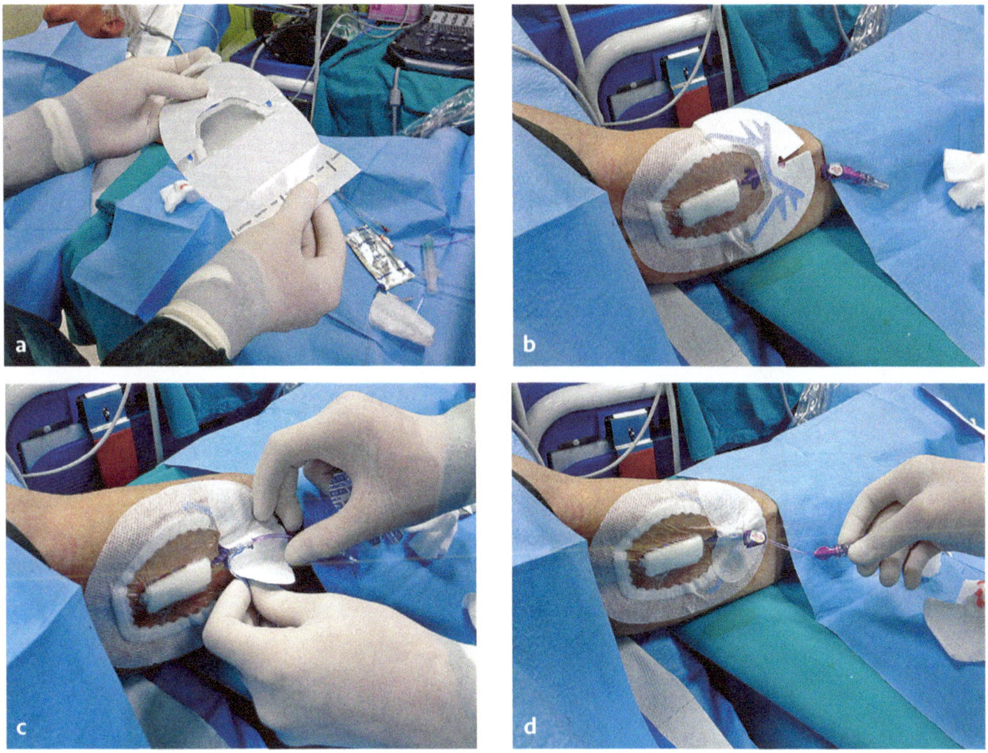

Figure **3.20**

two devices in one; it is obviously necessary a high familiarity with the application technique in order to be able to best benefit from the effectiveness of the attachment system (Figure 3.20).

- Finally, in the case tunneled-cuffed PICCs (TCC-type Pro-Lines), it must be remembered that, as with all cuffed devices, such as cuffed CICCs and cuffed FICCs, the cuff must be placed in the tunnelled tract at least 2 cm away from the exit site. Otherwise, if the cuff is placed too close to the exit site, the catheter will be very likely displaced when the cuff is rejected out of the tunnel.

At the same time, however, the operators in charge of managing the PICC dressing will need to comply with the following recommendations.

- When changing the dressing, the transparent dressing and the skin-adhesive sutureless device (StatLock or similar) must be removed with the utmost care following the manufacturer's instructions, to avoid displacing the catheter. If a Biopatch was applied, it should be carefully removed without detaching the catheter from the exit site. In case of a subcutaneously anchored system like SecuraCath, transparent dressing (or any sponge dressing) removal is easier and with no risk of displacement.

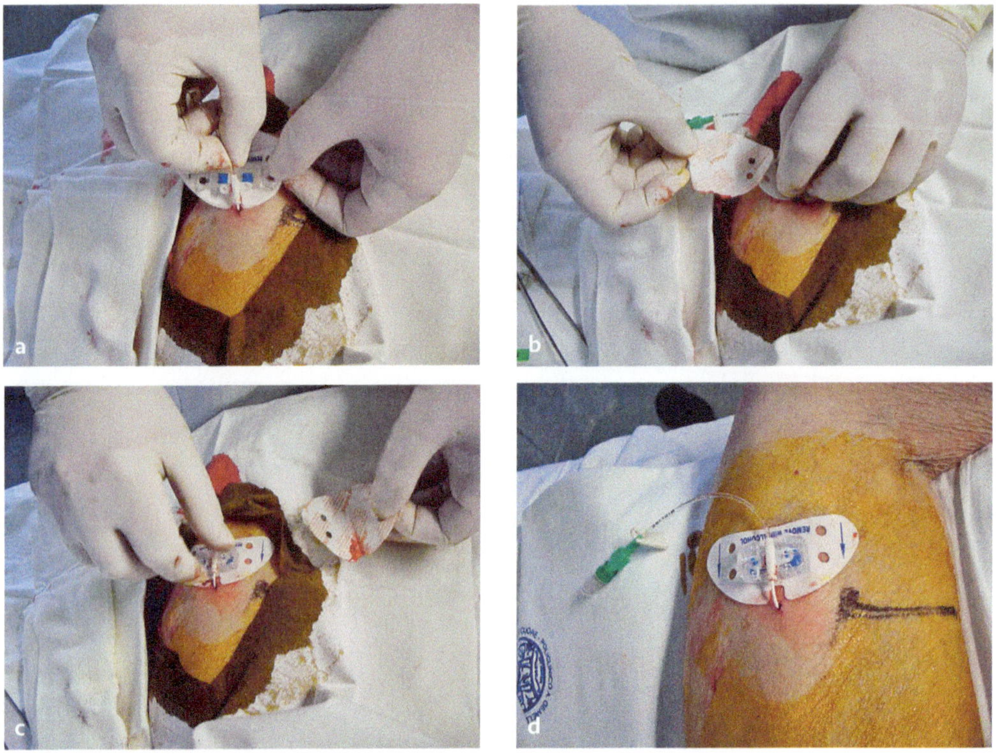

Figure **3.21**

- Similar care should be taken while repositioning skin adhesive sutureless devices (Stat-Lock or similar) (Figure 3.21). As previously explained, however, the SecuraCath does not require periodic replacement.
- Finally, the personnel in charge of line management should instruct the patient and/or caregiver on the need to avoid movements or traumas that may increase the risk of displacement.

Besides dislodgement of the extravascular tract of the catheter, which unfortunately is rather frequent, it is also worth mentioning a less frequent complication, i.e. the displacement of the intravascular tract without displacement of the extravascular tract (intravascular migration of the tip). The PICC tip that was originally positioned correctly can, in fact, move unexpectedly. This often happens in the ipsilateral jugular vein, where the risk of venous thrombosis is significantly increased. Such tip migration is particularly frequent in catheters whose tip is positioned too high in the superior cava ("too short" PICC) and in very thin catheters and/or made of silicone: a trigger factor is a repeated increase of the intrathoracic pressure, due to coughing or crying, as typically occurs in children. The best prevention method for this complication lies (1) in placing the PICC tip in the right location, close to the cavoatrial junction and (2) in giving preference to power injectable PICCs in polyurethane rather than silicone catheters, which are more susceptible to tip migration.

Practical protocol of exit site dressing

Careful monitoring of PICC or Midline exit site is vital for defining the appropriate time for dressing, at least in hospitalised patients. This monitoring consists of daily inspecting or palpating the point where the catheter exits from the skin, without removing the dressing, in addition to an inspection of the dressing itself. Such monitoring practice aims at checking the dressing condition and early detecting local signs or symptoms of infection (erythema, exudation, pain, etc.).

If the dressing has become detached, soiled or wet, and if local inflammation is suspected on palpation, the dressing must be changed.

A most careful inspection of the exit site after removing the dressing will enable to quantify the extent of local inflammation, preferably using a visual score such as the Visual Exit-site Score (Table 3.1).

When no pathological alterations are suspected, the dressing shall be replaced in accordance at scheduled intervals (that is, every week for dressings with transparent membranes). A practical protocol for applying dressing to the exit site must include:

- removal of the old dressing;
- removal of the chlorhexidine-releasing sponge (if present);
- removal of the sutureless device (Figure 3.22);
- skin antisepsis of the exit site and the area immediately around it;
- application of a new sutureless device;
- application of a new chlorhexidine-releasing sponge, if necessary;
- application of the new dressing.

The correct dressing technique naturally involves the strictest asepsis technique, in accordance to a procedure that must include, in sequence, the following:

- hand hygiene;
- clean, non-sterile gloves;
- old dressing removal with appropriate technique (in the case of transparent dressing, it is necessary to pay particular attention to using the technique of stretching the dressing starting from the sides, to allow air under the dressing and facilitate removal without catheter displacement);

Table 3.1 Visual Exit-site Score
Score 0 Healthy, intact skin with no sign of inflammation
Score 1 Hyperaemia <1 cm around the exit site, with or without exudate
Score 2 Hyperaemia >1 cm around the exit site, with or without exudate
Score 3 Hyperaemia, secretion, pus, with or without exudate

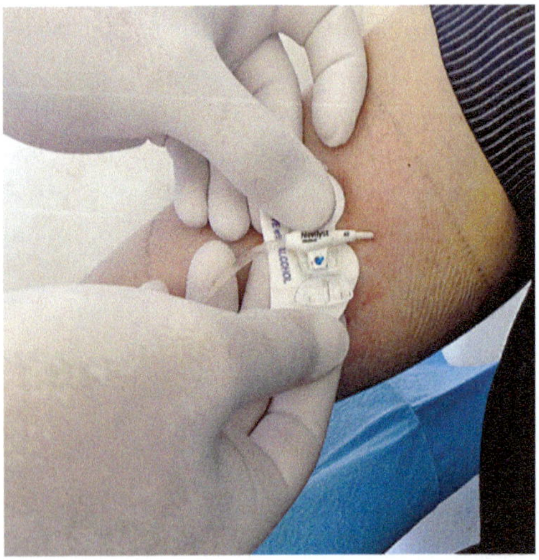

Figure **3.22**

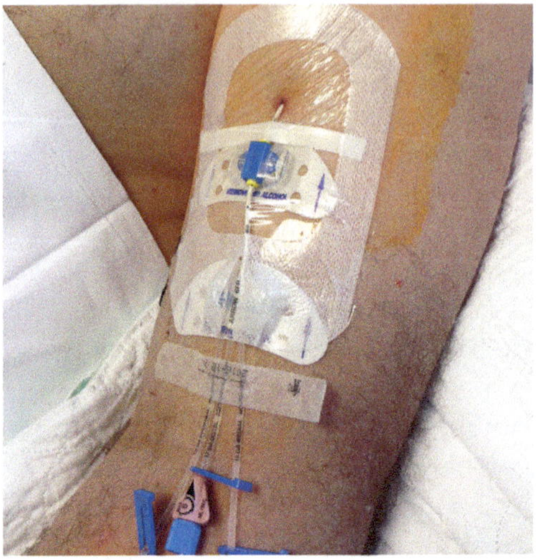

Figure **3.23**

- removal of the Biopatch, if present;
- removal of the sutureless device with appropriate technique (this is obviously not performed if the catheter is secured by a subcutaneously anchored device like SecuraCath);
- removal of clean gloves;
- repeated hand hygiene;
- sterile gloves;
- cleansing and antisepsis of the exit site and the surrounding area, with 2% chlorhexidine gluconate in isopropyl alcohol delivered through single-dose, disposable sterile applicators;
- application of the new sutureless device (this is clearly not performed if the catheter is attached with SecuraCath);
- application of the new biopatch, if indicated;
- application of the new semipermeable transparent dressing;
- annotation of the date on the dressing;
- registration of the dressing.

It is important to note: (1) that transparent membrane should be the default dressing (Figure 3.23) (gauze dressings should only be used in special cases, such as secretion, blood or hyperhidrosis at the exit site, and for limited periods); (2) that the decision whether or not to use the Biopatch (or other continuous chlorhexidine release system) is based on the policy of the operating unit; (3) that the SecuraCath will only be used in a selected population of patients at high risk of displacement, unfit for the use of traditional sutureless devices.

Recommendations for periodic dressing replacement

As recommended by the EPIC 2014 guidelines and as previously mentioned, under ideal conditions, the exit site of any venous catheter (central or peripheral) including PICCs or Midlines should be covered and protected with a semipermeable transparent dressing with high level of transpiration. This type of dressing (1) enables exit site inspection; (2) contributes to stabilising the catheter more effectively than other types of dressing and avoiding the “in-and-out” movement of the catheter that favours infections and thrombosis; and (3) keeps the exit site dry.
The semipermeable dressing must be replaced every seven days and whenever it detaches, or if there is humidity underneath.
Alternatively, and as a second choice, in the case of known intolerance to semipermeable transparent dressings, the exit site can be covered with gauze dressings that should be replaced every 48 hours, or immediately as they become soiled, detached or wet.
In the case of relevant sweating or bleeding or exudation of serum from the exit site, gauze dressings should be used. As mentioned previously, they must be replaced every 48 hours, or whenever they are soiled, detached or wet, or anytime it is necessary to inspect the exit site.
In the aforementioned cases (sweating, bleeding, etc.), as soon as the problem is resolved, the exit site must be covered again with semipermeable, transparent dressings. While it is not possible to formulate recommendations on the need to cover a fully healed insertion site of tunneled-cuffed PICCs, coverage is regarded as preferable, at least for protecting the catheter from any accidental traction.

Infusion line management

Washing protocol and system closure

PICC and Midlines patency, as with any other venous catheters used for infusion purposes (and not for dialysis or apheresis) is not ensured by heparinization but by applying a proper protocol of catheter flushing and locking.
The efficacy of heparin and other substances with anticoagulant action, such as citrate, has, in fact, only been demonstrated for vascular devices used for blood exchange procedures (haemodialysis, apheresis, diafiltration, etc.): this is not surprising, given that blood flows continuously through these catheters. On the other hand, there is no convincing scientific evidence on the supposed efficacy of heparin or citrate in maintaining the patency of catheters used for infusion, blood sampling or haemodynamic monitoring. In fact, it has been demonstrated that PICC and Midline patency (as with CICCs, TCCs and ports) is based essentially on a proper protocol of saline solution flushing. Gravity flushing is not effective: guidelines recommend active flushing by means of a 10-mL syringe, to be performed by hand using the so-called *push/pause,* or *start and stop* technique, that is, in steps of 2-3 mL each. Flushing must be performed during line opening before and after every infusion. In adults, flushing of central lines should be performed with 10 mL of saline solution. A flushing procedure with 20 mL

of saline solution is recommended in special conditions, such as after blood sampling, blood/blood product infusion, lipid-based parenteral nutrition infusion, or contrast medium injection.

Besides this good flushing practice *(flush)*, it is also advisable to close every system lumen with saline solution *(lock)* at the end each use. For all short-, medium- or long-term venous accesses, both peripheral and central (including needle cannulas, long peripheral cannulas, Midlines, PICCs, CICCs, ports, PICC-ports and TCCs), there is no evidence of efficacy for the use of *lock* with heparin solutions and it should be therefore avoided.

Together with saline flushing and locking, another essential element for maintaining PICC and Midline patency is the correct use of valve caps (Needle Free Connectors, NFC). Negative, neutral or positive pressure NFCs are available. In negative pressure NFCs (although it would be more correct to say negative "displacement"), when disconnecting the syringe or the infusion line from the NFC, an internal displacement of fluid occurs and causes a backflow of blood inside the catheter (Figure 3.24); to avoid this backflow, which may occlude the distal end of the catheter, it is necessary to clamp the catheter before disconnecting the syringe, and then leave it clamped. This manoeuvre implies some risk of error and leaving the catheter clamped carries the risk of damaging the catheter in the long run (not to mention the fact that some PICCs, being valved, are not furnished with clamping mechanisms). To prevent the backflow of blood inside the system, it is therefore necessary to use neutral or positive displacement NFCs. As we will discuss below, positive displacement NFCs should be used with caution because some types of NFCs have been associated with an increased risk of infection for unclear reasons that are probably connected to the device having reservoirs in which bacterial proliferation is possible. For this reason, many guidelines (including the GAVeCeLT recommendations) recommend the use of neutral displacement NFCs (Figure 3.25). When it is not possible to exploit the action of these neutral

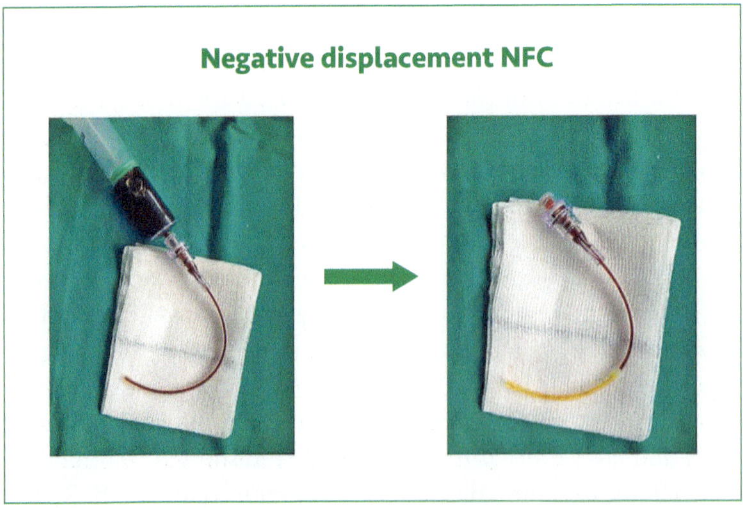

Figure **3.24**

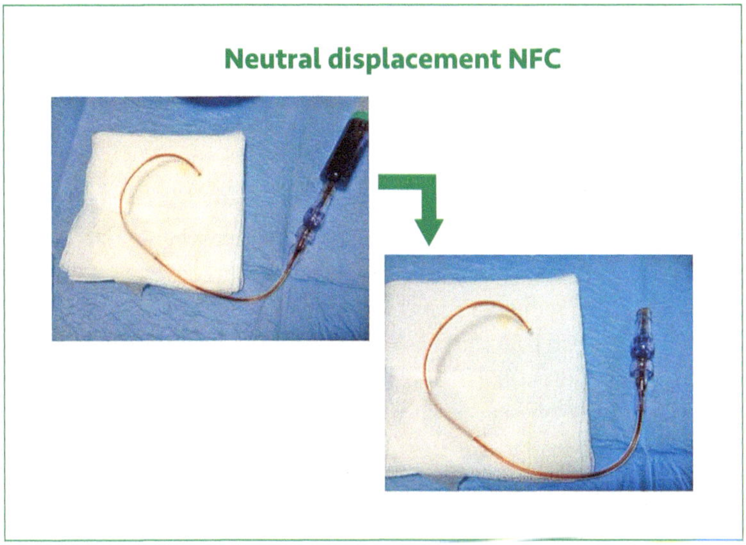

Figure **3.25**

or positive displacement caps (for example, when a Huber needle is removed from a PICC-port), the removal manoeuvre should be performed so to leave some "positive pressure" inside the system.

Recommendations for infusion line periodic replacement

Generally, venous catheter routine replacement at scheduled intervals does not reduce the risk of bacteraemic infections and therefore it is not recommended.
The replacement of a venous short-, medium- or long-term catheter, either peripheral or central, should be considered only on the basis of clinical indications.
It is, however, important to plan infusions line replacements (infusion sets, ramps, extensions, stopcocks and everything that is not part of the PICC or Midline) at a preset frequency.
Infusion lines that are used continuously (typically, in-hospital settings) must be replaced every 96 hours. If, however, they have been used for blood or blood product infusions, they must be replaced immediately at the end of the infusion and, in any event, every 8 hours. If the infusion lines have been used for administering parenteral nutrition containing lipids or other lipid solutions, they must be replaced every 24 hours. Infusion lines used for chemotherapy administration must be replaced and disposed of in accordance with hospital policies.
The optimal frequency for replacing infusion lines used for discontinuous administration (typically, extra-hospital settings) is an unresolved problem. It seems safe, however, to replace the infusion line at the end of each infusion cycle. All the aforementioned indications are valid, with the exception of cases in which the infusion set manufacturer specifically indicates a different replacement frequency.

Hub and connection management

An essential role in hub and connection management is played by how the so-called "valve caps" (Needle Free Connector, NFC) are selected and used.

Generally, all accesses to the infusion line (so-called *hubs*) must preferably be closed with NFCs, rather than with standard caps.

NFCs guarantee a greater safety for the operator during intravenous infusions administered through vascular catheters, if compared to needle-based access, and if correctly selected and used they are potentially effective in reducing the entry of germs in the system and in preventing venous catheter occlusions by reducing or eliminating the backflow when infusion lines are disconnected. As suggested by the most recent guidelines on the prevention of catheter-related infections (EPIC 2014), the use of NFCs can reduce bacterial colonisation more effectively than standard caps. Even though the latter must be constantly replaced on every hub after each use, this is not always the case. As already mentioned, however, the use of positive displacement NFCs (Figure 3.26) could, on the contrary, favour the bacterial contamination of the infusion line.

On the other hand, the use of negative displacement NFCs is associated with the hazard of blood backflow into the system and therefore with the risk of occlusion.

In conclusion, neutral displacement NFCs are to be preferred.

From a structural point of view, NFCs with the following characteristics should be preferred: (1) a luer-lock type of connection with the infusion lines; (2) a smooth and even outer surface (especially in the connecting septum) so that it can be disinfected as effectively as possible; (3) minimal inner dead space; and (4) a laminar-type internal flow or a least turbulent flow possible. Venous catheter access by means of the connection of infusion lines to NFCs must be carried out with aseptic technique. NFC disinfection

Positive displacement NFC

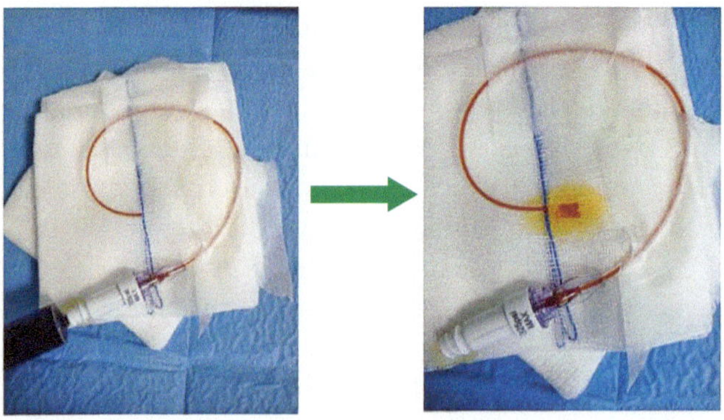

Figure **3.26**

must be performed by vigorously scrubbing their surface for at least 15 seconds with wipes soaked in 2% chlorhexidine in isopropyl alcohol before and after accessing the system. In both cases, a *no touch* technique must be guaranteed. Therefore, the proper venous catheter access through NFCs demands that operators perform this procedure, in sequence:

- hand hygiene;
- clean, non-sterile gloves;
- vigorous scrubbing of the outer surface of the NFC for 15 seconds using a gauze wipe soaked in 2% chlorhexidine in 70% isopropyl alcohol before and after access to the system, avoiding touching the connecting surfaces after disinfectant application;
- connection of the infusion line;
- final hand hygiene.

When disconnecting infusion lines, operators must follow this procedure:

- hand hygiene;
- clean, non sterile gloves;
- disconnection of the infusion lines and disposal in accordance with the hospital policy;
- disinfection of the NFC according to the methods indicated previously (or replacement, with the same frequency indicated for replacing the infusion sets);
- after cleaning or replacing the NFC, flushing with at least 10 mL of saline solution (20 mL after infusions of blood, blood products or parenteral nutrition containing lipids) using a *start and stop* technique;
- routine hand-washing.

Special devices for the passive and continuous disinfection of NFCs have been recently marketed, ensuring greater effectiveness and certainly greater compliance by operators. They are called *port protectors* (caps containing a sponge soaked in 70% isopropyl alcohol) (Figures 3.27 and 3.28) and are applied to the NFC when the infusion lines are discon-

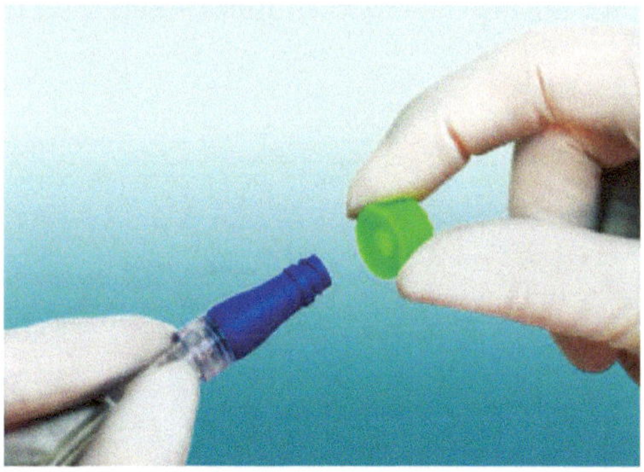

Figure **3.27**

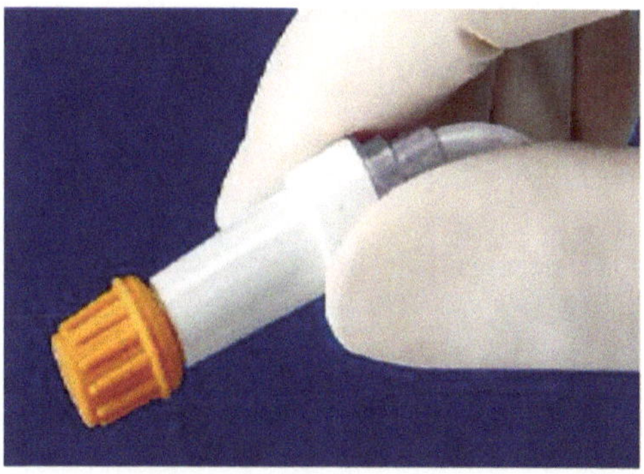

Figure **3.28**

nected: once in place, they ensure a disinfecting action that starts rapidly and last for seven days. When the infusion line needs to be accessed, the *port protector* is removed and the line connected, without the need to disinfect the NFC.
The sequence for accessing the infusion lines can be broken into the following steps:

- hand hygiene;
- clean, non-sterile gloves;
- removal of the *port protector* from the NFC;
- connection of the infusion line to the NFC;
- final hand hygiene.

The disconnecting sequence is the same:

- hand hygiene;
- clean, non-sterile gloves;
- disconnection of the infusion lines and disposal in accordance with the hospital policy;
- flushing with at least 10 mL of saline solution (20 mL after infusions of blood, blood products or parenteral nutrition containing lipids), using the *start and stop* technique;
- placement of a new *port protector* on the NFC;
- routine hand hygiene.

PICC-port management must follow specific recommendations:

- skin antisepsis before positioning Huber's needle must be carried out with 2% chlorhexidine gluconate in 70% isopropyl alcohol;
- sterile gloves must be worn for performing Huber's needle insertion;
- Huber's needle must be removed as soon as it is no longer necessary and, in any event, it must be replaced no more than seven days after insertion;
- Huber's needle must be covered and stabilised with a transparent semipermeable dressing;
- Huber's needle must be closed with an NFC, which should be replaced in accordance with the criteria indicated above.

When not in use, the PICC-port should be flushed and locked with saline solution as indicated above every 3-4 weeks.
Tunneled-cuffed PICCs must also be closed with an NFC, which should be replaced in accordance with the aforementioned criteria.

Recommendations for preventing and treating late complications

Disinfection of the exit site

Exit site infection a rather frequent phenomenon, which can compromise the PICC or Midline *in situ* duration and even cause bacteraemic catheter infection.

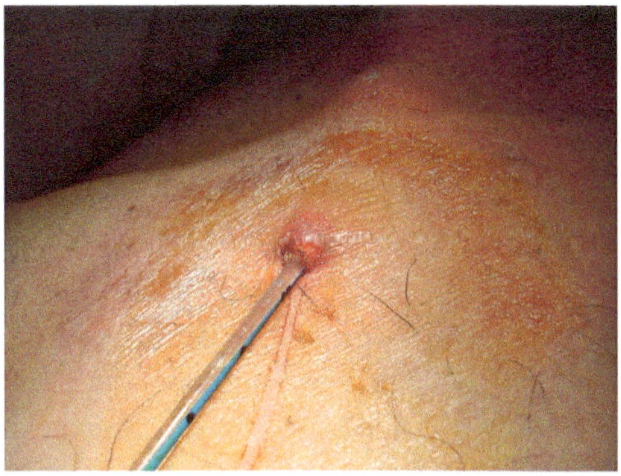

Figure **3.29**

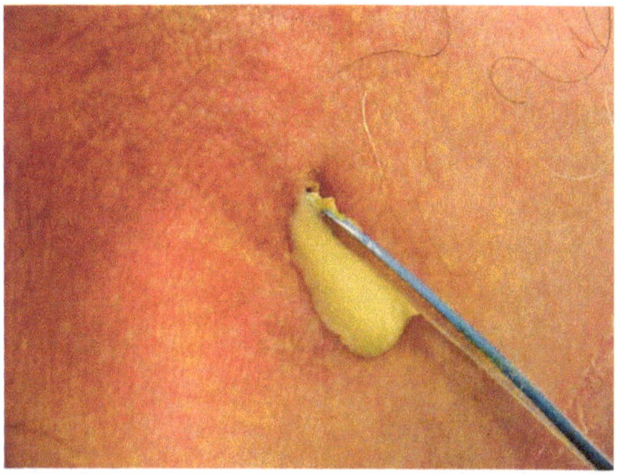

Figure **3.30**

Early diagnosis is based on exit site monitoring, to be performed on a daily basis in hospitalised patients and with a planned frequency (to be defined case-by-case) in patients being treated at home, as outpatients or at day hospital. Daily monitoring implies inspection or palpation of the exit site, even though daily inspection is not essential (sometimes it may be impossible to inspect the site directly, either due to a chlorhexidine releasing sponge dressing or the temporary presence of a gauze dressing): obviously, the detection of pain on palpation may require dressing removal and exit site inspection.

A diagnosis of exit site infection is based on signs of inflammation (reddening, hardening, secretion) at the site of the cutaneous breach from which the catheter exits (Figure 3.29). The use of a visual scale of inflammation, like the one previously mentioned (Visual Exit-site Score), would be pointless in this case.

A manifest infection of the exit site (Figure 3.30) is an automatic indication for the removal of PICCs or Midlines (except tunneled PICCs), due to the very high risk that the local infection could be complicated by catheter-related bacteraemic infection. In case of cuffed and uncuffed tunneled PICCs, where the exit site is far from the entry site of the catheter in the vein, it is possible to try to treat the infection with systemic antibiotic treatment and daily dressing change (local antisepsis with 2% chlorhexidine+ daily dressing with gauze dressing). Should there be evidence or the suspicion that the infection has not improved with conservative treatment, the PICC should in any case be removed.

The correct prevention of local exit site infection is obviously based on a correct dressing procedure of the exit site (see earlier in this chapter). A specific case of local infection is cutaneous/subcutaneous infection at the pocket of the PICC-port: in this case, the removal of the system is almost always indicated.

Bacteraemic infection

While CLABSI (Central Line Associated Bloodstream Infection, i.e. a bacteraemic infection in a patient with a central venous catheter) is an epidemiological concept, from the clinical point of view it is more appropriate to focus on CRBSI (Catheter Related Blood Stream Infection, i.e. a bacteraemic infection caused by central venous catheter). CLABSI indicates any bacteraemic infection that occurs in a patient with a central venous catheter, whereas CRBSI, in its correct sense, refers to bacteraemic infections in which the catheter is actually responsible for systemic infection. It should be underlined that the mere presence of bacteria inside the catheter is not a symptom of infection: such cases are referred to as catheter "colonisation".

The appropriate diagnosis of CRBSI cannot therefore be based either on mere detection of signs of infection (fever, leucocytosis) in a patient with a PICC or Midline, or on the findings of positive blood culture (bacteraemia) in a patient with a venous catheter. For a correct diagnosis of "true" CRBSI, the same germ cultivated in the blood must also be present in the culture of the catheter tip (or, in any event, of the intravascular tract). This would theoretically imply the need to always remove the catheter and cultivate it to obtain a certain diagnosis. In practice, according to the international guidelines (see IDSA 2009 guidelines), it is possible to formulate an accurate diagnosis of CRBSI even without the removal and direct culture of the catheter, using instead the paired cultures method (that is: simultaneous blood culture of the blood taken from the catheter + blood culture of a peripheral vein blood). In case of a suspected infection from a PICC, blood cultures should be performed simultaneously from the PICC ("central" blood) and from a peripheral vein ("peripheral" blood). The diagnosis of CRBSI is based essentially on a comparison between the time of positivisation of the "central" blood culture and the time of positivisation of the "peripheral" blood culture: the method is called the Delayed Time to Positivity (DTP) and is inexpensive and simple to perform, as long as the microbiology laboratory of the hospital is collaborating. Depending on the result, different situations may occur (Figure 3.31):

- both blood cultures are negative: there is no evidence of bacteraemic infection;
- only the "peripheral" blood culture is positive or the "peripheral" blood culture becomes positive at least two hours before the "central" blood culture: the bacteraemia is not caused by the PICC;
- only the "central" blood culture is positive: there is no evidence of bacteraemia or CRBSI, but the PICC is colonised;
- both blood cultures are positive but the "central" becomes positive at least two hours before the peripheral: CRBSI is confirmed (bacteraemic infection directly caused by the catheter).

If the bacteraemia is unrelated to the catheter, finding the source of the infection and initiating targeted antibiotic treatment are indicated, while the PICC should not be removed as it will be used for administering the antibiotic treatment.

If the bacteraemia is related to the PICC (CRBSI), there is always an indication for the removal of the PICC (even in the case of a Midline, a TCC or a PICC-port) and to initiate a targeted antibiotic treatment, preferably through a new peripheral access. It is almost never indicated to attempt to "save" or "renew" the PICC through systemic antibiotic treatments or local intracatheter treatments (so-called *antibiotic lock therapy*): in most cases, the removal (and any repositioning later, once the infection has been resolved) is associated with a better clinical outcome and savings in terms of resources.

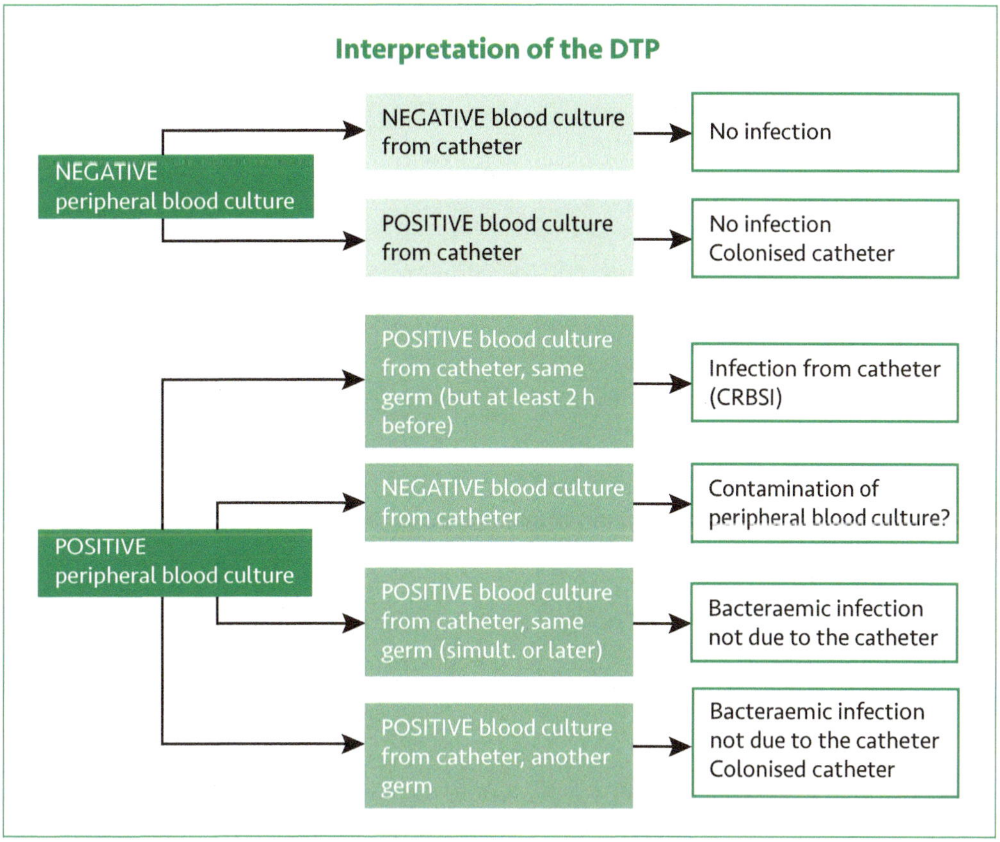

Figure **3.31**

The mere presence of catheter "colonisation" without any associated infection must be assessed case-by-case: the decision on whether to remove the PICC or not will depend on the type of germ, the clinical situation, the actual need for the PICC and the possibility/feasibility of new venous accesses.

The prevention of catheter-related infections is based on a series of recommendations that are summarised in the GAVeCeLT *bundle* for the prevention of infections of short to medium term central venous catheters (CICCs and PICCs). These recommendations regard both the insertion phase and the management phase (Table 3.2), and can be summarised in seven steps:

1. asepsis during the insertion (hand hygiene, maximum barrier precautions, skin antisepsis with 2% chlorhexidine in alcohol);
2. rational selection of the exit site (for PICCs means primarily the recommendation to obtain an exit site in Dawson's green area);
3. ultrasound-guided venipuncture;
4. asepsis during management (hand hygiene, skin antisepsis with 2% chlorhexidine in alcohol during dressing change, use of chlorhexidine releasing sponges, disinfection of the NFCs with chlorhexidine before accessing the infusion line);

Table 3.2 Bundlefor the prevention of infections from central venous access (GAVeCeLT2008)
1. Hand hygiene, maximum barrier precautions and skin antisepsis with 2% chlorhexidine during the insertion
2. Rational choice of the exit site (in order of preference: mid-third of upper arm, infraclavicular region, supraclavicular, neck, groin)
3. Ultrasound-guided venipuncture
4. 2% chlorhexidine for continuous and discontinuous skin antisepsis of the exit site, and for disinfection of the NFCs
5. Securement with sutureless systems
6. Use of the transparent, semipermeable dressings, where possible
7. Immediate removal of a central access that is no longer necessary

5. use of sutureless devices;
6. use of transparent dressings, where possible;
7. immediate removal of a PICC or CICC as soon as it is no longer required.

In addition to this *bundle*, established in 2008, we can now add the use of *port protectors* (recently introduced in clinical practice) as an effective system recommended for continuous ("passive" or "automatic") disinfection of the NFC when the connection is not in use. Currently, the actual indication for the use of antibacterial/antiseptic lock for infection prevention in PICCs (prophylactic *lock*, not to be confused with the aforementioned *antibiotic lock therapy)* is yet to be defined. The *lock* of venous catheters with antibiotic drugs (*antibiotic lock prophylaxis*) has been proven effective in preventing CRBSI in patients with catheters for dialysis and in patients with a history of repeated episodes of catheter-related infection, despite full adherence to the aseptic technique. Evidence for routine use of this type of prophylactic is rather weak, however, considering the potential disadvantages (high cost, risk of allergic reactions, risk of developing bacterial resistance to antibiotics). Accordingly, venous catheter *lock* with antibiotic substances must not be used routinely, even though it is taken into consideration by the Atlanta CDC guidelines. More interesting and promising is the *lock* with antibacterial substances with biofilm properties, such as citrate or taurolidine. Although high quality evidence is still lacking, it is highly probable that, in the near future, high-risk situations will be identified for catheter-related infections in which a preventive *lock* with citrate or taurolidine is used, even in association.

Catheter-related venous thrombosis

Definition

Catheter-related venous thrombosis means that the tract of vein in which the catheter is inserted presents a venous thrombosis originating from an endothelial lesion caused either by the penetration of the catheter in the vein or by mechanical and/or chemical trauma caused by the tip of the catheter on the venous endothelium. Venous thrombosis must be distinguished from occlusion of the lumen caused by clots and from the so-called

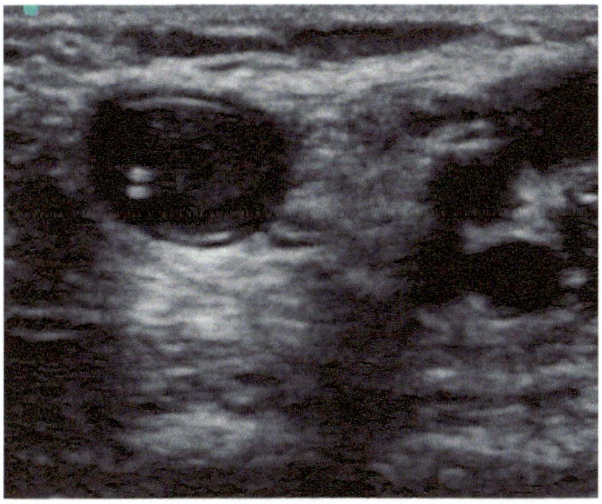

Figure **3.32**

“fibrin sleeve”, which is actually a fibroblast sheath that gradually tends to cover the catheter in the intravascular tract, and which should be interpreted as a blood tissue reaction to a foreign body.

Therefore, events often grouped under the term “catheter-related thrombosis” can be classified as follows.

- *Fibroblast sheath* (the so-called *fibrin sleeve*): at ultrasound exam, it presents as a sleeve around the catheter outer surface, at any point of its course; typically, it does not adhere to the endothelium walls but can cover the entire catheter length, interfering with its functioning (this occurs especially with closed end valved PICCs or Midlines and even more so with long peripheral cannulas). During catheter removal, it can often be detected floating inside the vein’s lumen by ultrasound. It does not carry risks of pulmonary embolism.
- *“Peripheral” or “proximal” venous thrombosis* (i.e., close to the catheter point of entry in the vein, or more precisely in the basilic-brachial-axillary tract, in the case of PICCs) (Figure 3.32). This type of thrombosis can be vessel-occlusive or non-occlusive and its etiopathogenesis can be recognised in the endothelial trauma at the point of venous cannulation (for example, after difficult or “problematic” venipuncture) or due to inequality between the cannulated vein diameter and the catheter diameter (if the catheter occupies more than a third of the diameter of the vein, the blood flow will be reduced and the risk of thrombosis increased).
- *“Central” or “distal” venous thrombosis* (close to the catheter tip). In the case of PICCs, this type of thrombosis typically involves the superior vena cava and/or the innominate veins; the etiopathogenesis often lies in an incorrect central position (for example, when the tip is too far from the cavoatrial junction and/or in direct contact with the venous wall, causing mechanical and/or chemical damage). When occlusive, it is associated with a superior cava syndrome.

Diagnosis

The diagnosis of thrombosis related to PICCs or Midlines is essentially based on a clinical suspicion (pain or oedema in the arm concerned) (Figure 3.33), which must then be confirmed with a thorough ultrasound examination. The use of Doppler echocardi-

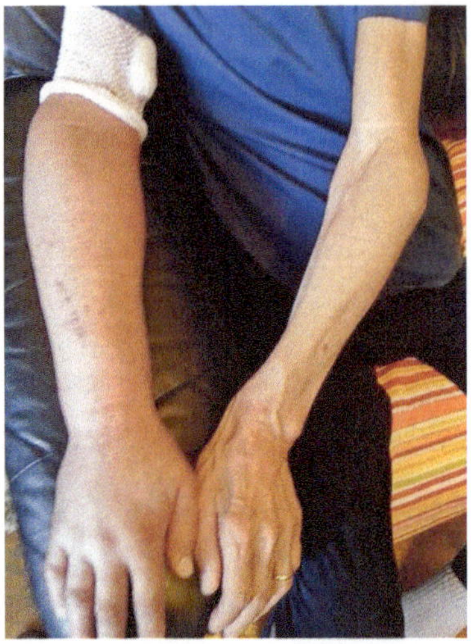

Figure **3.33**

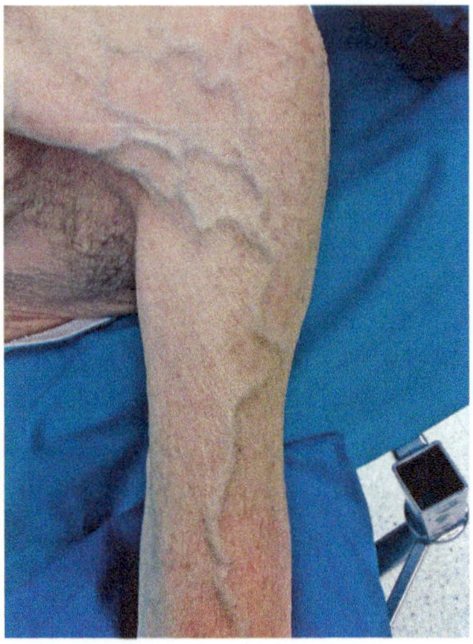

Figure **3.34**

ography is important but not essential, given that the diagnosis of limb thrombosis can be formulated very reliably and accurately through the so-called CUS (Compression Ultrasonography) based on the degree of non-compressibility of the thrombosed vessel compared to the vessel containing fluid blood. Ultrasound examination produces a direct view on the thrombus in the form of a hyperechoic structure partially or completely occupying the lumen only a few days after the formation of the thrombus: a "fresh" thrombus of recent formation is as anechoic as fluid blood.

The ultrasound examination therefore enables to identify thrombosis, to classify it as occlusive or non-occlusive, and to assess its extent (i.e., whether limited only to the brachial tract of the PICC/Midline or also extending to axillary vein in the infraclavicular region or to supraclavicular region veins). The presence of an occlusive or particularly extensive thrombosis is usually associated with clinical symptoms, and sometimes collateral venous circles may appear (such as, for example, in the case of a complete obstruction of the axillary-subclavian tract) (Figure 3.34). Many non-occlusive thromboses limited to the veins of the arm are often asymptomatic or oligosymptomatic and may constitute an incidental finding during ultrasound examinations performed for removing PICCs or for other reasons.

The involvement of veins in the supraclavicular area (subclavian, internal jugular, external jugular, innominate) indicates greater thrombosis severity and indicates the need to perform a CT scan with contrast medium to visualise the superior vena cava.

"Distal" venous thrombosis located near the catheter's tip (nearly always secondary to malpositioning) is the most difficult to diagnose: it is often suspected in a malfunctioning PICC. This malfunction is often manifesting as a PWO (Persistent Withdrawal Occlusion) or the ability to infuse but not aspirate.

There are various explanations for a PICC PWO:

- distal valve malfunctioning (a frequent occurrence with the Groshong PICC);
- presence of a fibroblast sheath;
- malpositioned tip (on the wall or wedged in a secondary vein);
- presence of a thrombus at the catheter's tip (often in association with a malpositioned PICC, for example too short).

In these cases, a diagnosis can be formulated through a cathetergram *(line-o-gram)*, a radiological study following infusion of contrast medium within the catheter. It will then be possible to visualise the malpositioned and/or fibroblast sheath (with typical "double contour" image of the catheter) and/or the presence of central thrombosis.
It is important to underline that, in the case of a proximal thrombosis from a PICC (even if symptomatic), the catheter is usually functioning well, while a distal thrombosis is associated with catheter malfunctioning.
In some rare cases, the presence of symptoms that are highly suggestive of thrombosis (swelling and pain in the arm) is not associated with ultrasound evidence of thrombosis. In these cases, it can be assumed that the PICC/Midline can interfere directly or indirectly with the lymphatic backflow of the arm. No specific treatment is indicated, other than raising the concerned arm and a mild antiedemigenous treatment.
The presence of a fibroblast sheath (paraphysiological phenomenon) is often an incidental finding that, however, inexpert ultrasound operators can mistaken for catheter-related thrombosis, even though these phenomena have a different pathogenesis.

Treatment

The presence of asymptomatic thrombosis related to a PICC/Midline, associated with a properly functioning catheter, is not an indication for the removal of the device, as typically, this will be a non-occlusive thrombosis limited to the veins of the arm. The indication for anticoagulation treatment is questionable and, while it can be taken into consideration, it should be established on a case-by-case basis. The catheter can be used normally.
The presence of symptomatic thrombosis related to a PICC/Midline (typically, occlusive and/or extensive thrombosis in the veins of the infra- or supraclavicular region) is always an indication for anticoagulant treatment (an appropriate dose of low-molecular-weight heparin, for example, 100 units/kg/12 h, in the absence of contraindications). In the case of extensive thrombosis of the veins in the supraclavicular area, performing an angiography-CT scan is essential to fully assess the clinical situation. Antibiotic treatment is usually not indicated, while the administration of anti-inflammatory drugs may be beneficial. In this type of patient, the PICC is usually functioning well while the Midline is not. It is, in any event, hazardous (and pointless) to remove the device: the removal of a catheter with recent thrombosis can be associated with mobilisation of the thrombus and risk of pulmonary embolism. As a matter of fact, removing the catheter does not seem to accelerate the thrombus resolution in any way, which is, however, favoured by a prompt administration of low-molecular-weight heparin. Catheter removal is indicated in the case (albeit very rare) that the thrombosis is associated with a documented cath-

eter-related infection or when the catheter is no longer beneficial or can no longer be used, as long as the thrombus is sufficiently stabilised. The latter detail is difficult to define precisely: certainly, a catheter with hyperechoic thrombus, and/or that occurred at least 7 days earlier, and/or with clearly good adhesion to the venous wall during the ultrasound examination can be removed relatively safely. On the contrary, if the catheter is forming an anechoic or hyperechoic thrombus, and/or occurred a few days earlier, and/or is apparently "floating" on ultrasound examination, its removal may be associated with a significant risk of pulmonary embolism.
Whether the catheter is removed or remains in place, anticoagulant treatment must be continued for several months. The specific period for continuing anticoagulant treatment has not yet been fully defined but certainly spans for the entire duration of device use. In certain cases, it may be advisable to switch from treatment with subcutaneous heparin to dicumarol taken orally.

Prevention

Catheter-related venous thrombosis is only partially preventable since the patient's tendency to thrombophilia, be it congenital (due to congenital conditions, often hereditary) or acquired (linked to an underlying disease or, more rarely, to treatments), plays an essential role.
Based-evidence recommendations, however, can reduce the risk of catheter-related thrombosis (Table 3.3):

- select a silicone or polyurethane catheter rather than a Teflon or polyethylene one;
- avoid placing a PICC/Midline close to or on the same side as a recent venous thrombosis;
- select a vein with a calibre at least three times the catheter calibre (i.e., 4 Fr catheters require veins of at least 12 Fr = 4 mm diameter, 5 Fr catheters require veins of at least 15 Fr = 5 mm etc.);
- in the case of PICCs or in-dwelling peripheral venous catheters (long peripheral cannulas and Midlines), always use ultrasound-guided venipuncture in order to minimise the trauma arising from the procedure;
- in the case of PICCs, ensure that the catheter tip is correctly positioned close to the cavoatrial junction and turned downwards (the intracavitary ECG method allows to verify the tip position intraprocedurally for maximum safety, accuracy and cost-effectiveness);

Table 3.3 Recommendations for preventing thrombosis from central venous catheter (GAVeCeLT 2012)
1. Check that the vein calibre is sufficient for the catheter calibre
2. Use ultrasound-guided venipuncture
3. Check that the catheter tip is close to the cavoatrial junction
4. Adequately stabilise the catheter (appropriate exit-site + *sutureless device* + transparent dressing)

- in the case of any venous access, either peripheral (needle cannulas, long peripheral cannulas, Midlines, etc.) or central (PICC), it is important to secure the catheter in order to minimise or eliminate any movement around the exit site, considering that catheter friction against the endothelium of the cannulated vein is another potential cause of thrombosis. Strategies to reduce catheter mobility include: rational exit site selection, appropriate securement with a *sutureless* system with cutaneous adhesion or subcutaneous anchorage, use of cyanoacrylate glue, if necessary, and, finally, the preferential use of semipermeable adhesive transparent dressings;
- prophylaxis with subcutaneous low-molecular-weight heparin (100 units/kg/day) is only indicated in selected patients (previous catheter-related venous thrombosis, congenital thrombophilia, history of venous thrombosis of various types in patients suffering from diseases known to be associated with thrombotic risk, etc.).

Fibroblast sheath

As already mentioned, the fibroblast sheath (often improperly called *"fibrin sleeve"*) is a paraphysiological reaction to the presence of an intravascular device. This is an actual "reaction to a foreign body", that is, the physiopathological response of the blood tissue to the presence of a catheter (Figure 3.35). The most reputable theories suggest that the external surface of the catheter acts as a foreign body and is covered by a circulating hepatic protein, called fibronectin, that attracts circulating macrophages (or perhaps macrophages originating in the endothelium). These then adhere to the catheter surface and differentiate in fibroblasts, forming a net of cells that soon transforms into connective tissue.

The forming of the sheath is therefore a phenomenon that, both in its pathogenesis and its histological structure, is fundamentally different from venous thrombosis.

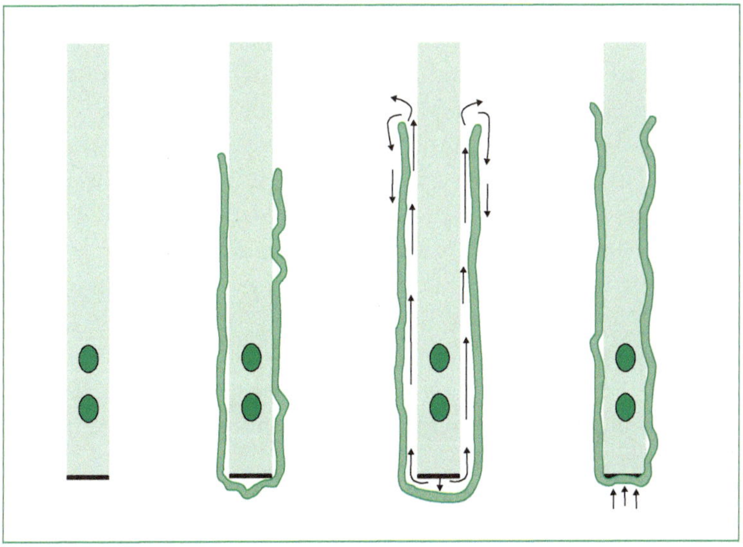

Figure **3.35**

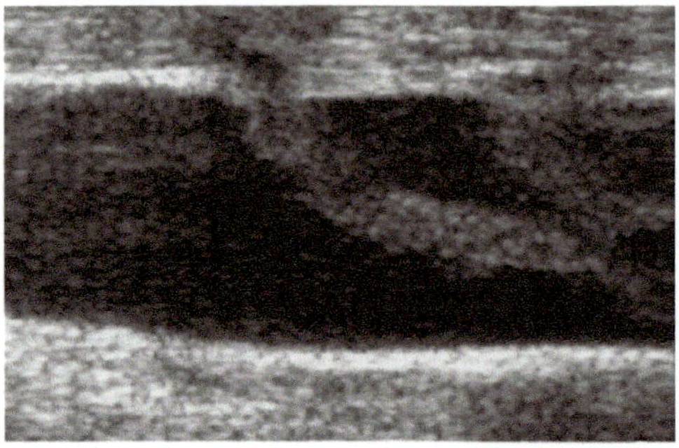

Figure **3.36**

A fibroblast sheath may be assumed to inevitably cover any intravascular device that has been in place for at least several consecutive days to some degree. In specific clinical situations and patients, this sheath is more marked and more evident with ultrasound, though the cause is unknown. In most cases, the fibroblast sheath is not probably associated with any sign of device malfunctioning. Sometimes, this is identified as an incidental ultrasound finding after the removal of a central venous catheter (Figure 3.36): at the time of the removal, the sheath persists in the intravascular tract for a short period (possibly 24-48 hours) and is then reabsorbed in the vascular wall.
While this condition is mostly asymptomatic, the sheath can sometimes interfere with the functioning of a PICC/Midline, especially in the following situations:

- In the case of a PICC or Midline with Groshong-type valved end, it is highly likely for the fibroblast sheath to interfere with the valve. The malfunction presents itself as the previously-described PWO; in such cases, it must be decided whether to remove the catheter or continue to use it for infusion only. Heparin or thrombolytic infusion is ineffective and makes no sense, as the sheath is made of connective tissue. The best prophylaxis procedure is obviously to avoid the use of distal valved catheters (the alleged clinical benefits of which have never been demonstrated).
- In the case of Midline or mini-Midline, even with open tip, the formation of a fibroblast sheath can cause device malfunctioning, typically associated with leakage of infused fluid from the exit site around the catheter. The phenomenon is more likely with long peripheral cannulas (so-called mini-Midlines) than with traditional *(midclavicular)* Midlines, due to the different tip location. The presence of the tip in a small vein of the arm, at a short distance from the exit site, makes it possible for the fibroblast sheath to form earlier and more completely encompass the tip; obviously, the phenomenon frequency will increase when the catheter remains in place for long periods, while it will be highly improbable in peripheral accesses that remain in place only for a few days.
- For open-tip PICCs, secondary malfunctioning from fibroblast sheath is very rare; some data suggest that the formation of a "symptomatic" sheath is more likely in PICCs that are too short or malpositioned (with the tip in an innominate vein or in the upper third of the superior cava).
- Finally, small-diameter PICCs used in paediatric patients (3 Fr) are more sensitive to the negative effects of the fibroblast sheath.

Lumen occlusion

Occlusion of the lumen of a venous catheter may have different causes: clots after blood withdrawals or infusion of blood or blood products (Figure 3.37), lipid aggregates during of parenteral nutrition with lipids, drug precipitates often after simultaneous, or almost simultaneous, infusion of incompatible drugs, contrast medium after execution of CT or MRI scans that use particularly viscous contrast media (Figure 3.38).

The basic recommendations for preventing occlusions are given above and are summarised in the GAVeCeLT recommendations (Table 3.4).

The occlusion may be complete or partial; one particular type of partial occlusion is the aforementioned PWO, when the catheter infuses but does not aspirate, particularly common with closed-end catheters (Figure 3.39).

The specific occlusion type can be diagnosed primarily taking into account the patient's medical history: an unexpected difficulty in performing the infusion after blood sampling, contrast media infusion or incompatible drug cocktail infusion leaves little doubt about the etiopathogenesis; equally, a difficulty in performing the infusion that presents slowly and gradually in a catheter used for parenteral nutrition will clearly be due to the progressive accumulation of lipid aggregates inside the lumen.

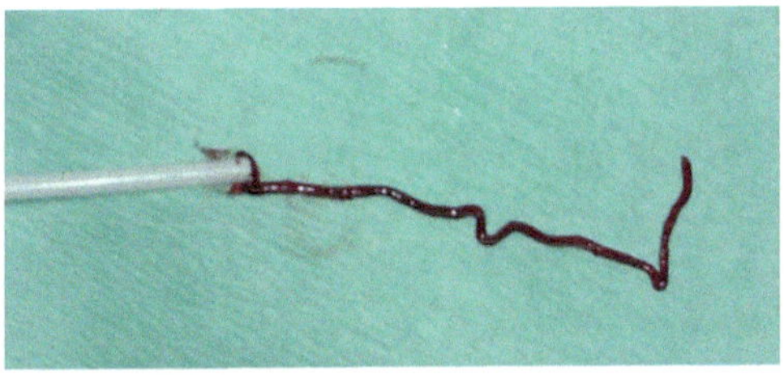

Figure **3.37**

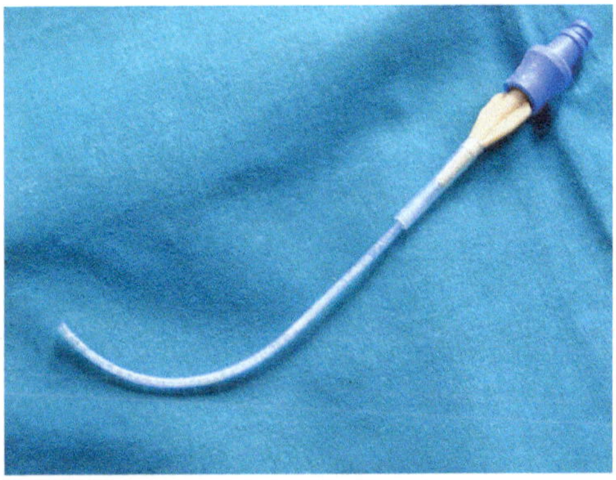

Figure **3.38**

Table 3.4 Bundle for the prevention of occlusions of venous access (adult patient) (GAVeCeLT 2012)

1. Flush with the *push/pause* method with 10 mL of saline solution before and after each infusion
2. Flush with the *push/pause* method with 20 mL of saline solution after infusion of blood products, lipids or contrast medium, or after blood sampling
3. Lock the system with saline solution only, unless heparinisation is expressly not recommended by the device manufacturer
4. Avoid backflow on disconnection of the system by using a "neutral" pressure NFC for external catheters, both valved and not valved, leaving positive pressure during the removal of the Huber from the port

If the obstruction involves a long peripheral cannula, it is advisable to remove the device at once. If the obstruction concerns usable PICCs or Midlines, it is advisable, on the other hand, to try to unblock it.
In the case of partial or complete catheter occlusion, saline solution must be used in the first attempts at unblocking it. If the catheter (PICC or Midline) is of silicone or polyurethane material, but it is not *power injectable*, 10 mL syringes must be used to unblock it hydraulically to avoid excess pressure in the system. If the PICC or Midline is *power injectable*, 5 mL or 2 mL syringes can also be used, as they apply greater pressure: such pressure will, in any event, be lower than 325 PSI (which is the pressure resistance limit for *power injectable* catheters). If the PICC or Midline is *power injectable,* there is a good chance that the unblocking procedure will be effective. Usually, the procedure involves repeated infusion of a few millimetres of saline solution under pressure, preceded by pumping or small, rapid movements of aspiration/infusion, in order to mobilise the aggregates that obstruct the lumen. Reinserting stylets or metal guidewires is never recommended since the risk of creating structural lesions in the catheter is high.
Should the hydraulic manoeuvres not be sufficient (typically, in silicone catheters or, in any event, in not power injectable catheters), it is wise to use an "unblocking" solution.
The nature of the "unblocking" solution must be established on the basis of the assumed etiopathogenesis: if an obstruction due to clots is suspected, a thrombolytic will be used (urokinase 10,000 units /mL or rTPA 2 mg/mL); in the case of a lipid obstruction, 50-70% ethanol must be used; in the case of obstruction from contrast medium for CT or MRI, molar bicarbonate (8.5%) will be employed; if the obstruction is probably due to precipitate of drugs with low pH, an acidifying solution will be used (HC1 0, 1N), or basifying (NaOH 0, 1N) solution in the case of high pH drugs. If the obstruction is only partial, the unblocking solution inserted will equal the dead space of the catheter (for example, 1.5-2 mL) and will be left to act for at least 30 minutes: the procedure should be repeated 3-4 times in a period of 2-3 hours. If, on the other hand, the obstruction is complete, the unblocking solution should be inserted "passively" with the two-syringe method (Figure 3.40): the PICC is connected to a three-way stopcock connected to two 10 mL syringes, one empty and one filled with the unblocking solution. Operating the stopcock so that only the empty syringe is connected with the catheter, aspirate with

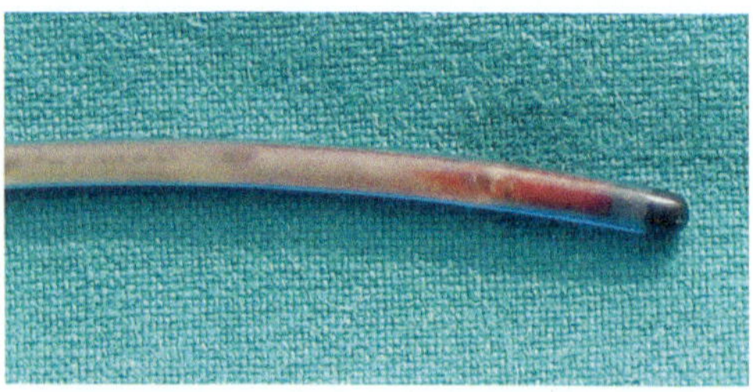

Figure **3.39**

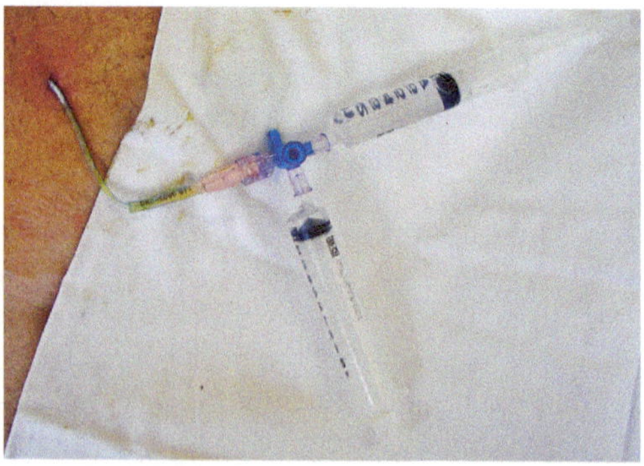

Figure **3.40**

the syringe in order to create a void inside the system: then, while still aspirating, the stopcock is switched so that the catheter aspirates the unblocking solution within it. This procedure is repeated every 15-30 minutes, aspirating with the empty syringe until the blood flow confirms the system is unblocked. This technique is beneficial as no pressure is created within the catheter as the unblocking solution gradually acts inside it.

If these procedures do not succeed and if the PICC/Midline is still clinically necessary, replacement over guidewire can be performed. After checking that there is no sign of thrombosis along the catheter, the sterile field is prepared and the catheter is partially retracted and trimmed. Then the metal guidewire is inserted, the final fragment of catheter is removed and the new catheter is inserted after disinfection. When the obstruction is complete and irreversible, and the metal guide cannot pass inside the catheter, complete removal of the device and its insertion *ex novo* elsewhere is necessary.

As mentioned, occlusion prevention is based essentially on a proper flushing protocol with saline, through hand-operated syringe with the *push/pause* technique, to be performed before and after every infusion. In adults, flushing with 10 mL saline solution are recommended under normal conditions, while 20 mL flushing is suggested after blood sampling or blood/blood product, lipid or contrast medium infusions. Besides this good flushing practice, it is also advisable to lock every lumen of the system with saline solution after each use. The use of lock solutions with anticoagulant properties (for example, heparin) is useful only in catheters used for haemodialysis or apheresis. For all short-, medium- or long-term venous accesses (including PICCs, CICCs, ports, PICC-ports and TCCs), there is no evidence for heparinised solution effectiveness and this practice should be abandoned. Neutral displacement valve caps (NFC) are equally essential in preventing occlusions, in order to avoid the backflow of blood inside the catheter when the infusion line is disconnected. When it is not possible to exploit the action of these neutral displacement caps (for example, while removing a Huber needle from a port), it is necessary to use procedures that leave a "positive pressure" inside the system.

Extra- or intravascular rupture of the tract

Ruptures of the extra- or intravascular tract may be due to inappropriate flushing manoeuvres at high pressures, or to the inadequate use of non-*power injectable* catheters for contrast medium high-pressure infusion, or inappropriate dressing removal with scissors or sharp objects. The rupture of a central venous access always results either in its complete removal or replacement over guidewire. The prevention of ruptures is mainly based on the use of external central venous catheters (PICCs, Midlines, TCCs) preferably *power-injectable* in third-generation polyurethane rather than standard polyurethane or silicone. Compared to polyurethane PICCs (both power injectable and regular), silicone PICCs are significantly associated with a higher risk of ruptures both of the external and internal tracts.

Table 3.5 illustrates GAVeCeLT recommendations for mechanical complication prevention (ruptures and displacements). It should be remembered that one of the basic principles for preventing catheter displacements and ruptures is employing *power injectable* PICCs in third-generation polyurethane: these are more resistant than silicone ones,

Table 3.5 Recommendations for mechanical complications prevention (ruptures, displacements) (GAVeCeLT 2012)

1. Use catheters in *power-injectable* polyurethane
2. Do not use sharp objects (scissors, etc.) when changing the dressing
3. Adequately stabilise the catheter
   - appropriate *exit-site*
   - *sutureless device*
   - transparent dressing

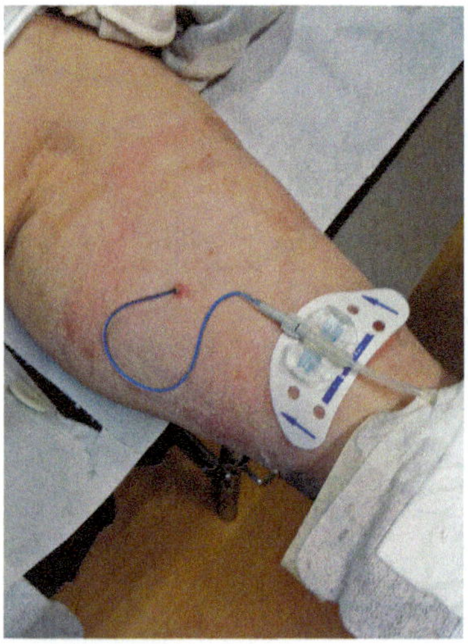

Figure **3.41**

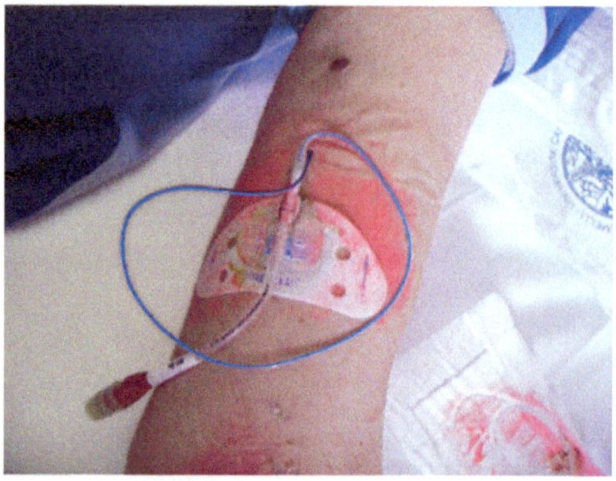

Figure **3.42**

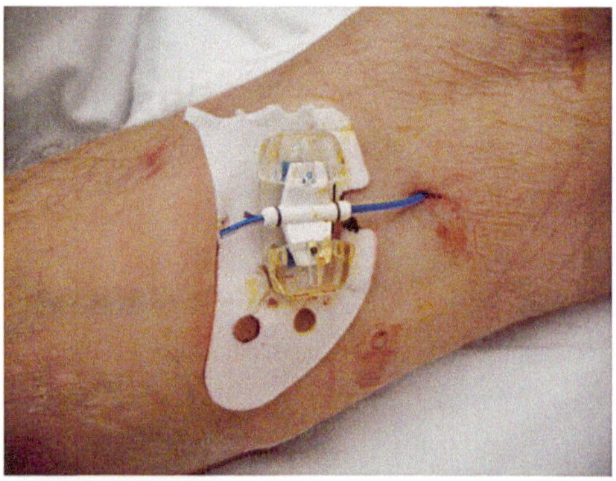

Figure **3.43**

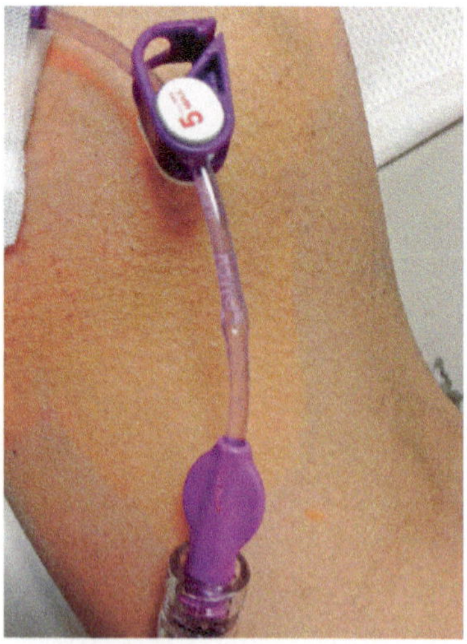

Figure **3.44**

which are much more susceptible to displacement (Figure 3.41 and 3.42) and ruptures (Figure 3.43). Another simple and important recommendation is avoiding to keep the catheter clamped: the clamp should only be used during valve cap replacement or catheter temporary opening. The clamp damages the catheter extension in the clamped tract (Figure 3.44) in the long run.

CHAPTER 4

Removal and replacement

PICC and Midline removal

Indications

Peripheral or central venous access devices should be removed only when they are no longer useful or adequate for their purpose, or in case of complications whose treatment requires their removal.

As regards PICCs and Midlines, there are various reasons for removal (Table 4.1): (1) end of use; (2) the device is inadequate for the planned clinical use; (3) infectious complications; (4) occlusive complications; (5) mechanical complications; (6) thrombotic complications; (7) malfunction.

A PICC may be removed at the end of use, for example, if it was inserted in a patient due to undergo surgery, for infusing intravenous treatment in the perioperative period: as soon as the patient resumes regular water, food and medicine oral intake, the PICC should be removed. All international guidelines (SHEA, EPIC, CDC) recommend that any central venous catheter that is no longer necessary should be promptly removed.

A Midline placed in-hospital for fluid infusion for the purpose of hydration is an example of removal due to inappropriateness. If, during the clinical course of the patient, a hyperosmolar parenteral nutrition is later found to be necessary, this would be a specific indication for the application of a central venous line and Midline removal.

Removal due to infective complications is probably one of the most frequent causes for the early removal of a PICC before treatment is completed. International guidelines recommend the removal of a PICC or Midline whenever the exit site is infected (Figure 4.1): in these conditions, the risk of an actual infection of the catheter through extraluminal contamination deriving from skin infection is deemed to be very high. The

Table 4.1 Indications for PICC and Midline removal
• Device no longer necessary • Device no longer appropriate • Infection • Irreversible occlusion • Mechanical damage • Venous thrombosis with malfunction • Malfunction due to fibroblast sheath or other causes

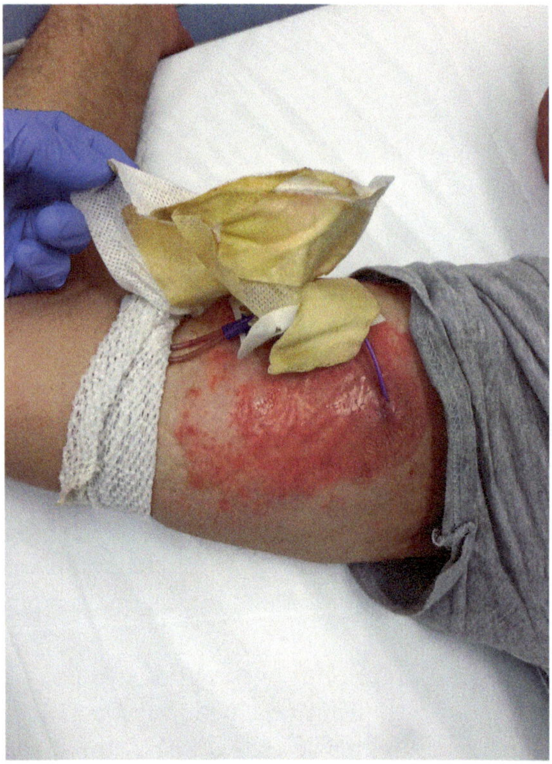

Figure **4.1**

non-infectious inflammation of the exit site (simple erythema, or "0 score" according to the Visual Exit-site Score; see Table 3.1) (Figure 4.2) does not constitute an indication for removal, but only for local surveillance. In the case of a tunneled PICC, uncomplicated infection at the exit site does not necessarily indicate removal since, in this case, the tunneling protects the catheter from extraluminal contamination. The suppurative infection of a PICC-port pocket or the infection of a tunneled PICC tunnel indicates immediate system removal. The most frequent case, however, is removal due to catheter-related bacteraemia infection (CRBSI), though the mere presence of fever in patients with PICC or Midline should not be considered an automatic indication for removal. Indeed, a

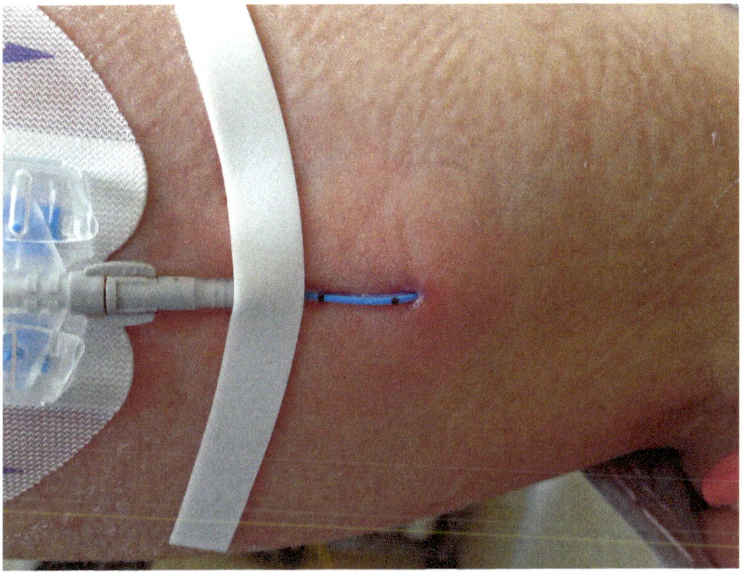

Figure **4.2**

central venous access removal on the basis of mere suspicion, where no adequate diagnosis of infection has been formulated, has been seen to lead to the removal of an "innocent" catheter in more than half of the cases. Removal should usually only be performed after a diagnosis of CRBSI obtained using the Delayed Time to Positivity (DTP) method described above. If no proper diagnosis of CRBSI is available (or when a simple colonisation of the system has occurred), the removal decision should be taken on a case-by-case basis.

A lumen occlusion (or one of the lumina) that resists hydraulic and chemical unblocking procedures constitutes an indication for device removal. Today, however, device removal should rarely justified by occlusive complications, as most lumen occlusions can be prevented through appropriate saline flushing and treated successfully by hydraulic or chemical disobstruction. In particular, the use of power-injectable polyurethane PICCs and Midlines reduces the risk of occlusion and increases the likelihood of successful hydraulic disobstruction. Silicone PICCs and Midlines (the use of which, as mentioned above, has no clear indication in clinical practice any longer) tend to occlude more often and are particularly difficult to unblock. In this case, hydraulic disobstruction should be carried out with 10 mL syringes or larger, with a less effective pressor response, due to the fragility of the silicone material.

Device removal due to mechanical complications is indicated in the following cases: (1) structural damage to the external part of the device, if direct repair or guidewire replacement are not possible; (2) structural damage of the device in its intravascular tract; (3) displacement of a PICC that cannot be replaced over guidewire; (4) erosion of the skin above the reservoir of a PICC-port or above the subcutaneous tract of a tunneled PICC.

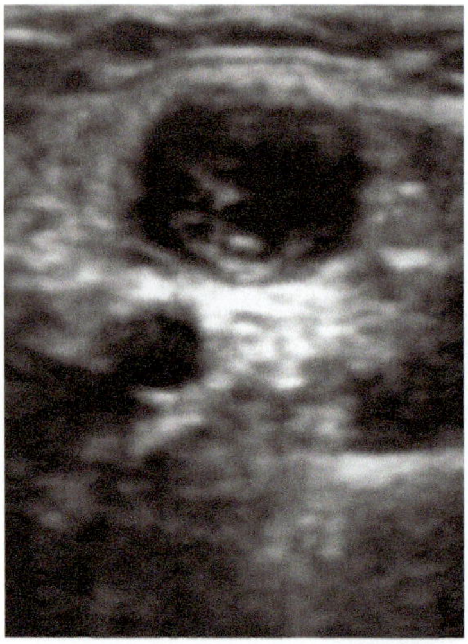

Figure **4.3**

In the case of catheter-related venous thrombosis (Figure 4.3), as mentioned above, the device removal is highly contraindicated in the case of recent thrombosis (less than 72 hours) and should be carried out with great caution and only if absolutely necessary (for example: suspicion of associated CRBSI; persistence/aggravation of symptoms despite an anticoagulant treatment) many days after the thrombotic event and the start of the anticoagulant treatment. As a general rule, the removal of a thrombosed PICC in the brachial tract is less dangerous than the removal of a PICC associated with thrombosis of the central veins (subclavian, innominate etc.). Before any removal, the absence of floating thrombi should be verified by ultrasound and/or radiological means. The most favourable situation is that of "old" already fibrotic thrombus adherent to the wall: on ultrasound examination shows them as hyperechoic thrombi with good vessel wall-adhesion. Leaving a thrombosed PICC in place even for weeks is, in fact, common practice, considering that (1) the PICC removal does not accelerate the resolution of the thrombosis, and (2) in most cases, the thrombosed PICC is well functioning and can be used safely.

Another cause of removal is a malfunction not caused by lumen occlusion or structural damage, but by other complications such as secondary malposition (so-called *tip migration*), where the PICC tip is in an incorrect position that is not favourable for the infusion/aspiration, or fibroblast sheath (often mistakenly called "fibrin sheath"), the diagnosis of which usually requires a radiological exam after injection of a contrast medium into the catheter *(line-o-gram)*. The fibroblast sheath is a frequent cause for PWO-type malfunction (Persistent Withdrawal Obstruction) in PICCs with Groshong-type distal valve. Moreover, it is a frequent cause of Midline malfunction (in particular the shorter "mini-Midlines") and is typically characterized by infusion fluid leakage from the exit site and around the catheter. While a secondary malposition can sometimes be treated replacing the guidewire, a fibroblast sheath that interferes with the functionality of the device is almost inevitably an indication for system removal.

Recommendations

Only trained personnel should perform removal procedures, when appropriate. Ultrasound examination of the veins of the arm and chest along the trajectory of the PICC/Midline (Figure 4.4) should ideally be performed after removal, so to exclude the presence of thrombosis, which could also be asymptomatic. The pre-removal ultrasound examination becomes mandatory in case of clinical suspicion of thrombosis (oedema, arm pain). The removal procedure should start by removing the dressing and the sutureless device using clean, non-sterile gloves (after proper hand hygiene). After skin antisepsis with 2% chlorhexidine, the catheter is slowly drawn out of the skin until complete removal. Routine culture of the tip of the removed catheter is not indicated. Bleeding from the exit site is infrequent and often minimal and can be stopped by gentle active compression for a couple of minutes or preferably by local application of cyanoacrylate glue. Difficulty in removing the catheter is a relatively frequent event with small calibre epicutaneo-cava catheters, while it is quite rare in the case of PICCs and usually secondary to the fibroblastic sheath surrounding the catheter. In most cases, applying a slow constant pressure helps overcoming the resistance. Caution must be used in the case of silicone catheters: while polyurethane (especially third generation) is quite resistant and hardly breaks, Groshong-type silicone PICCs are fragile and can deform and break if subject to excessive traction.

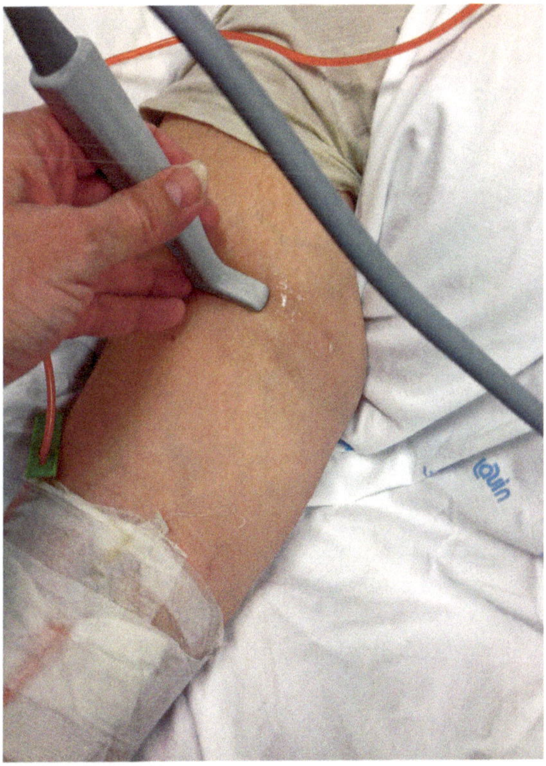

Figure **4.4**

In case of non-tunneled CICC removal, the risk of gas embolism exists, therefore placing the patient in a supine position and continue compression long after the catheter removal is recommended. Such recommendation does not apply to PICCs, since the venous pressure at arm level is never negative, not even during forced inspiration.
Uncuffed tunneled PICC removal does not usually lead to any difficulties: the catheter is mobilised and withdrawn easily out of the exit site.
Tunneled-cuffed PICC or PICC-port removal will obviously require a small cutaneous incision in order to mobilise the cuff or the reservoir, respectively. In case of tunneled-cuffed PICCs, the exact subcutaneous position of the cuff may be identified using ultrasound; then, following local anaesthesia, a small transversal incision is made at the cuff site. Once the cuff is mobilised, the entire catheter can be easily extracted. In the case of a PICC-port, a cut must be made along the incision line of the reservoir pocket: the system is removed by identifying the connection between the reservoir and the catheter first, then extracting the catheter and finally removing the reservoir. Both procedures obviously require 2% chlorhexidine for skin antisepsis and an appropriate local anaesthetic for infiltration (for example, with 0.75% ropivacaine).

PICC and Midline guidewire replacement

Indications

In certain situations, guidewire replacement is quite an effective alternative to removal and reinsertion in another site.
Typical indications for guidewire replacement are lumen occlusion and mechanical complications (Table 4.2). However, it is contraindicated in thrombotic and infective complications (Table 4.3). In particular, guidewire replacement of any central venous catheter to prevent and/or diagnose catheter-related infections should be avoided: the preventive replacement with a new catheter has been shown to be ineffective in reducing the infective risks while the diagnosis of CRBSI should now be carried out with the DTP method described above.

Table 4.2 Indications for PICC and Midline guidewire replacement
• Mechanical damage of the extravascular tract • Secondary malpositioning (displacement or *tip migration*) • Malfunction from partial intraluminal occlusion • Replacement with more appropriate device

Table 4.3 Contraindications for PICC and Midline guidewire replacement
• Certain or suspected infection • Venous thrombosis at any point along the catheter • Malfunction due to the presence of fibroblastic sheath

Indications for guidewire replacement are the following:

- unrepairable structural damage of the external tract of a PICC/Midline catheter;
- PICC tip dislodgement due to a partial accidental device removal; as mentioned above, when the displaced tract exceeds 4 cm (Figure 4.5), it is mandatory to remove or replace the device, even without further radiologic control, since it is certain that the tip is no longer in a central position, while if the dislodgement is suspected or minimal (Figure 4.6), the actual position of the tip should be assessed performing a chest x-ray;
- PICC tip dislodgement due to tip migration (secondary malposition)
- complete or partial intraluminal occlusion that cannot be resolved with hydraulic or chemical unblocking methods;
- replacement of a Midline catheter with a PICC catheter, when the former device has become inappropriate for the intended use (for example, due to a switch to intravenous treatments that require a central line).

Malfunction due to fibroblast sheath (radiologically documented by means of *line-o-gram*) does not constitute so much an indication for guidewire replacement as for system removal, due to the high risk of complications during replacement and fibroblast sheath recurrence on the new catheter.
Structural damage of the PICC intravascular tract (radiologically documented by means of *line-o-gram*) does not constitute so much an indication for guidewire replacement as for system removal, due to the high risk of the damage being worsened by the guide passing through, with possible embolization of catheter fragments.

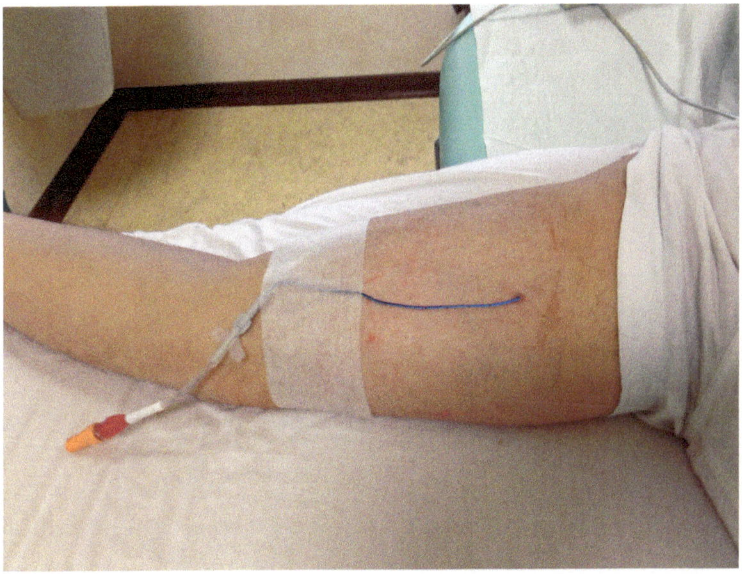

Figure **4.5**

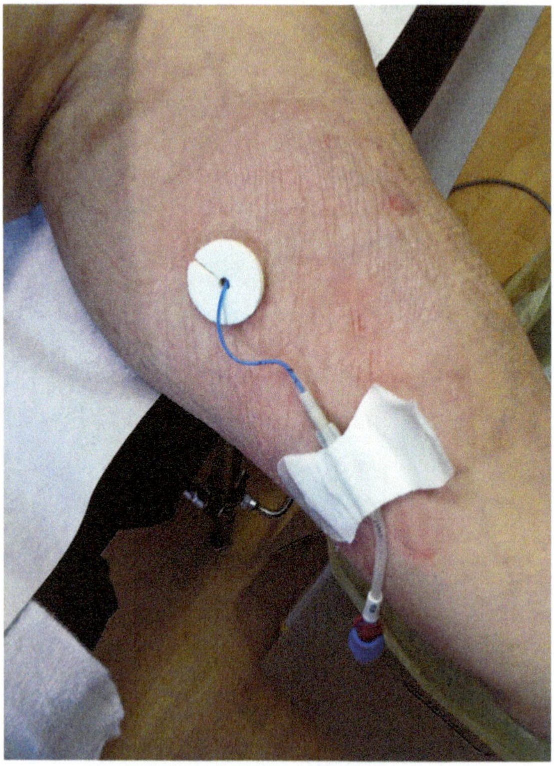

Figure **4.6**

Recommendations

PICC or Midline guidewire replacement should always be performed by expert personnel and after carefully excluding of the presence of catheter-related thrombosis by ultrasound examination. The presence of thrombosis or suspected thrombosis is a contraindication for the performance of the procedure.

Guidewire replacement should never be performed by introducing the guidewire into the catheter hub, but according to the procedure described below:

- ultrasound examination of the veins of the arm and the supraclavicular-infraclavicular veins (axillary, subclavian, internal jugular, innominate) in order to exclude the presence of thrombosis; the examination should be carried both at the brachial level (Figure 4.7) and at the subclavian level (Figure 4.8), as well as in long axis (Figure 4.9), whenever necessary;
- hand hygiene and clean, non-sterile gloves;
- dressing and securement device removal;
- wearing sterile gloves, prepare the sterile field by disinfecting the skin with 2% chlorhexidine in 70% IPA;
- after pulling out a sufficient tract of catheter (proportionally to the length of the guidewire to insert), the catheter is trimmed at a point that was previously established inside the vein;

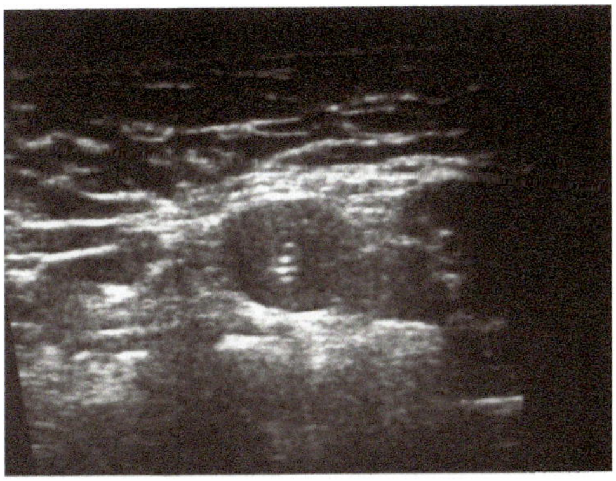

Figure **4.7**

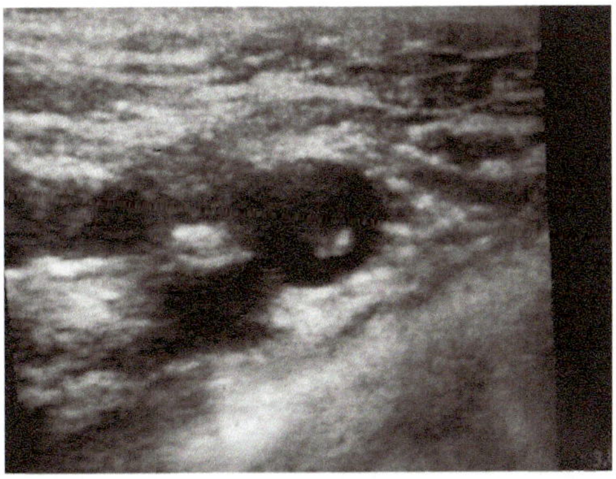

Figure **4.8**

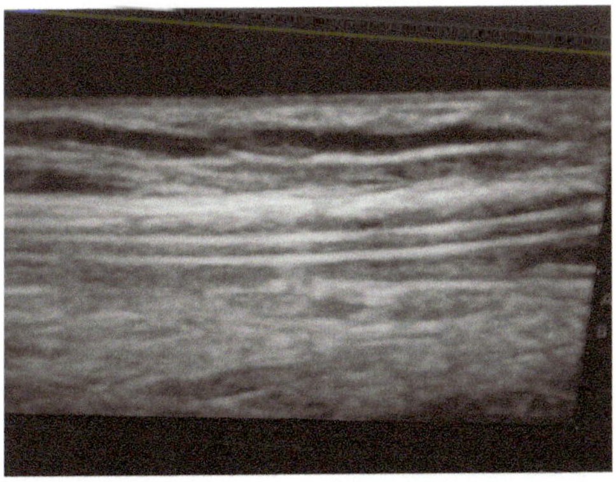

Figure **4.9**

- the guidewire is threaded into the catheter for a sufficient tract, so to pass the distal end of the catheter; then the catheter is slowly removed, leaving the guidewire in place;
- at this time, it is recommended to discard the gloves, wear new sterile gloves and disinfect the area around the exit site again using 2% chlorhexidine in 70% IPA;
- a micro introducer/dilator is inserted over the guidewire; then the procedure continues as if it were a new insertion (including accurate tip positioning with the tip location method as with intracavitary ECG).

Among the difficulties that may arise during guidewire replacement, it should be remembered that it can sometimes be hard or impossible to insert the metal guide in the catheter: the lumina of a 4 Fr bi-lumen catheter can be too thin for letting the metal guide commonly used for PICCs and Midlines (0.018" diameter) through; the catheter may be completely obstructed and/or bent, so that guidewire passage encounters an insurmountable resistance; the presence of a Groshong-type distal valve, especially if already malfunctioning, can sometimes block the complete passage of the guide.

Intraluminal obstructions are not necessarily a contraindication for guidewire replacement: while it is true that the passage of the guide can mobilise the material occluding the lumen (clots, biofilm, drug precipitates, etc.), it is also true that the injection of inert material previously contained in the lumen into the circulation has never been reported to cause complications. It is necessary to underline that the material occluding the lumen is never a real thrombus (by definition, thrombosis occurs only inside the intravascular system) and cannot cause the clinical syndrome known as pulmonary embolism. Nonetheless, the mobilisation of intraluminal inert material colonised by microorganisms or with pyrogenic action (cellular debris, protein byproducts or lipid breakdown, etc.) can cause symptoms such as fever or shivering, that are usually transitory.

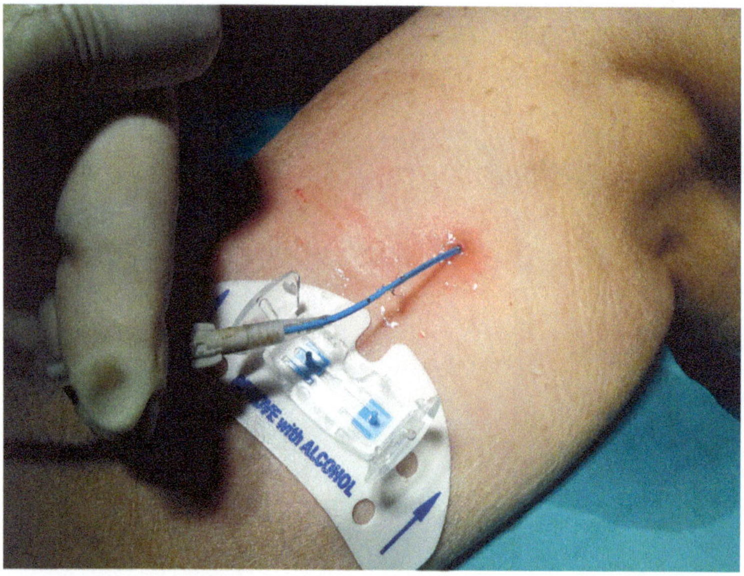

Figure **4.10**

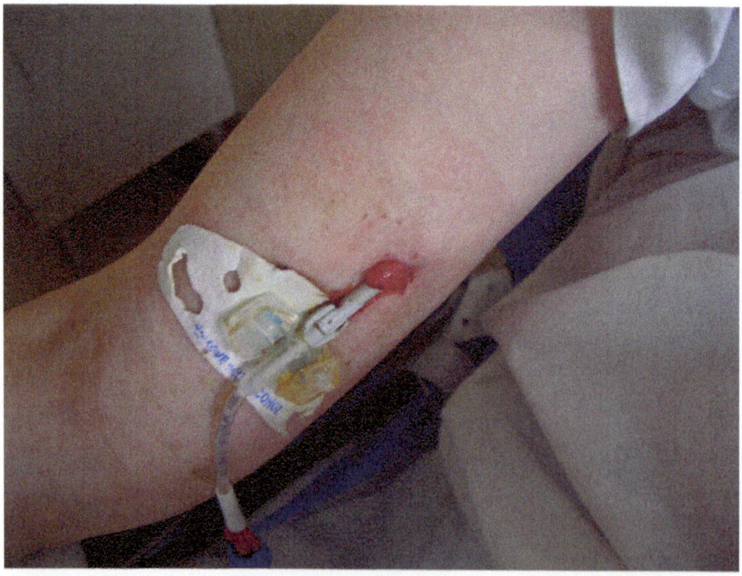

Figure **4.11**

A suspected exit site infection is an obvious contraindication to guidewire replacement (Figure 4.10). The presence of a granuloma at the insertion site (quite a rare occurrence) (Figure 4.11), even in the absence of exit site infection, may be a contraindication for the procedure.

It is worth remembering that for a safe procedure performance, it is advisable not only to exclude the presence of thrombosis and apply the recommendations for infection prevention as described above, but also to be aware of the length of the catheter to replace and of the length of the guidewire. The guidewire must be long enough to extend at least 10-20 cm further than the tract of catheter that it will replace, to avoid the risk of drawing out the catheter and guidewire simultaneously, or worse, of accidental embolizing the guidewire into the vascular system. During the entire catheter removal procedure, the operator should control the proximal end of the guidewire.

If the PICC to be replaced is tunneled (uncuffed), there are no contraindications for guidewire replacement, as long as the tunneled tract is shorter than the micro introducer-dilator that is inserted over the guidewire.

The guided replacement of cuffed PICCs or PICC-ports is theoretically possible with certain adaptations, but it is generally too complex to be recommended in clinical practice.

CHAPTER 5

Materials and technical aspects

Choice of materials

The choice of materials for PICC and Midline insertion and management is crucial for the successful clinical outcome of the device. It can be confidently stated that what specifically qualifies an expert operator is the ability to select the most appropriate materials and methods.

Some of the fundamental points on material selection will be analysed below.

Catheter

A series of characteristics (Table 5.1) must be considered to select a specific type of PICC (or Midline), one of the most important being the device material.

Silicone is often described as the most biocompatible material, but third-generation polyurethanes (which were introduced at the end of the 1990s) have demonstrated similar performance in terms of duration and infection and thrombosis incidence. When comparing the risk of complications with silicone or polyurethane, there are no evident benefits in using silicone PICCs.

As regards the risk of infection, comparison studies between silicone and first-generation polyurethane conducted in the 1970s and 1980s produced contradictory results. In the last fifteen years, however, no clinical study has shown differences between the two materials in terms of risk of infection, with the exception of a clinical study comparing polyurethane and silicone valved catheters, which observed a lower risk of infection for polyurethane catheters. In fact, current guidelines issued by the most important scientific societies (EPIC, ESPEN, CDC) advise against the use of polyvinyl chloride or polyethylene catheters only, underlining that silicone and polyurethane show no provable difference in terms of infections. The risk of infection is obviously linked to many different

Table 5.1 PICC specifications
• Material • Calibre • Number of lumina • Centimetre marking • Stylet • Special features – *reverse tapering* – proximal or distal valves – specialised tip – possibility of proximal *trimming*

factors (training of the staff in charge of inserting and managing the PICC, appropriate device indication, application of correct insertion and management protocols, etc.).
Clinical and experimental studies carried out three decades ago and investigating the risk of thrombosis comparing silicone, first-generation polyurethane and polyethylene, produced contrasting results, that favoured both silicone and polyurethane. In the last fifteen years, no clinical study has identified any difference between these two materials in terms of thrombotic risk. According to the most recent guidelines on the prevention of catheter-related venous thrombosis (see Appendix IV), silicone vs. polyurethane catheters show no differences in terms of risk of thrombosis: venous thrombosis is definitely related to many other factors (patient's thrombophilia, selected PICC diameter compared to cannulated vein diameter, PICC insertion technique, catheter tip position, adequate technique of securement to the skin, etc.).
However, there are differences between silicone and polyurethane in terms of risk of mechanical complications (ruptures and displacements): indeed, all the clinical studies carried out in the last twenty years have unequivocally shown a greater incidence of these complications in silicone PICCs. This result appears is highly expected, as silicone is more fragile if compared to polyurethane and third-generation polyurethane, in particular.
Even though more than 20 years ago, one study suggested that polyurethane may be less susceptible to the risk of occlusion than silicone, most clinical studies carried out in more recent times have shown no statistically significant difference in terms of lumen occlusion, irrespective of a valve being present (see below). The risk of occlusion seems to be associated with factors that are connected to PICC management, among which the adoption of a correct *flush* and *lock* protocol is the most relevant.
As the above information indicate, evidently silicone PICCs have no advantages over polyurethane PICCs in terms of the risk of thrombotic or infective complications, but are certainly more exposed to complications from displacement or rupture of the extra- or intravascular tract.
As for clinical *performance*, many studies have shown that first-generation polyurethane PICCs are associated with higher flows than silicone PICCs. In recent times, the avail-

ability of power injectable PICCs made in third-generation polyurethane has further expanded the clinical use of PICCs, ensuring high flows (up to 2 mL/sec), the possibility of injecting contrast medium for radiological exams, reliable assessment of central venous pressure, the guarantee of maximum resistance to mechanical traumas, as well as an easier disobstruction.

One last point to be considered is the potential risk of interaction between polyurethane and certain antiblastic drugs (such as taxols) that are administered in alcohol solution. While it is theoretically true that polyurethanes are more susceptible than silicone to the effect of alcohol, it should be emphasised that actual damage to catheters has never been demonstrated, either *in vivo* or *in vitro*. A high quality *in vitro* study conducted by the Maki group showed that exposure for long periods (up to 10 weeks) to 70% concentrations of ethanol led to minimal to no impact on first-generation polyurethane or silicone catheter structure, without any significant difference between the two materials. Third-generation polyurethanes (such as those of power injectable PICCs), in particular, have a known resistance to alcohol (as certified in the manufacturers' information leaflets). A recent *in vitro* study on five different types of third-generation polyurethanes (Tecoflex, Tecothane, Carbothane, Pellethane, Chronoflex) revealed no significant structural alterations after 90 days of exposure to highly concentrated alcohol solutions.

In conclusion, there is no evidence that silicone PICCs have any advantages or any preferential indication over polyurethane PICCs. Other evidence indicate that the use of silicone PICCs can limit device performance and increase the risk of mechanical complications. Today, third-generation polyurethane power injectable PICCs ensure maximum safety and cost-effectiveness under any clinical conditions. It is no coincidence that the vast majority of PICCs (85%) currently used on the USA market, primarily for chemotherapy purposes, are made of this material.

Valves represent another potentially controversial aspect in PICC selection. Both silicone and polyurethane PICCs integrate proximal or distal valves in their structure. Specifically, non-valved open-tip PICCs, open-tip PICCs with proximal valve and closed-tip PICCs with Groshong-type distal valve (the latter entirely made of silicone) are available on the market.

In the past, these valves were considered useful for preventing occlusive complications and improving central venous catheter management. Prospective controlled studies on long-term central venous access have shown that valved catheter, both as ports and cuffed tunneled catheters, are useless: the presence of a valve, indeed, seems to be associated with a greater incidence of malfunctions and mechanical complications. As for PICCs, literature presents even more evidence on this matter.

In the past fifteen years, many randomized studies have shown: (1) that the use of a polyurethane PICC with proximal valve does not have any advantage over non-valved PICCs in terms of risk of occlusion; (2) that there are no differences in terms of occlusions when comparing polyurethane PICCs with proximal valve to silicone PICCs with distal valve (apart from an obviously greater incidence of mechanical complications in silicone PICCs); (3) that there are no differences in terms of complications between non-valved power injectable PICCs and those integrating a proximal valve; (4) that there are no

significant differences between silicone PICCs silicone with distal valve and non-valved polyurethane PICCs.
A few years ago, two non-randomized prospective studies showed no significant differences between third-generation polyurethane non-valved PICCs, standard polyurethane non-valved PICCs and silicone PICCs with distal valves, in terms of occlusions or infections, although in both studies silicone catheters showed a greater incidence of mechanical complications.
Finally, in the last two years, two interesting randomized studies have compared three groups of PICCs: non-valved polyurethane PICCs *versus* polyurethane PICCs with proximal valve *versus* silicone PICCs with distal valve in the first study, and power injectable PICCs with PASV-type proximal valve *versus* power injectable PICCs with SOLO-type proximal valve *versus* non-valved power injectable PICCs in the second study. In neither study, conducted respectively on 102 and 160 patients, was it possible to demonstrate any advantage connected to any type of valve. It is interesting to underline that, in the light of what the latest guidelines (EPIC 2014) recommend, in the last study cited no catheter was closed with heparinized solution, irrespective of the presence of a valve.
In conclusion, there is no clinical reason nor scientific rationale for preferring the use of a valved PICC, whatever the type of valve. Both valved and non-valved PICCs show the same risk of lumen occlusions: This complication can be adequately prevented not by using a *lock* with heparin but by adopting an adequate flushing protocol with saline solution before and after every infusion.
Choosing between valved and non-valved PICCs still has consequences from the clinical point of view: selecting a catheter with a distal valve (necessarily in silicone) leads to a greater risk of mechanical complications; moreover, valved PICCs are never cost-effective since their additional cost is not justified by clinical benefits.
The best PICC today, in terms of safety, cost-effectiveness and the ability to be implanted in any patient in any clinical situation, is therefore (Figure 5.1):

- power injectable;
- in third-generation polyurethane;
- open tip;
- non-valved.

This type of PICC is available in various calibres (from 3 Fr and 6 Fr) and with different numbers of lumina (from one to three). Considering the clinical performance and the average calibre of the veins of the arms, in non-intensive care adult patients 4 Fr single-lumen and 5 Fr double-lumen PICCs are most frequently used. In adult patients in intensive care 6 Fr triple-lumen PICCs are often indicated, while 3 Fr single-lumen or 4 Fr double-lumen PICCs are preferred in pediatric patients. In double-lumen PICCs, the two lumina have equal calibre, volume and clinical use. A double-lumen PICC with a distal lumen to be used as a PICC and a proximal lumen to be used as a Midline exist but is not commercially available yet (Figure 5.2). In the case of a triple-lumen, on the other hand, the three lumina are not equal, since only one is power injectable.

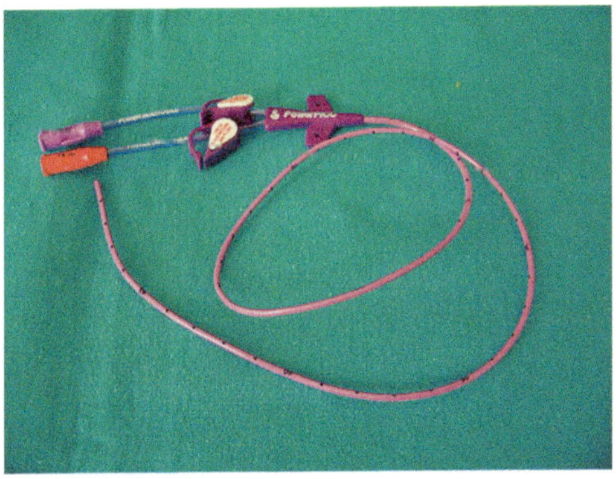

Figure **5.1**

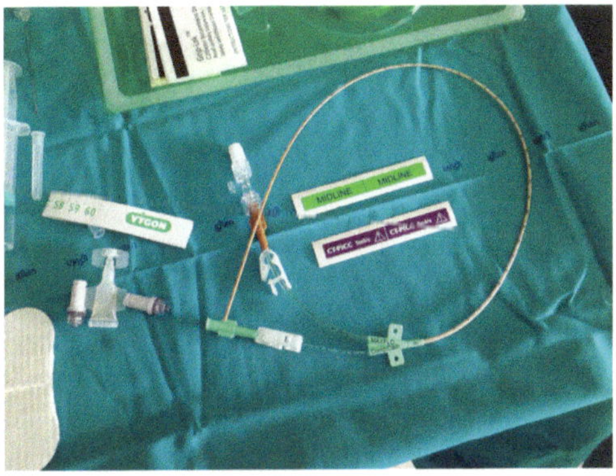

Figure **5.2**

As well as the calibre and the number of lumens, other features must be discussed.

- The PICC must be marked with a centimetre scale with clearly readable numbers.
- The stylet should preferably be integrated in the catheter (insertion at the time of use could risk damaging the catheter) and include an adequate blocking system, as the stylet is usually only partially pulled out, to allow the distal trimming of the catheter (see the insertion technique above), then blocked in accordance to the new length. An electrically conductive stylet can facilitate the intracavitary ECG method for assessing the tip position.
- Some PICCs have a reverse tapering, as their proximal tract diameter increases close to the securement wing. This structural characteristic was first introduced in PICCs for an easy handling of the external tract and may be useful to decrease bleeding at the exit site and reduce the risk of displacement. On the other hand, however, it could potentially be counterproductive in terms of thrombotic risk and can effectively be an obstacle in performing the tunneling procedure. In summary, while literature presents no certain data, today it seems advisable to prefer PICCs with minimal or no reverse tapering (= or <2 cm).
- Polyurethane PICCs have recently been introduced. They provide proximal rather than distal trimming (Easy PICCs) (Figure 5.3), which represents a significant advantage when adopting the intracavitary ECG technique: it is, in fact, possible to easily decide the length of the intravascular tract by ECG method and only later adjust the trimming of the catheter. This excludes the risk of trimming the catheter too short, after wrongly estimating the length needed. This is especially true for PICCs to be used in pediatric patients, where estimates based on surface landmarks are rather imprecise.
- After trimming the catheter, it is necessary to connect it to the securement wing (as in silicone PICCs with distal valve, for which proximal trimming is mandatory).

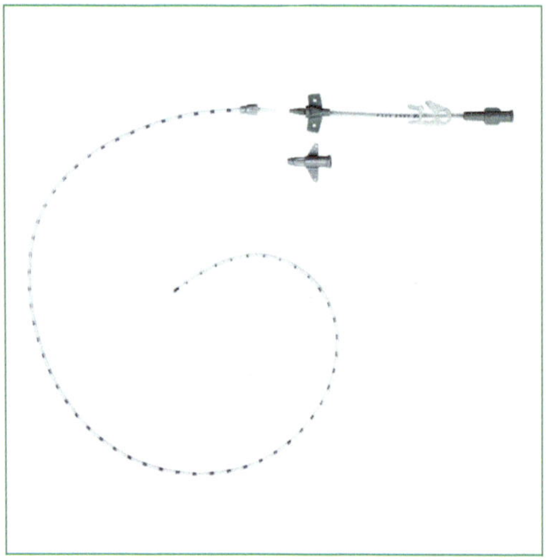

Figure **5.3**

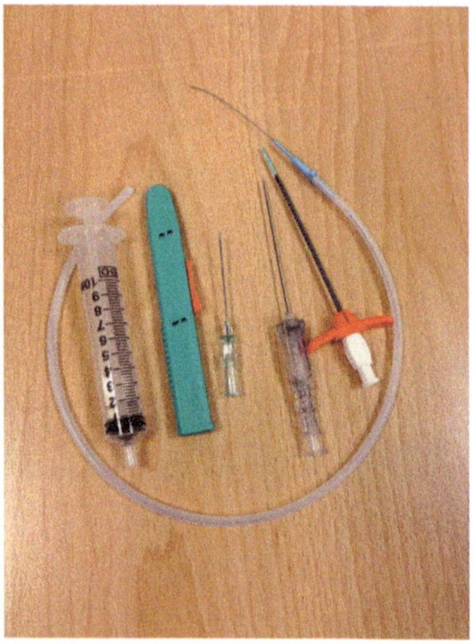

Figure **5.4**

- There are also PICCs with "specialised" tip (Blue Tip) that offer the option of entirely avoiding trimming: PICCs of the estimated length must be chosen in advance (for example: 40, 45 or 50 cm) in order to avoid leaving a long extracutaneous tract. In many cases, however, it is recommended to use these PICCs in the traditional way, i.e. trimming them distally and sacrificing the tip, as the risk of wrongly assessing the catheter length is very high and the advantages of the "specialised" tip are only theoretical and have never been clinically demonstrated.

Micro-introduction kit

A good micro-introduction kit (Figure 5.4) is one of the basic prerequisites for the success of the insertion. If the guidewire tip is not sufficiently flexible or the introducer-dilator is not stiff enough or has inadequate tapering, the insertion can be severely compromised even when performed by expert operators.
In summary, micro-introduction kit items should have the following specifications:

- needle: 21 G, with echogenic tip, sufficiently rigid and sharp (Figure 5.5);
- guidewire (Figure 5.6): 0.018", in nitinol with a straight but flexible tip (*floppy straight tip*), shorter than 50 cm; guides that are too long bear the danger of contaminating the operating field and/or causing cardiac arrhythmias;
- introducer-dilator (Figure 5.7): sufficiently rigid, with an adequate connection between the introducer and dilator and optimal tapering in the guidewire/dilator transition, as well as in the dilator/introducer transition, so to minimise trauma to the venous wall.

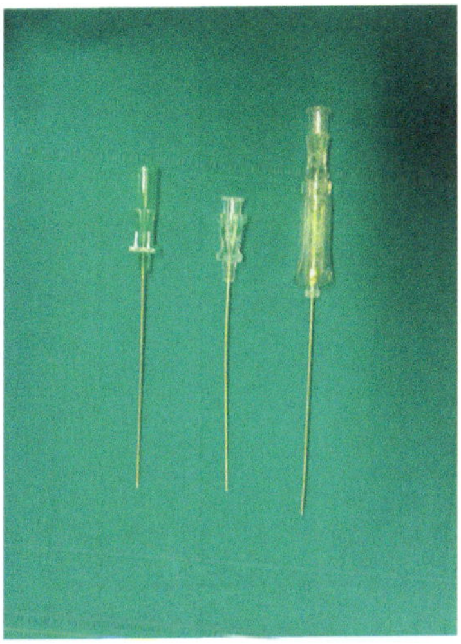

Figure **5.5**

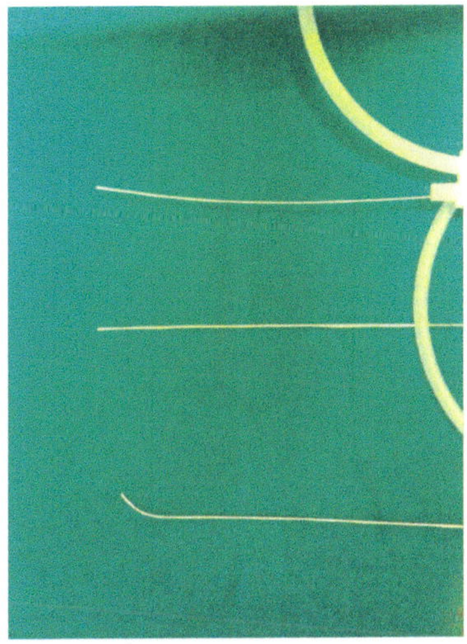

Figure **5.6**

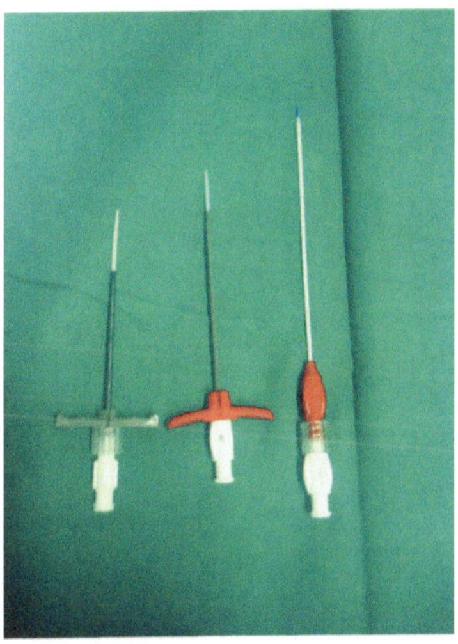

Figure **5.7**

Ultrasound

PICCs and Midlines are often inserted at the bedside and therefore a light, portable ultrasound device is needed, preferably with the following features (Figure 5.8):

- linear probe of sufficient wavelength (7-10 Mhz, for example) and not too large (26-38 mm, for example);
- good image definition: an indicator of the good quality of the image is the ability to easily identify the median nerve in the transversal scans of the upper arm; the mere ultrasound visualisation of veins and arteries (possible even with the simplest equipment) is not sufficient if we consider that the accidental puncture of the median nerve -

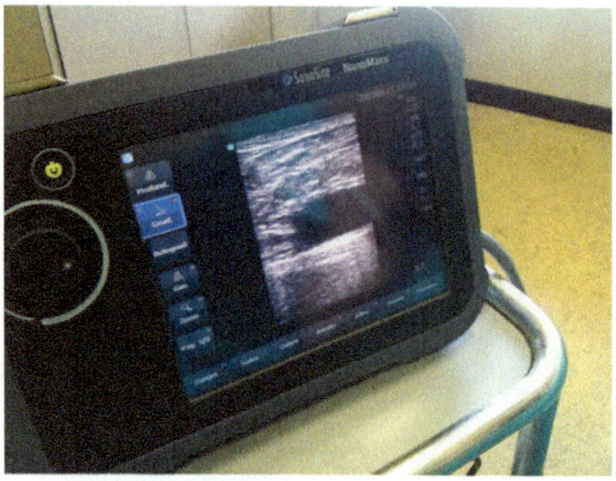

Figure **5.8**

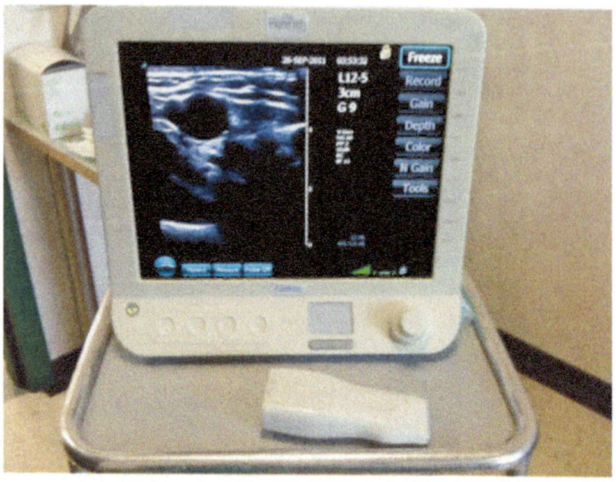

Figure **5.9**

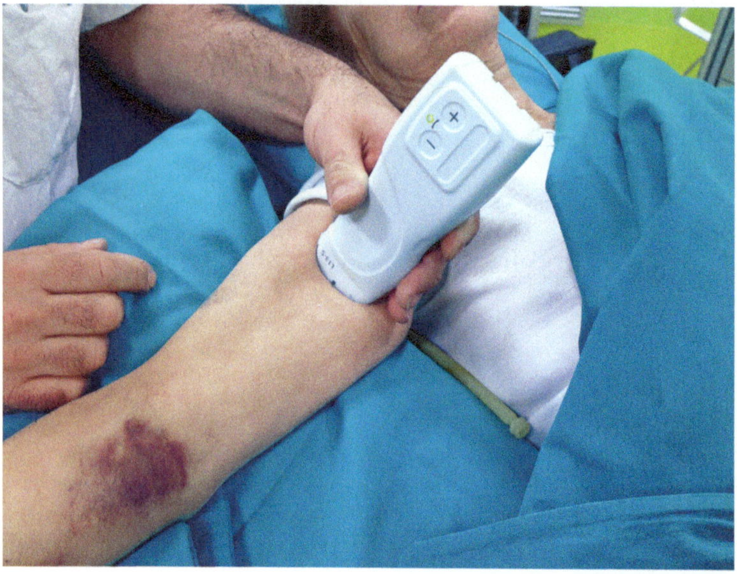

Figure **5.10**

the most feared complication associated with PICC insertion - can be easily prevented through an adequate ultrasound visualisation of the nerve;

- simple and easy to use controls: in most insertions, the operator will actually use only very few controls (depth, gain, freezing the image);
- the ultrasound device should be keyboard-less and the controls should be knob or touchscreen operated to prevent infection: keyboards on medical devices are an important route for microorganism transmission from one patient to another; therefore, as these devices will be used at the bedside, the risk of spreading pathogens is significant.

Colour Doppler must not necessarily be present, given that, in the vast majority of cases, PICC insertion and verification simply require a two-dimensional ultrasound scan. Even thrombosis of the veins of the arm and the infraclavicular region can be adequately diagnosed and assessed using the so-called *compression ultrasonography* (CUS), which identifies the thrombosed vein on the basis of its resistance to collapse under the pressure of the probe.
In recent times, ultrasound devices with *wireless* probes (Figure 5.9 and Figure 5.10) have been marketed, to further help maintain the sterility of the procedure and simplify operator handling during ultrasound-guided venipuncture.

Devices for intracavitary ECG technique

As already mentioned, accurate intraprocedural verification of the PICC tip position can be performed through intracavitary ECG technique with an ECG monitor and a sterile cable connecting the electrode and the catheter.
Two monitor types are allowed: a standard ECG monitor or a dedicated ECG monitor specifically designed for the intracavitary ECG technique. While the intracavitary ECG technique can be performed with any ECG monitor, it is undoubtedly easier if using the monitor of a defibrillator, as the signal is more stable and better protected from interference compared to any other monitor, the number of electrodes is limited (two surface electrodes + one intracavitary) and the system offers the option of immediately printing the trace for documentation purposes.
Among ECG monitors dedicated to intracavitary ECG technique, the first and most reliable is the Nautilus (Figure 5.11), also available as wireless device (Nautilus Delta) (Figure 5.12). The benefits of using a dedicated monitor are greater ease of use, extreme portability, protection from interference, easier interpretation of the P wave and the option of saving and printing for documentation purposes. As mentioned, other devices that associate *tip location* by intracavitary ECG technique to *tip navigation* obtained by means of electromagnetic (Sherlock 3CG) or Doppler (Vasonova VPS) method are avail-

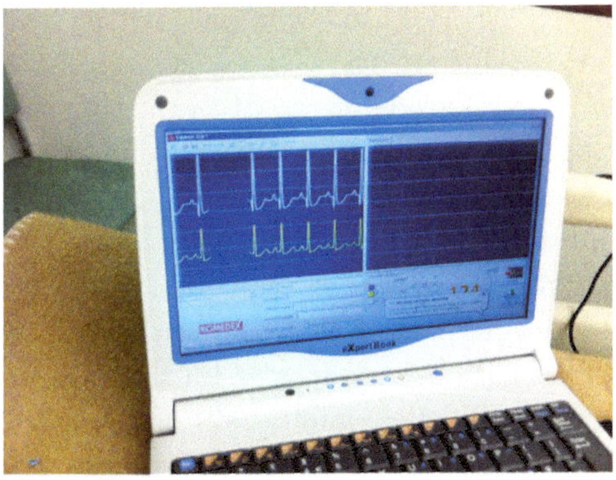

Figure **5.11**

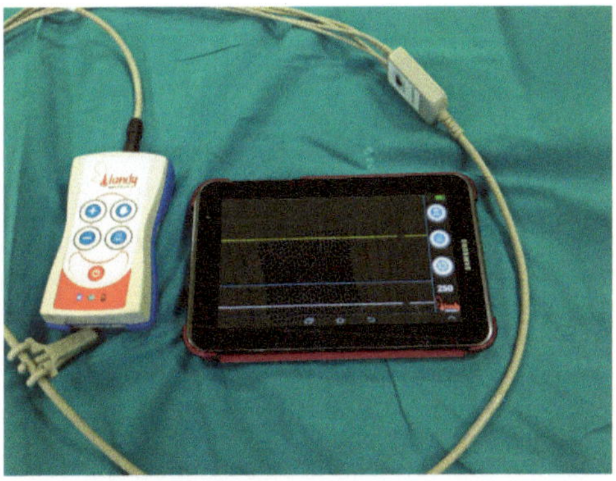

Figure **5.12**

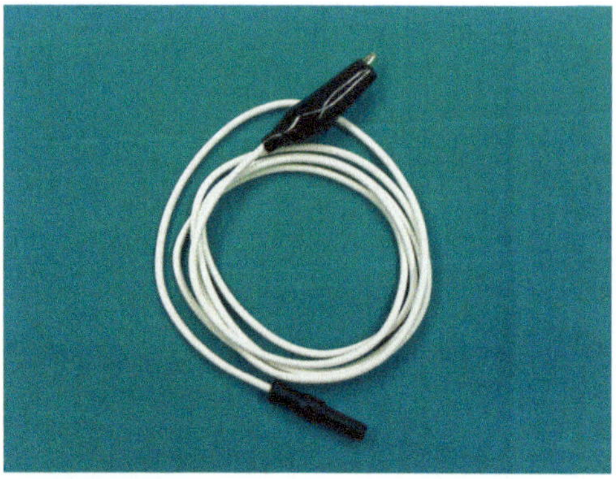

Figure **5.13**

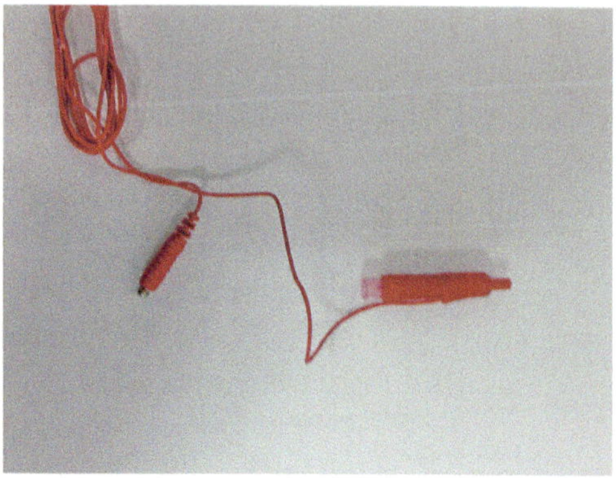

Figure **5.14**

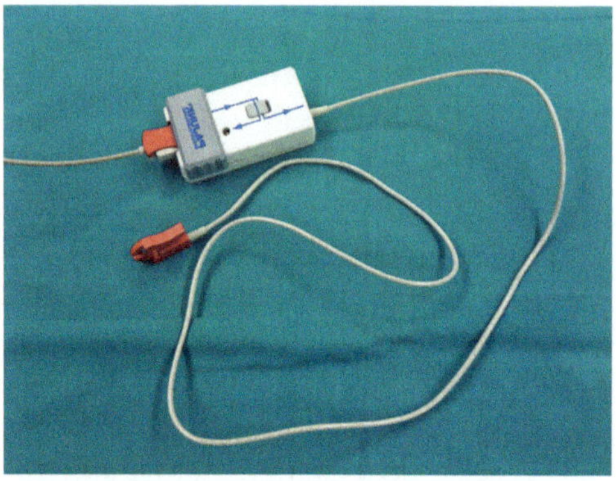

Figure **5.15**

able: currently, there is no clinical evidence that demonstrates any advantages of these "mixed" systems in terms of accuracy or cost-effectiveness compared to the simple intracavitary technique.

Electrode-catheter connection is at the core of the intracavitary ECG technique and requires a reliable electrical connection between the electrode of the ECG monitor and the column of saline filling the PICC. This can be obtained through a sterile cable (Figure 5.13), either directly (by means of a sort of button) or indirectly (by interposing a switch box) connected to the electrode on one end and to the catheter on the other end, either through a saline adapter (Figure 5.14) directly contacting the saline contained in the PICC, or by an alligator clip gripping the PICC stylet (which, in turn, is inserted into the saline filling the catheter). Different types of cables have been marketed for this purpose by several manufacturers (Vygon, Romedex, BBraun, Teleflex) and usually at a very low cost. There are also different brands of switch boxes that can be used, should the cable require an indirect connection to the ECG monitor (Figure 5.15).

Materials for exit site management

Among the materials used for managing the exit site (essential practice for preventing extraluminal contamination and displacement), the following are noted:

- *Antiseptic for disinfecting the skin:* the most effective disinfectant for the skin, according to all the most recent international guidelines, is 2% chlorhexidine in 70% isopropyl alcohol (IPA), as explained above. This antiseptic must strictly be considered as the first choice for all PICC and Midline insertions performed on adult and pediatric patients (the evidence in newborns is less unequivocal), as well as for skin disinfection when changing dressing. The use of less effective antiseptics (10% povidone-iodine) should only be considered in case of a known allergy of the patient to chlorhexidine (a very rare occurrence). EPIC guidelines recommend using 2% chlorhexidine alcohol solutions that are preferably (1) coloured; (2) sterile; (3) provided as single-dose dispenser (ChloraPrep type) (Figure 5.16).
- *Dressing:* as recommended by the 2014 EPIC guidelines, the first choice dressing for any venous access must be a semipermeable transparent polyurethane membrane. The use of gauze dressing must only be taken into consideration for limited periods in case of excessive local humidity (from perspiration, secretions and bleeding); any gauze dressing should be removed every 24-48 hours and, as soon as site is stable, it is advisable to use transparent dressings, to be replaced weekly. Dressing selection should consider the degree of membrane breathability: skin reddening conditions erroneously attributed to "allergic reaction" or "intolerance" to the membrane are actually secondary to a lack of transpiration. "Bordered" transparent membranes are usually more stable. Some transparent membranes integrate securement systems that can effectively replace the sutureless device in case of peripheral venous accesses inserted for limited time periods (needle cannulas, long peripheral cannulas and Midlines). Adhesive transparent dressings with chlorhexidine releasing hydrogel

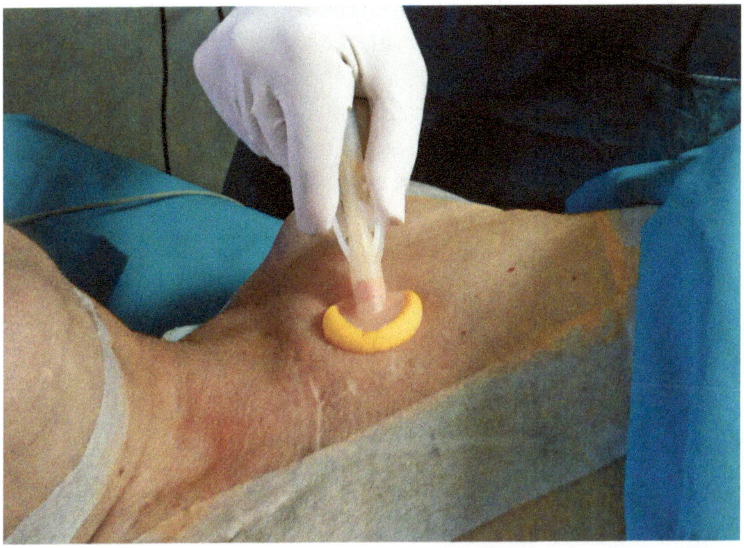

Figure **5.16**

are also available: their efficacy has been documented although they are not appropriate in conditions of excessive perspiration or humidity, as the release of chlorhexidine is no longer reliable and the dressing must be removed.

- *Chlorhexidine-releasing sponges:* numerous randomized studies in recent years have demonstrated the effectiveness of chlorhedixine-releasing polyurethane sponge dressings for the continuous disinfection of the exit site. This circular sponge is placed around the catheter at the exit site, below the transparent dressing, and should be replaced weekly. The sponge has great absorbent capacity that aids in keeping the skin environment beneath the dressing sufficiently dry.
- *Sutureless devices:* as explained above, no PICC or Midline (and no external vascular catheter of any type) should ever be attached to the skin by sutures. Today, sutureless skin adhesion systems (Statlock, GripLok, WingGuard) and subcutaneously anchored devices (SecuraCath) can be selected: the former have a much lower cost but must be replaced every week and can be ineffective in specific conditions (hyperhidrosis and abnormalities of the skin that prevent sufficient cutaneous adhesion; uncooperative patients, etc.), while subcutaneously anchored devices are more expensive but have the advantages of being placed just at the time of PICC insertion, and being effective in all situations, eliminating the risk of displacement consistently.
- *Cyanoacrylate glue:* although still not recommended by most international guidelines, the use of cyanoacrylate glue is spreading among PICC inserters as a highly effective aid in preventing bleeding at the exit site, reducing the risk of early device displacement and reducing the risk of extraluminal contamination of the catheter. The glue is actually applied in very small quantities (0.2-0.3 mL) around the exit site, specifically around the catheter in the point it exits from the skin, in order to "seal" the skin cut. So far, no adverse effects have been identified, either involving patient's skin or catheter materials. Cyanoacrylate glue should also be used for closing skin incisions performed to tunnel PICCs or for sealing the skin over a subcutaneously implanted PICC-port. Many glues are commercially available (Dermabond, Hystoacryl, etc.) with substantially the same specifications (Figures 5.17 and 5.18).

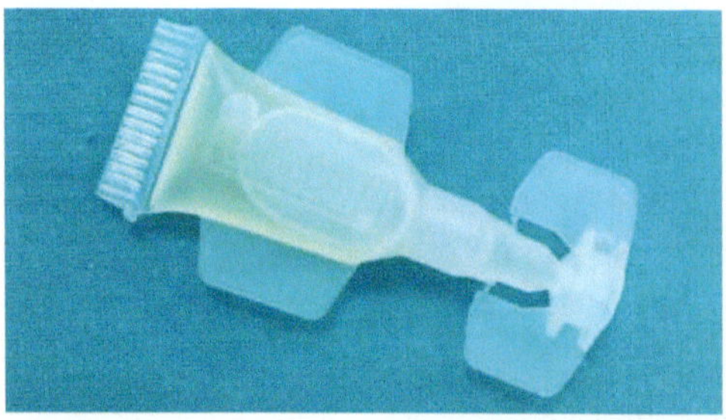

Figure **5.17**

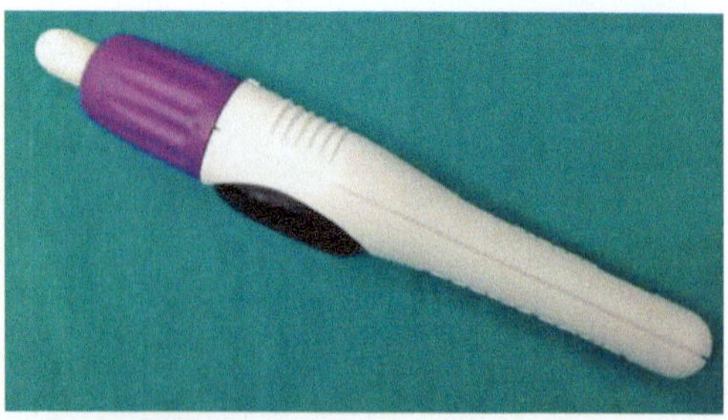

Figure **5.18**

Materials for infusion line management

Among the materials used for managing infusion lines (a fundamental point for the prevention of intraluminal contamination and lumen occlusion), the most importance choice concerns NFCs (Needle Free Connectors) or "valve caps".

As explained above, NFCs must be used to close infusion lines used occasionally: they should be applied to the catheter hub, if the catheter is not used continuously, or - in multilumen PICCs - on the hub of a catheter lumen temporarily not used, as well as on all ports of the infusion line that are used episodically (for example, on the port of a three-way stop-cock). Selecting the most appropriate NFC and its correct use is essential in preventing lumen occlusions and infective complications that could potentially be secondary to contamination by intraluminal route.

Originally, the introduction of NFCs in clinical practice had the goal to reduce the risks of accidental puncture of the operator or accidental contamination of the operator with infusions or biological fluids. This was achieved by creating a complete closure of infusion line access ports, which could be opened with a valve mechanism obtained through a simple septum with a central incision (the so-called *split septum*) or with a more complex internal mechanism (the so-called *mechanical valve*). It soon became clear that different NFC configurations implied different fluid behaviours within the catheter when the syringe was disconnected from the NFC. In some NFCs, in fact, at the time of disconnection, a negative displacement occurs, with blood backflow inside the catheter (so-called "negative pressure" NFCs). In this type of NFCs, it is therefore necessary to clamp the catheter before disconnecting the syringe and leave it clamped until reactivation of the infusion line. Later on, clinical practice witnessed the introduction of the so-called "neutral pressure" NFCs in which negative displacement within the catheter's lumen is absent or negligible during disconnection: these NFCs are therefore simpler and safer to use and do not require any catheter catheter clamping. Finally, the so-called "positive pressure" NFCs were also developed, in which a small amount of fluid is released inside the system at the time of disconnection. Although these NFCs should theoretically be more effective in preventing occlusions than neutral pressure ones, no clinical evidence has ever been obtained on this subject. Moreover, certain types of positive pressure NFCs have been associated with increased catheter-related infections, probably due to bacterial growth in small reservoirs located inside the NFC, that empty at the time of disconnection, creating a positive displacement of fluid.

In brief, literature has presented the following proven data:

- NFCs have been shown to be effective in protecting the operator;
- the use of NFCs is certainly associated with lower infective and obstructive complications if compared to the alternative option of closing every access port of the infusion lines with sterile caps that should be replaced every time the line is accessed;
- the use of negative displacement NFCs may increase the risk of obstructive complications;
- the use of positive displacement NFCs may increase the risk of infective complications.

In light of these considerations, neutral displacement NFCs applied to all access hubs not used continuously are recommended for the PICC and Midlines management. Among the neutral displacement NFCs available, those having least internal dead space, minimum internal flow turbulence and an easily disinfectable access surface are to be preferred. In fact, selecting an optimal NFC is not sufficient to prevent infective complications, unless accompanied by an appropriate policy of NFC disinfection on every use. This disinfection must be performed consistently and carefully before every access to the system, using an appropriate disinfectant (according to the EPIC guidelines, 2% chlorhexidine in isopropyl alcohol, although other guidelines also suggest the use of alcohol or povidone iodine), for an appropriate time (15 seconds). To simplify this procedure (in which a very low compliance is found among healthcare operators), various aids have been developed (readily available disinfectant wipes, cap applicators, etc.). In the last ten years, observational data have consistently shown, however, that such disinfection is disregarded or inadequately performed in the vast majority of cases, irrespective of the type of disinfectant or the method of application used. To fix this problem, disinfecting caps with 70% isopropyl alcohol (Curos; SwabCap; DualCap) have recently been marketed. If applied constantly on the NFC when the line is not used, they keep the access surface of the NFC "automatically" disinfected. These devices, called *port protectors*, have been shown to be very effective in reducing the risk of intraluminal contamination and are currently recommended by the 2014 SHEA guidelines.
A final controversial point concerning NFCs is replacement frequency. Although there is no firm evidence in the literature, it is generally advisable to replace NFCs connected to taps, ramps, etc., every 24 hours (or, in any case, when infusion lines are replaced); NFCs connected to catheters or unused lumina should be replaced when the lumen is periodically flushed, which usually happens weekly (such as, for example, with a PICC at home, which may not be used for many days).

Atypical applications of PICCs and Midlines

Although usually PICC and Midlines are indicated, as reported in the instructions for use provided by the manufacturer for example, for cannulating the veins of the arm (especially the basilic and brachial veins, but also the cephalic vein or the axillary vein within the upper arm), in some conditions these devices may be conveniently inserted in other central or peripheral veins, always using ultrasound for the puncture and cannulation of the vein. This is described as an *off-label* application of PICCs or Midlines (Table 5.2).

Insertion in the axillary vein

The deep veins of the arm may not always be available, either in the middle third (Dawson's green zone) or in the proximal third (yellow zone). This occurs, for example, in pediatric patients especially if very young, in severely malnourished adult patients or in

Table 5.2 *Off-label* PICC applications
• In axillary vein – in the axillary cavity (pediatric patients) – in the infraclavicular region • In external jugular vein – in the superficial tract (direct puncture) – in the deep tract (ultrasound-guidance) • In internal jugular vein • In subclavian vein • In innominate vein – ideal approach in newborns and infants • In femoral vein – always with tunneling

patients who have had repeated catheters inserted in the arm to the point of exhausting all possibilities for venous access. In some of these patients, it may be advantageous to puncture and cannulate the axillary vein, that runs from the arm to the clavicle (the axillary vein becomes the subclavian vein at the outer edge of the first rib or under the clavicle) and is accessible at any point of its course.

Inserting such devices in the axillary vein has a clear advantage: cannulating a large calibre vein is easier and the risk of thrombosis is reduced; axillary access also enables to insert a central venous catheter in patients without deep veins of sufficient calibre in the arm, while avoiding the placement a direct central venous catheter (CICC), the insertion of which can be associated with risks of accidental pleural or arterial puncture.

Whenever a vein in the axillary cavity (typically, in children) is to be punctured, tunneling is mandatory: it can be extended in the direction of the arm (with the exit site in Dawson's green zone) or along the thoracic wall (Figure 5.19). The exit site must necessarily lie in a clean zone that allows to apply a comfortable, stable dressing.

While in children the axillary vein can be identified by ultrasound, punctured and cannulated at almost every point of its course, in most adults the axillary vein is only accessible in the axillary cavity or in the infraclavicular area since it is fully covered by the pectoral muscle throughout the rest of its extrabrachial course. The ultrasound-guided insertion of a catheter used as a PICC in the axillary vein in the infraclavicular area (Figure 5.20) may be indicated in adult patients with bilateral contraindications to the insertion of a PICC in the arm. In fact, the central venous catheter inserted in this location is really a "CICC", according to the terminology explained above. The axillary vein insertion technique by infraclavicular approach is similar to that used for PICCs in the deep veins of the arm;

- selection of an adequate sized catheter (usually, any 4 Fr or 5 Fr catheter can easily be inserted since the axillary vein here always has a diameter >6 mm in adults);

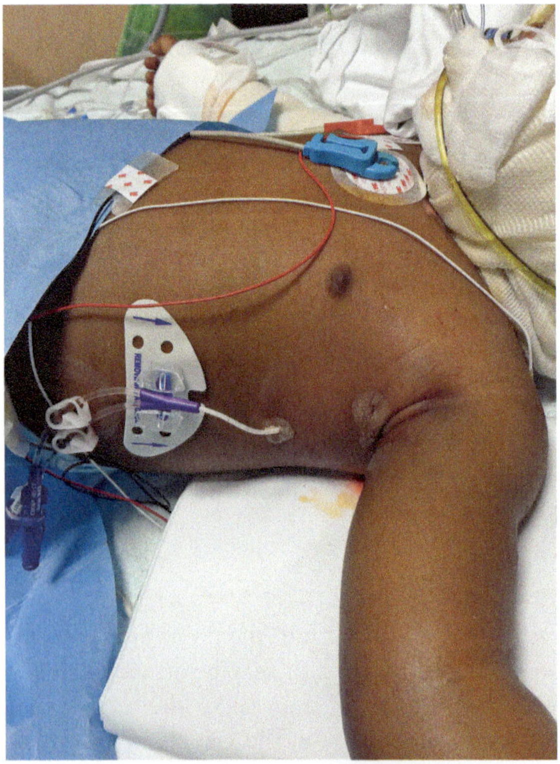

Figure **5.19**

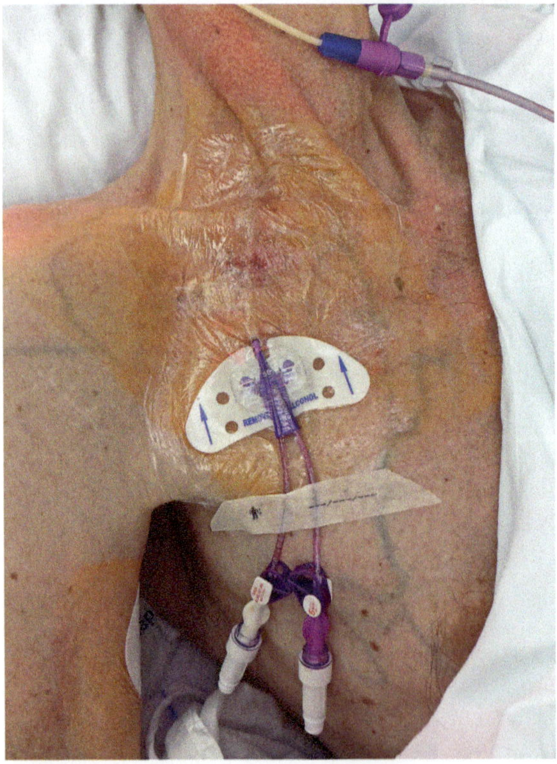

Figure **5.20**

- aseptic technique (hand hygiene, skin antisepsis with chlorhexidine, maximum barrier precautions);
- *out-of-plane* venipuncture with visualisation of the vein in short-axis (in expert hands, *in-plane* venipuncture can also be used, but in long-axis);
- catheter insertion using the micro-introducer technique with the modified Seldinger method;
- during the insertion of the catheter in the introducer, ultrasound scan of the supraclavicular area must be performed to check that the catheter is proceeding in the right direction (that is, towards the innominate and not towards the internal jugular vein);
- tip position verification through intracavitary ECG technique;
- treatment catheter securement with *sutureless* device.

Downward tunneling may sometimes be indicated even for infraclavicular approach to the axillary vein, for example, when the puncture site lies too close to a tracheotomy or to an area with skin alterations.
Contraindications to this approach are morbid obesity (in which the axillary vein is too deep), venous thrombosis of the axillary-subclavian-innominate ipsolateral axis, or difficult puncture due to a collapsed axillary vein (typically, in severe hypovolemia). In the case of an axillary vein that is small-sized or easily collapsible with breathing, it may be advisable to perform the venipuncture while keeping the patient's arm and bringing his/her shoulder slightly forward: this position releases the compression of the small pectoral muscle and the vein appears larger.
As mentioned above, a catheter inserted in this location cannot really be considered as a PICC (i.e., as a peripherally inserted central venous catheter) since the axillary infraclavicular approach is usually regarded as a 'central' approach. Notwithstanding this, in such cases the *off-label* application of a catheter marketed as a "PICC" rather than a traditional central venous catheter has many advantages:

- the micro-introduction kit usually provided inside PICC packaging has features that make it ideal for the puncture and cannulation of the axillary vein, such as a small 21 G echogenic needle (less traumatic than the 18 G – 19 G provided in the usual CICC kits) and a thin nitinol guide (0.018") with soft tip (*floppy straight tip*); the non-J soft tip is perfect for easily passing through the physiological curvature of the vein above the first rib, corresponding to the transition between the axillary and the subclavian vein;
- the length of catheters marketed as PICCs (50-60 cm) makes them suitable for any kind of tunneling and any type of patient: in fact, even in the absence of tunneling, the correct insertion of a central venous catheter in the left axillary vein requires a length of 22 - 27 cm (depending on the distance between the venipuncture site and the cavoatrial junction, variable according to the patient's constitution);
- furthermore, most catheters sold as CICCs are not certified for high-pressure resistance *(power injectability)*, unlike the majority of PICCs;
- finally, almost all the PICC kits contain accessories that are most useful for the insertion procedure (micro-introduction kit, *sutureless device,* valve caps, transparent dressing, etc.) and that are almost always excluded from traditional CICC kits.

All these factors increase the procedure safety and efficacy, therefore recommending *off-label* use of the catheters sold as PICCs for all situations in which a CICC in the axillary vein is required.

Insertion in the external jugular vein

The insertion of a PICC in the external jugular vein can be performed using two different techniques: (1) puncture and cannulation of the external jugular vein in the subcutaneous tract in the middle of the neck (by directly visualising the vein in its most superficial tract or by identifying the vein with NIR technology); or (2) ultrasound-guided puncture and cannulation of the external jugular vein in its deepest tract, shortly before the confluence with the subclavian vein:

1. the insertion of a PICC following puncture of the external jugular superficial tract can be performed both in children and adults, preferably using micro-introduction kits, but has various drawbacks that make it less desirable for the "classic" insertion in the middle third of the arm or in the infraclavicular area: firstly, the small calibre of the external jugular vein, its collapsibility and its winding course make the progression of the guidewire and/or catheter particularly difficult, and increase the risk of thrombosis; secondly, the exit site obtained with this puncture is far from being ideal (at mid-neck) and any tunneling procedure to move the exit site elsewhere can be difficult and uncomfortable for the patient;
2. the ultrasound-guided insertion of a PICC in the external jugular vein deepest tract is a technique that may be particularly useful in pediatric patients, where the external jugular often has a greater calibre than the subclavian vein. This procedure does not have the drawbacks described above for the puncture of the superficial tract (the calibre of the vein can be assessed by ultrasound, the vein is cannulated in its straightest tract, the exit site lies in the supraclavicular fossa and not in the middle of the neck, i.e. in a more favourable site) and can also be indicated in adults when axillary vein cannulation is contraindicated.

Insertion in the internal jugular vein

The insertion of a PICC in the internal jugular vein is another *off-label* application of these devices that can be adopted both in pediatric and adult patients. It has the same indications applying to the insertion in the axillary vein (that is: bilateral contraindication for the insertion of a PICC in the veins of the arm) but implies a less favourable exit site (supraclavicular fossa) compared to insertion in the axillary (infraclavicular region), unless tunneling is performed. The reasons for preferring the *off-label* insertion of a PICC as if it were a CICC, rather than inserting a central venous catheter specifically sold for this purpose are the same applying to insertion in the axillary vein.
When adopting this type of access, it is highly recommended to use the *in plane* ultrasound-guided venipuncture technique with visualisation of the internal jugular in short-axis.

Insertion in the subclavian vein

The insertion of a PICC in the subclavian vein is possible but rarely indicated and primarily in adult patients. The subclavian vein can be punctured and cannulated with ultrasound guidance almost exclusively applying a supraclavicular approach, with a more difficult and less safe technique than that needed for the ultrasound-guided cannulation of other, so-called "central" veins (axillary, external jugular, internal jugular, innominate). The exit site lies in the supraclavicular area.

Insertion in an innominate vein

The insertion of a PICC with ultrasound guidance technique in an innominate vein is a safe and easy technique for obtaining central venous access in newborns, infants and children with a contraindication for the insertion of a PICC in the arm.
In fact, newborns and infants often have very small veins in the arm (<3 mm), which cannot be used for the ultrasound-guided insertion of 3 Fr catheters or larger; at the same time, many of the so-called central veins (axillary, subclavian, external jugular, internal jugular) are too small or too difficult to cannulate at such an early age. The innominate vein – especially the right one – is always a good-sized vein that is easy to cannulate with ultrasound guidance in pediatric patients of any age, even in premature newborns with low weight at birth. As long as the innominate vein has at least a 3 mm calibre (as it is usually the case in all children and sometimes even in newborns weighing under 1 kg), it is possible to visualise it in long-axis behind the sternoclavicular joint, puncture it applying the *in plane* technique, and inserting a power injectable PICC of appropriate calibre (3 Fr or more, so to get an optimal flow performance).
In young patients, *off-label* use of PICCs to obtain a central venous route is ideal, if we consider the possible alternatives:

- the insertion of an ECC (epicutaneous-caval catheter, inserted in a peripheral superficial vein by direct vein visualisation or by using NIR technology) leads to: (1) unpredictable technical difficulties during catheter advancement, (2) potential difficulties in locating the catheter tip in a truly central position, (3) suboptimal clinical outcome, since EECs have a low flow (their calibre is between 1 Fr and 2.7 Fr and none of them is *power injectable)* and cannot be utilized for blood sampling or for haemodynamic monitoring;
- the insertion of a "traditional" central venous catheter marketed as a pediatric CICC will increase the general risk of the procedure and has less clinical efficiency, considering that these pediatric catheters are almost all technologically outdated: they are made of obsolete polyurethane, are not *power injectable,* do not have micro-introduction kits, are inserted with the direct Seldinger technique using non-echogenic, large calibre needles and big guidewires with J-tips (not recommended in pediatric age, since they obstruct the progression of the guide), and they are not suitable for tunneling.

The insertion of a PICC in the innominate vein of neonatal or pediatric patients is, on the other hand, free of significant risks of pneumothorax, accidental arterial puncture

or malpositioning, and can ensure a stable and safe central venous access with optimal clinical performance.
The insertion technique involves the following (Figures 5.21 – 5.25):

- sedation or general anaesthesia, depending on age and clinical conditions;
- ultrasound scan of all deep veins of the infra-/supraclavicular region, according to the RaCeVA protocol (Rapid Central Vein Assessment; see Table 2.2), in order to confirm the venous approach selected and check the vein calibre;
- selecting power injectable PICCs of an appropriate calibre for the vein and with a sufficient number of lumina required for the treatment (in pediatric age, the choice usually falls on single-lumen 3 Fr or double-lumen 4 Fr catheters);
- aseptic technique, as previously described (hand hygiene, skin disinfection with 2% chlorhexidine in 70% IPA, maximum barrier precautions);
- *in plane* venipuncture of the innominate vein in long-axis, so to enter the innominate vein coaxially to the main axis of the vein, maintaining control of the needle tip; the skin is usually punctured at the angle between clavicle and the sternocleidomastoid muscle;
- insertion of the micro guidewire (in nitinol, with *floppy straight tip*) and removal of the needle;
- small skin incision and insertion of the micro-introducer/dilator over the guidewire:
- insertion of the catheter into the introducer after removal of guidewire and dilator.

The entire procedure is performed under ultrasound control, that should be performed not only during the venipuncture but also later, so to check the intravascular position and direction of the guidewire, the micro-introducer and finally the catheter itself.

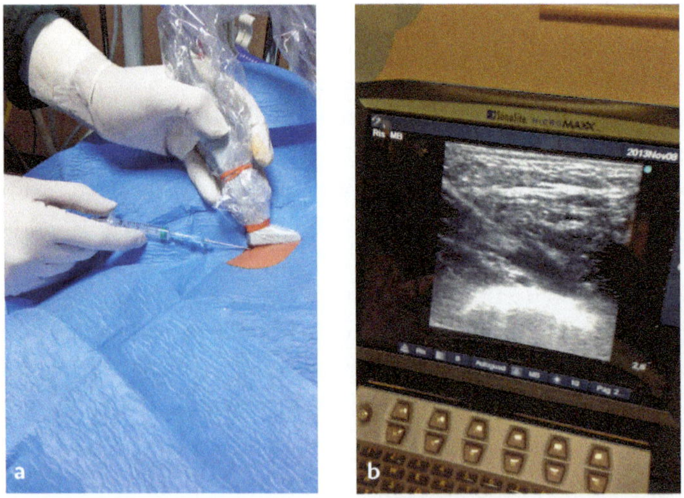

Figure **5.21**

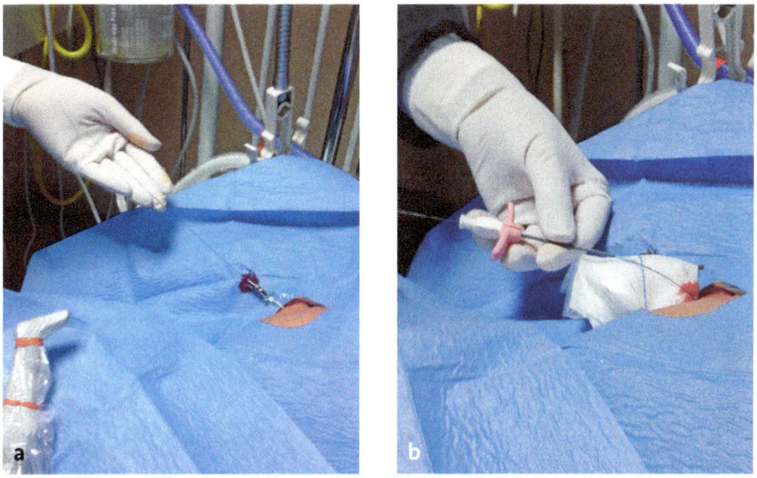

Figure **5.22**

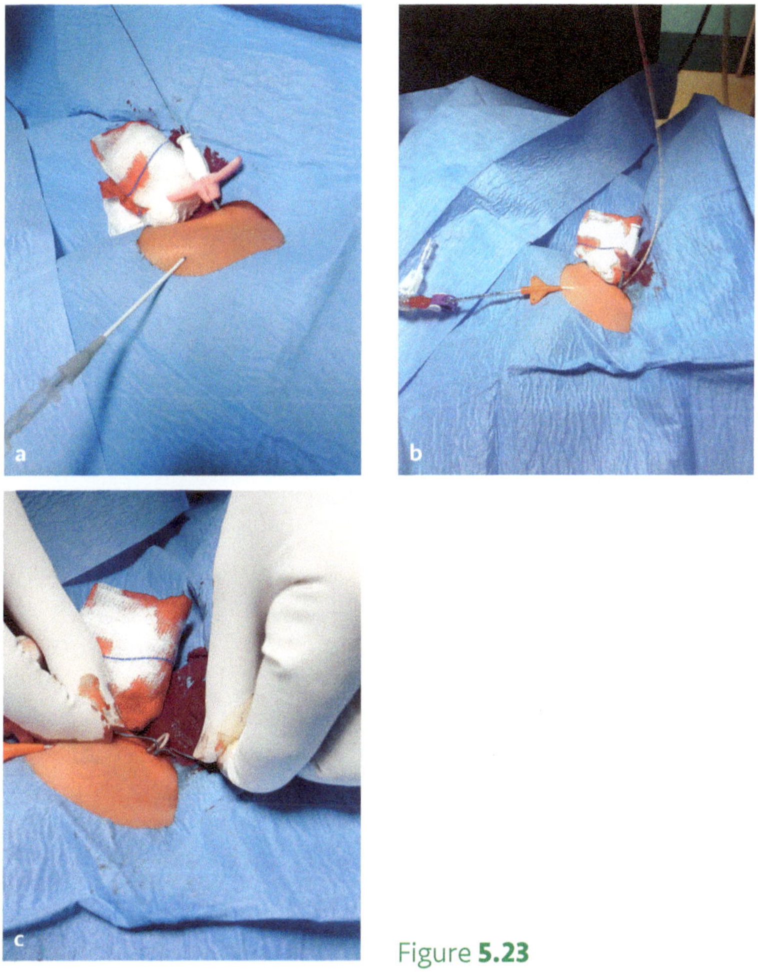

Figure **5.23**

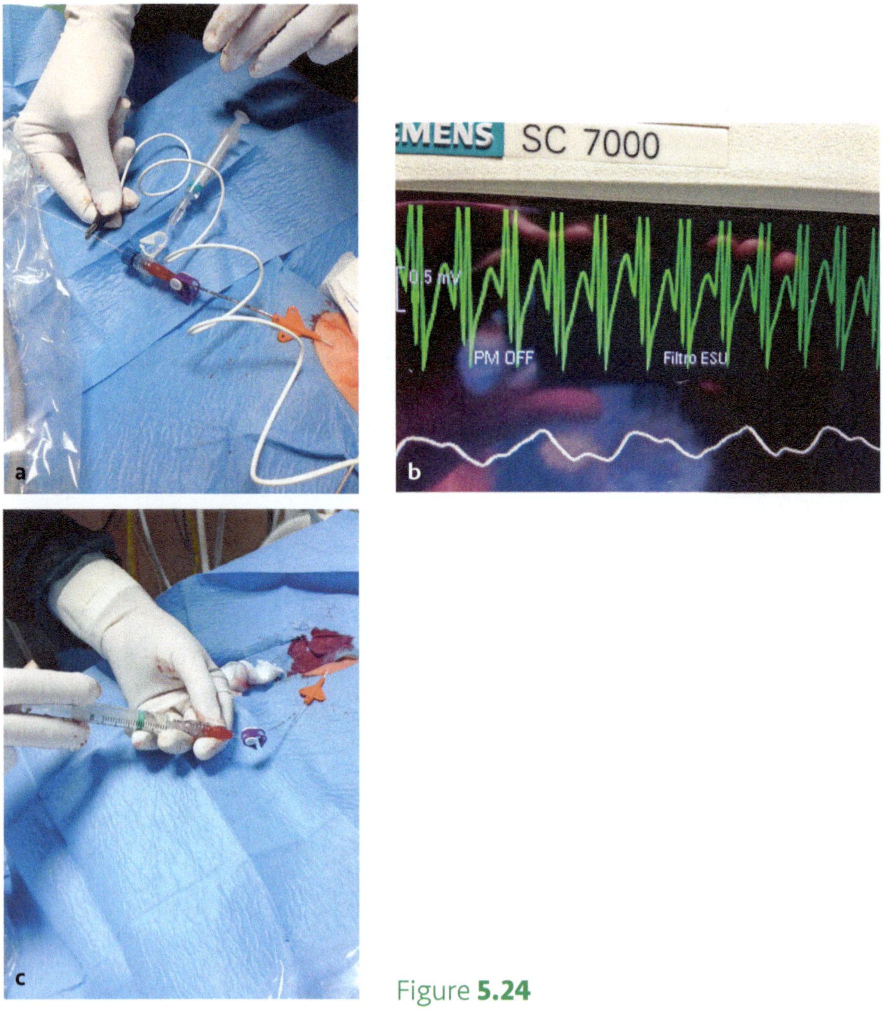

Figure **5.24**

In most newborns and infants, it is advisable to tunnel the catheter in order to avoid leaving an exit site at the crease of the neck. The tunneling must be planned so to obtain an appropriate exit site in the infraclavicular area, passing the catheter through a subcutaneous tunnel that runs from the planned exit site (below the clavicle) to the site of venipuncture (above the clavicle); the catheter is then inserted into the vein through the introducer (so-called "anterograde" tunneling). The subcutaneous tunnel can be created by inserting the catheter into a 14 G or 16 G cannula, or by pulling the catheter under the skin using a specific tunneling tool. The tip position is then assessed applying the intracavitary ECG method:

- the catheter is tunneled and then trimmed so to get the desired length, as estimated from surface landmarks (in newborns and infants, the surface landmark of the

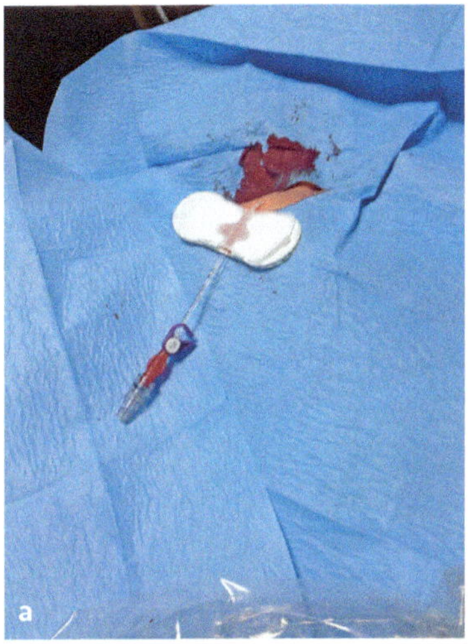

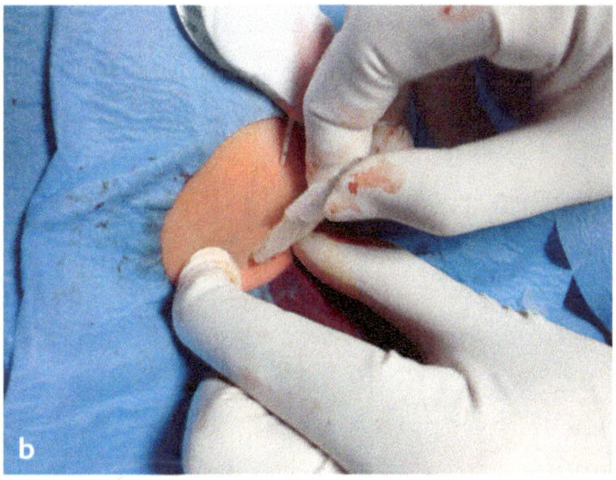

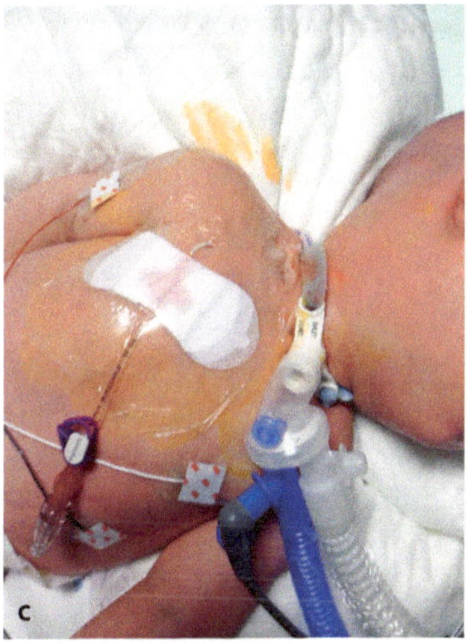

Figure **5.25**

cavoatrial junction is the intermediate point between the jugulum and the xiphoid apophysis; in children – as in adults – it is the third intercostal space on the right parasternal line);

- the catheter is then inserted into the introducer and the position of the tip adjusted using the intracavitary ECG method (maximum P wave = cavoatrial junction).

At the end of the procedure, the catheter is secured by means of: (1) sutureless device; (2) cyanoacrylate glue to close the puncture site and seal the exit site; (3) transparent dressing.

The *off-label* insertion of an ultrasound-guided PICC in the innominate vein, with catheter tunneling to the infraclavicular area, can also be indicated in adults when the deep veins of the arm are not feasible and the axillary vein is difficult to puncture.

Insertion in the femoral vein

PICCs are ideal to obtain an elective venous access to the inferior vena cava.

We have already explained that there are substantially two indications for femoral venous access (FICC): (1) the need for emergency venous access for infusions or dialysis/apheretic procedures (non-tunneled FICC); (2) the need for short-medium term venous access for patients with contraindication to the use of veins in the neck and upper limbs, due to obstruction of the superior vena cava (tunneled FICC).

In the second case, the *off-label* use of PICCs is ideal: doubt has also been raised over whether this is truly an *off-label* use, considering that the femoral vein is mainly regarded as a peripheral vein. Certainly, the elective insertion of a venous catheter in the femoral vein always requires tunneling, at least in adult patients, given the high risk of infection of the inguinal area. Considering the catheter length required for tunneling plus its intravascular tract, it is clear that among all short and medium term devices PICCs are the only ones having a sufficient length for this procedure.

The definition of such access as "central" is debatable, considering that the position of the tip in the inferior vena cava is not unanimously considered "central" (a definition that only refers to the position in proximity to the cavoatrial junction), even though it can certainly be used for infusing intravenous treatments that require a central route (vesicant and irritant drugs with pH >9 or <5, etc.).

The following steps are needed to insert a tunneled PICC in the femoral vein:

- Ultrasound scan of both inguinal regions to identify the best side for venipuncture.
- Preparation of the field according to the usual aseptic technique.
- Ultrasound-guided venipuncture of the femoral vein visualised in short-axis, using the *out of plane* technique; it is usually recommended to puncture the vein close to the iliac-femoral passage, right above the confluence of the saphenous vein.
- Insertion of the nitinol guidewire and removal of the needle.
- At this point, an anterograde tunneling of the catheter is performed, which should be a "double" tunneling: first, from the planned exit site (for example in the peri-umbilical region) to an intermediate point on the inguinal line, laterally at the puncture site; then, from this intermediate point to the puncture site; the purpose of this "double" tunneling is to prevent the catheter from bending at more than 90°.
- The catheter is passed into the subcutaneous tissue using an appropriate metal tunneler, until it emerges from the puncture site, close to the guidewire.
- The catheter is then trimmed to the desired length (adding the length of the double tunneling to the length of the intravascular tract required; the latter can be estimated by measuring the distance between the puncture site and the umbilicus, since the umbilicus corresponds to the surface landmark of the central portion of the inferior vena cava).
- The introducer-dilator is then inserted over the guidewire.
- After removing the dilator and the guidewire, the catheter is inserted into the introducer.

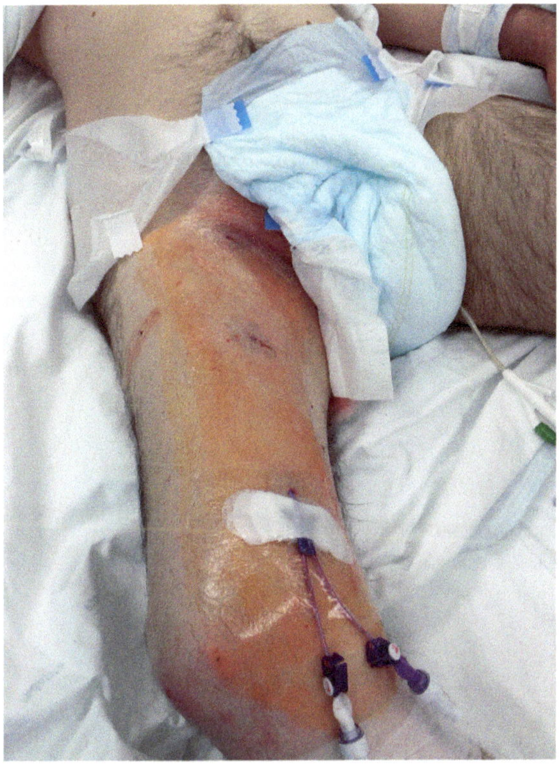

Figure **5.26**

- The catheter is finally secured using a sutureless device.
- Cyanoacrylate glue is used to close the puncture site and the intermediate tunneling site, as well as to seal the exit site.

In particular cases, straight tunneling downwards may be indicated in order to obtain an exit site a little above the knee (Figure 5.26): this tunneling is advisable in agitated, uncooperative patients (elderly patients suffering from dementia or very young children) who may accidentally pull out the catheter.
One particular PICC insertion in the inferior cava consists of ultrasound-guided cannulation of the saphenous vein; this option is very rarely advantageous, however, since this vein is very small in pediatric age and too susceptible to thrombosis in adult patients.

When and how to tunnel PICCs

As mentioned, the traditional PICC insertion technique is based on the identification of a deep vein in the middle third of the arm, in the so-called "green zone" according to the Zone Insertion Method (ZIM) described by Dawson. In some conditions, however, at this level there are no veins large enough to receive catheters of the desired diameter (it should be remembered that the insertion of a 3 Fr catheter requires a vein of at least

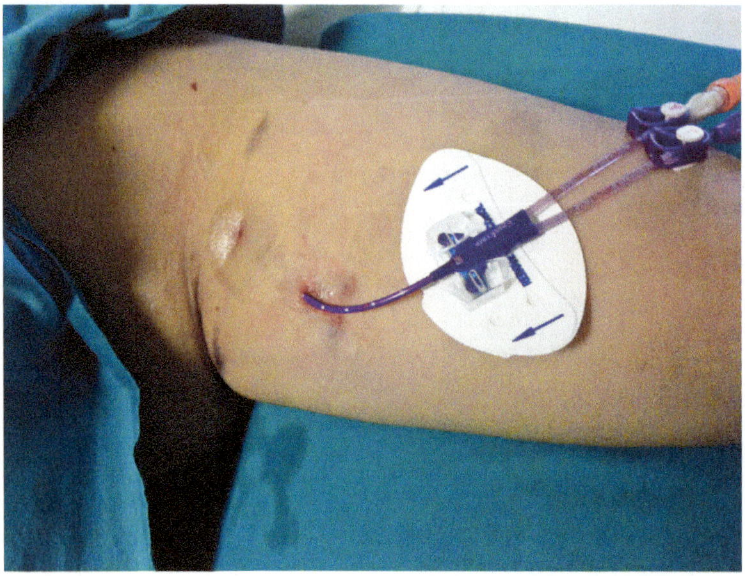

Figure **5.27**

3 mm, a 4 Fr catheter requires a vein of at least 4 mm, etc.). In these situations where the only vein of appropriate calibre can be found in the proximal third of the arm (Dawson's yellow zone), it is appropriate/advisable to tunnel the catheter so as to move the exit site to the green zone, far from the puncture site (Figure 5.27).

Tunneling is also indicated in specific *off-label* PICC applications: when catheters are inserted in the femoral vein, it is mandatory in order to avoid an exit site in the inguinal region; it is recommended in "central" insertions usually associated with an exit site in the supraclavicular area (puncture of the subclavian, external jugular, internal jugular or innominate vein), when an infraclavicular exit site is preferable. In special cases (skin alterations or the presence of a tracheotomy), it may also be indicated after axillary venipuncture, so to move the exit site far from the clavicle.

Please note that tunneling has two positive effects on the risk of infections: an indirect effect described above (the emergence of the catheter is moved to a more favourable area of the skin) and a "direct" effect (the tunnel creates a barrier against contamination by extraluminal route, since it moves the catheter entry point in the vein far from the skin). The latter makes tunneling particularly important for CICCs and FICCs, which when tunneled should be considered as medium-term venous access devices.

In addition to the effect on infective complications, tunneling also expands the indications for PICCs and reduce the thrombotic risk, since it also enables PICC to be inserted in patients with very small veins in the middle third of the arm, where the insertion of a PICC would be unthinkable or associated with a high risk of thrombosis. Tunneling does not necessarily imply that the catheter (PICC, CICC or FICC) is cuffed: a Dacron cuff is an additional, structural feature that increases the chances of catheter stabilisation. The simultaneous presence of tunneling (for preventing infections from extralu-

minal contamination) and a cuff (for stabilisation) transforms the device into a long-term venous access device.
From a technical standpoint, a few centimetres of tunneling (such as that required for moving the exit site from the yellow to the green zone, for example) can be performed with a 14 G (for catheters from 4 Fr to 5 Fr) or 16 G needle cannula (for 3 Fr catheters) (Figure 5.28). Soon after inserting the guidewire in the vein, the cutaneous breach is enlarged, and a point is marked in the green zone where the exit site is planned: after a subcutaneous injection of a few millilitres of local anaesthetic (0.75% ropivacaine, for example) a small incision with the tip of a scalpel blade is performed in this site. A needle cannula is then inserted until it emerges from the cutaneous breach, in correspondence with the puncture site. After removing the needle, the catheter is advanced through the cannula, which is then removed. After the subcutaneous passage, the catheter is inserted in the micro-introducer/dilator (so-called anterograde tunneling: that is, the catheter is first inserted in the tunnel and then in the vein). Cyanoacrylate glue is used both to close the puncture site and to seal the exit site.
For longer tunneling, we can use specific tunnelers marketed by several brands: some of them are long needle cannulas in which the cannula can be removed with a *peel-away* system (Figure 5.29); others are proper metal tunnelers (Figure 5.30), usually 12-15 cm

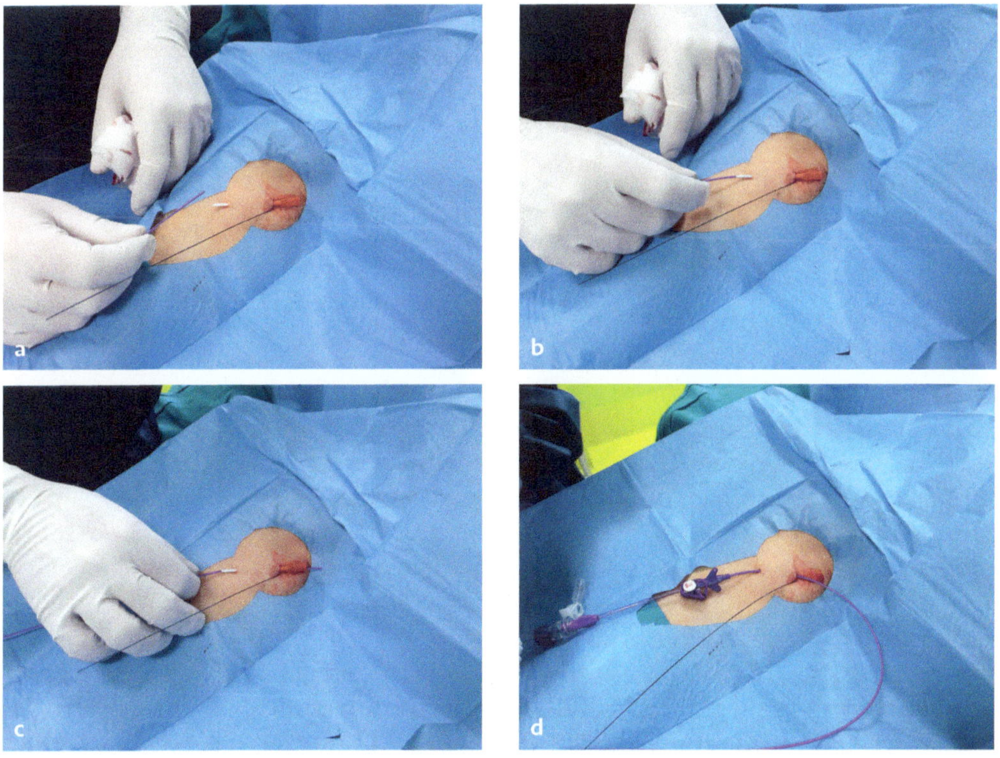

Figure **5.28**

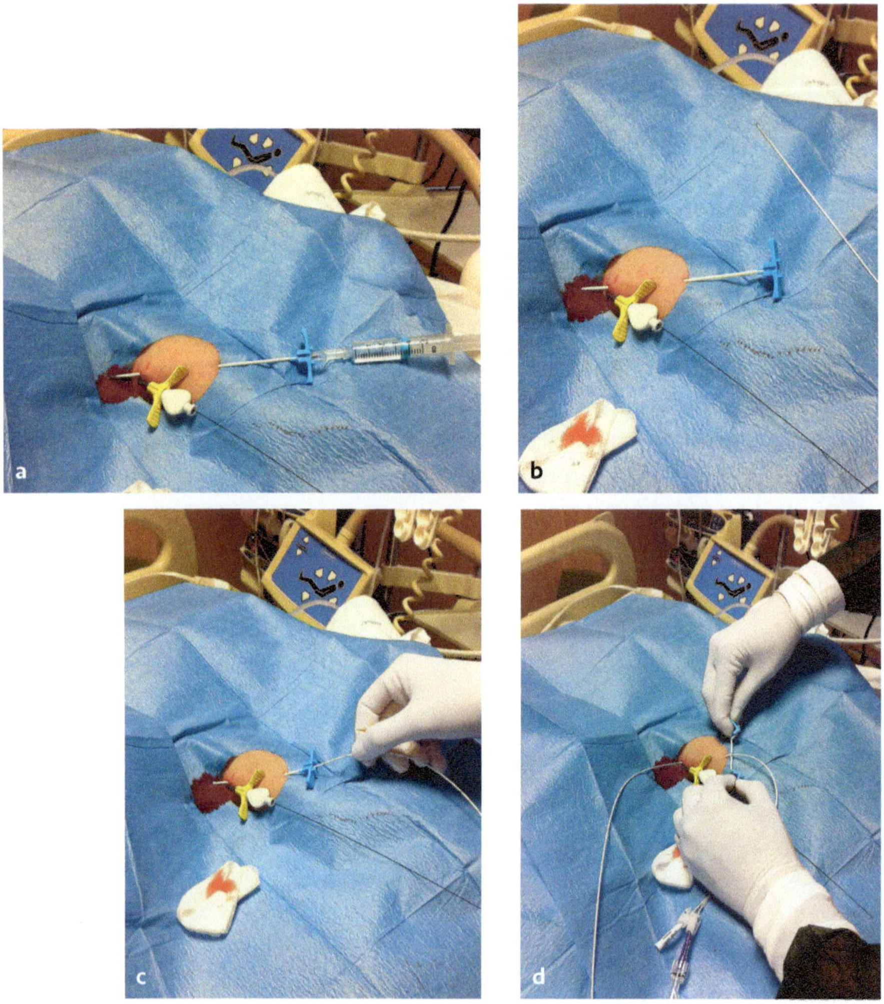

Figure **5.29**

long, and are furnished with a proximal end that, when connected to the catheter tip, enables it to be drawn into the subcutaneous tunnel created by the tunneler (Figure 5.31 – 5.33). Anterograde tunneling is mandatory for most PICCs designed for distal *trimming* or not to be trimmed. PICCs designed for proximal *trimming* (Groshong PICCs or Easy PICCs) can, however, be tunneled by retrograde route (before insertion of the catheter in the vein through the introducer and then tunneling from the suture point to the exit site).

The tunneling technique is simple to learn and is not associated to any significant complication. Specifically, the incidence of haematomas in the tunnel site is very rare, especially if the subcutaneous tissue is expanded by infusing local anaesthetic and/or saline before the passage of the tunneler to reduce the trauma.

Table 5.3 summarises the most important indications for tunneling.

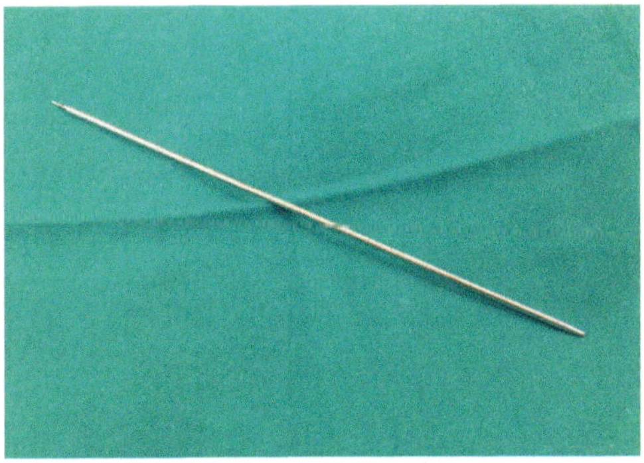

Figure **5.30**

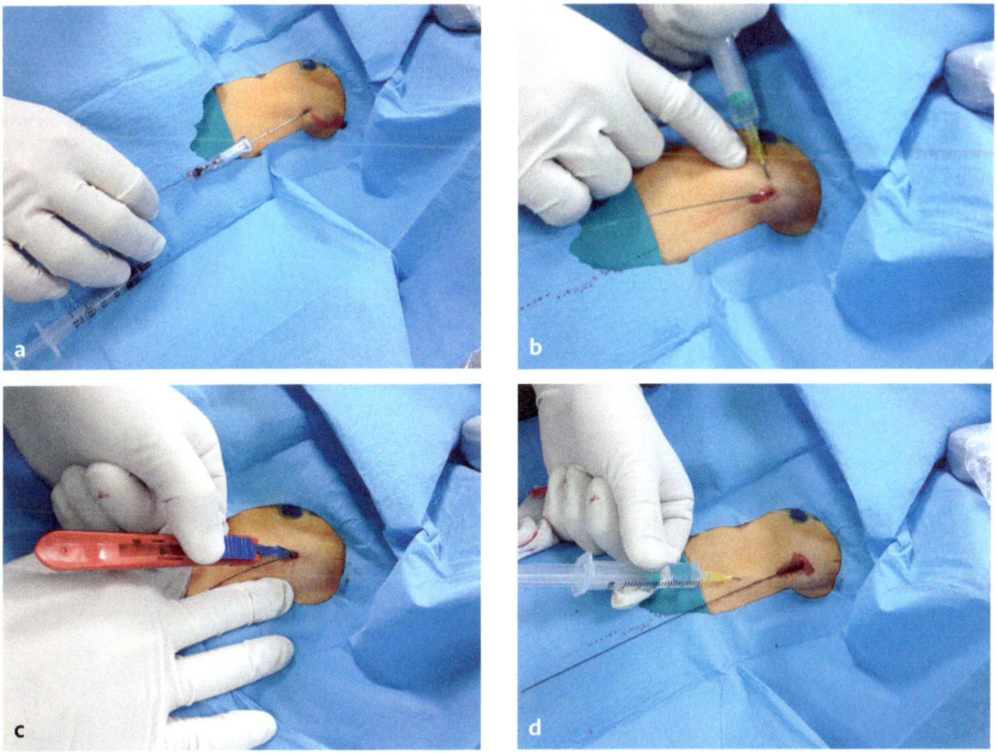

Figure **5.31**

Table 5.3 Mandatory indications for tunneling
• After "high" puncture of the veins of the arm (in Dawson's yellow zone) • After puncture of the axillary vein in the axillary cavity • After supraclavicular puncture (innominate vein) in newborns and children • After cannulation of the femoral vein in adult patients

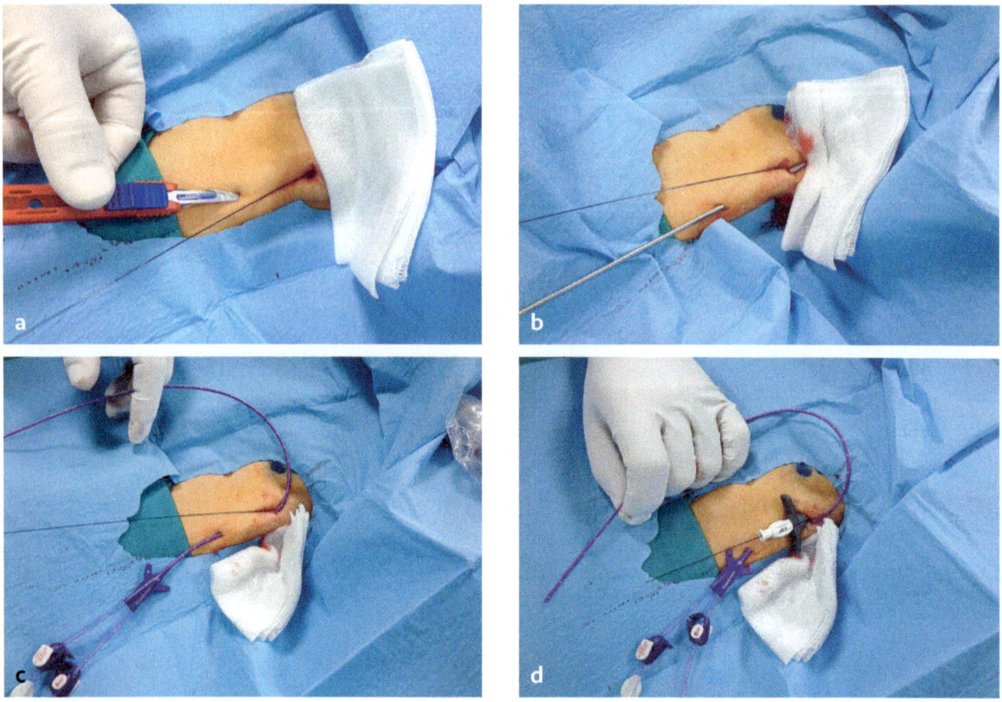

Figure **5.32**

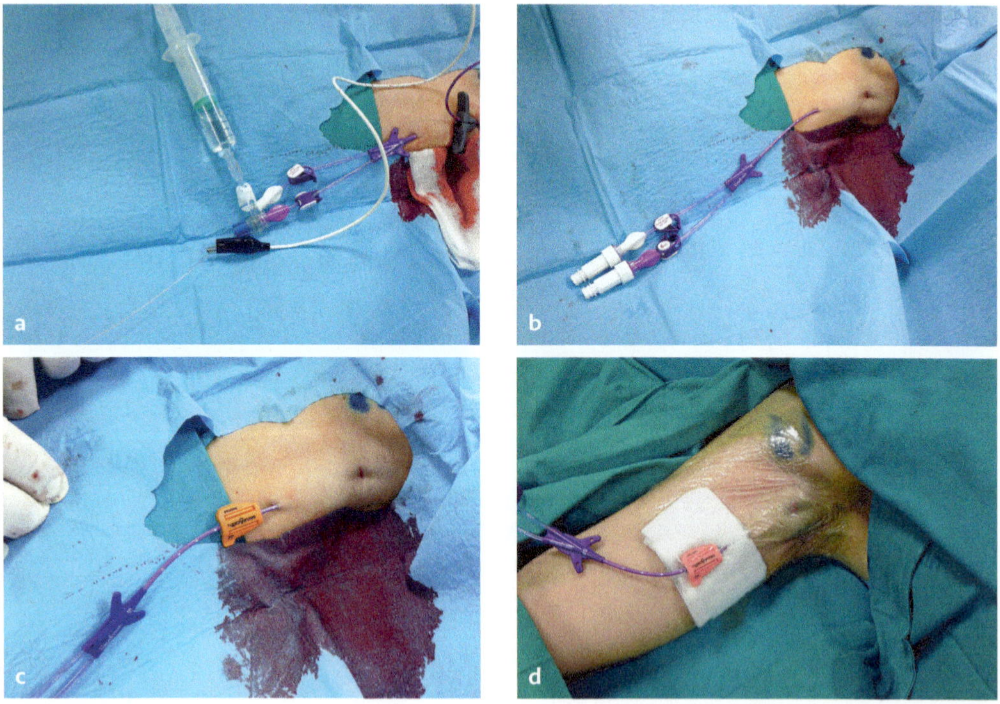

Figure **5.33**

Cuffed PICCs

In recent times, cuffed PICCs designed for tunneling have been marketed (Figure 5.34). Tunneling will therefore be mandatory with cuffed PICCs, even if there is a vein of adequate size in the green zone.
As described above, every cuffed/tunneled device should be considered appropriate for long-term use in extra-hospital setting. Therefore, the actual indication for cuffed PICCs is the planning of a long-term venous access (for more than 4-6 months) to be used frequently (more than once a week, such as in patients with parenteral nutrition for an indefinite period, for example). Their clinical use is too recent to judge whether their safety and efficacy performance is comparable to that of cuffed CICCs, which are typically used in this type of patients. Another possible indication of these devices is for home care patients who are candidates for a PICC but are at high risk of displacement of the system and/or at high risk of infection, since the simultaneous presence of the cuff and tunneling has a protective effect on both. Cuffed PICCs are power injectable and made of third-generation polyurethane; the cuff is usually located at 5-7 cm from the securement wing. The insertion technique is the one described above for tunneled PICCs, the only difference being that it is necessary to carefully plan the length of the tunnel so that the cuff will lie within the tunnel at least 2 cm from the exit site. If the cuff is mistakenly inserted too close to the cutaneous breach, it is probable that, sooner or later, it will be gradually expelled out of the skin, with a significant increase of the risk of displacement and infection.
When frequent long-term access is required, cuffed PICCs can be inserted in the femoral vein or in veins of the supra-infraclavicular area (Figures 5.35-5.39). Cuffed catheters currently available on the market (cuffed Groshong, Hickman, Broviac, Leonard) have numerous disadvantages: they are made of silicone (and therefore susceptible to mechanical damage and malpositioning), are not power injectable, do not allow for high flows or allow them only by using large calibres, are not supplied with micro-introduction kits and are often difficult to secure since they do not have a wing. Given the above conditions, they do not have any advantages over cuffed polyurethane PICCs: as explained above, silicone has no advantages in terms of biocompatibility and there is no evidence

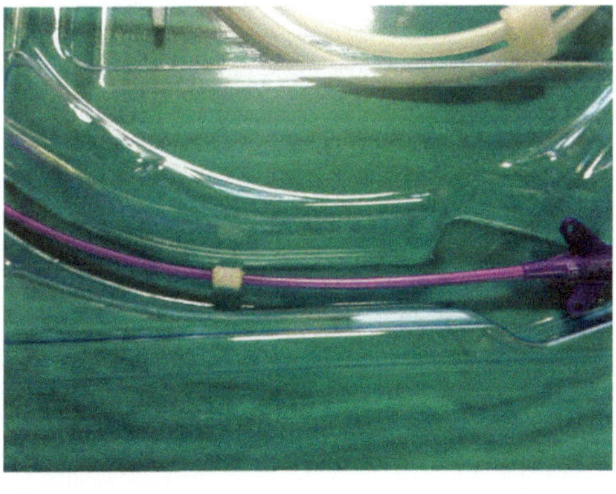

Figure **5.34**

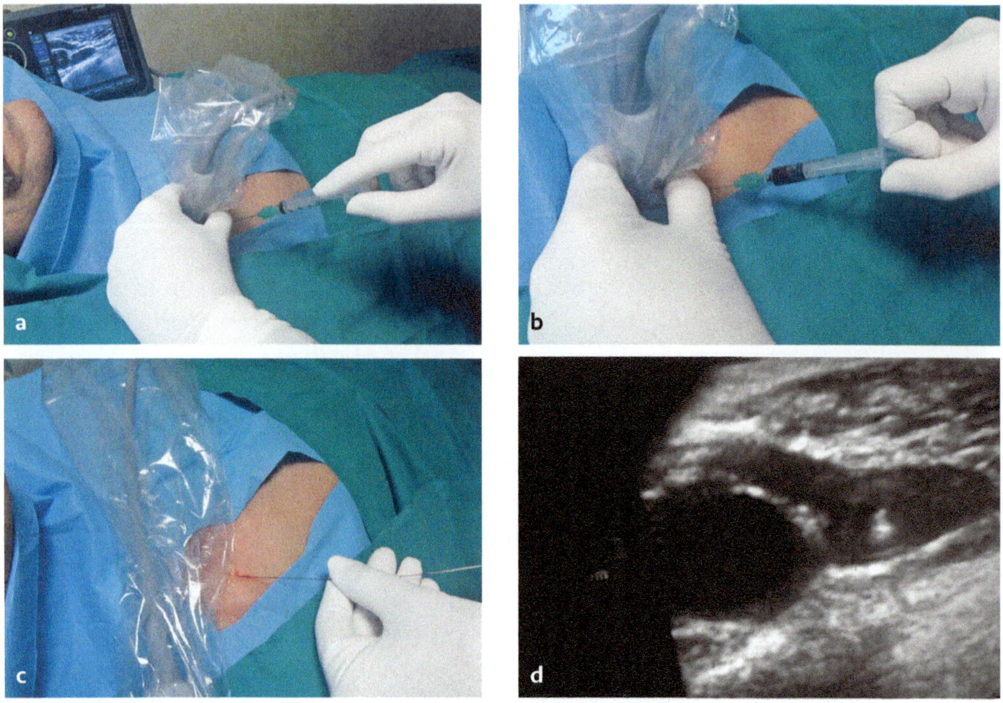

Figure **5.35**

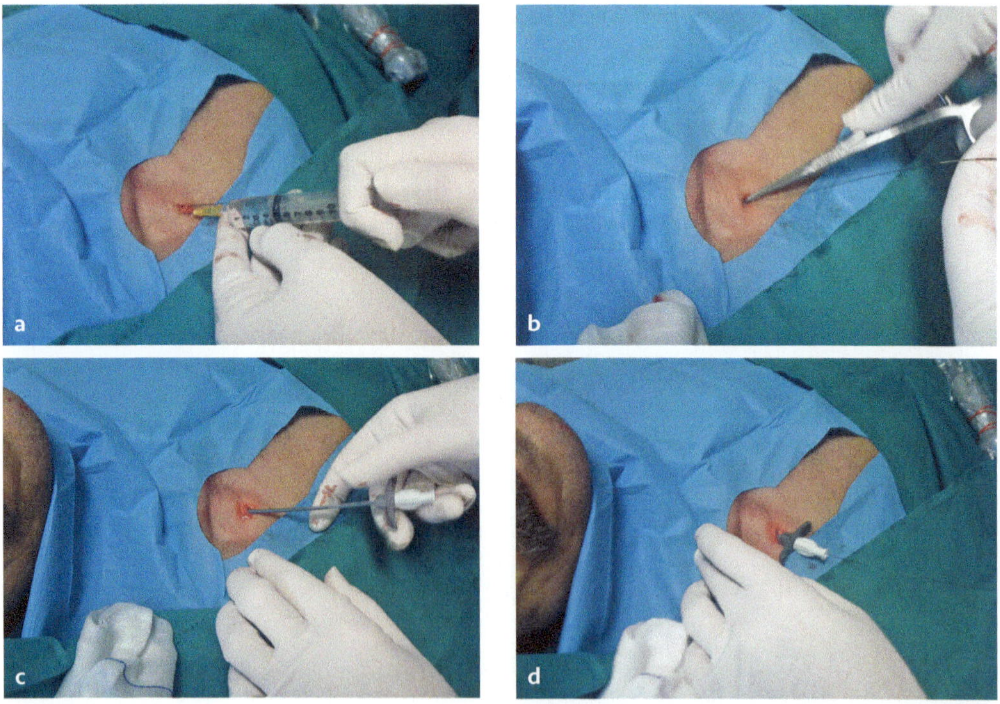

Figure **5.36**

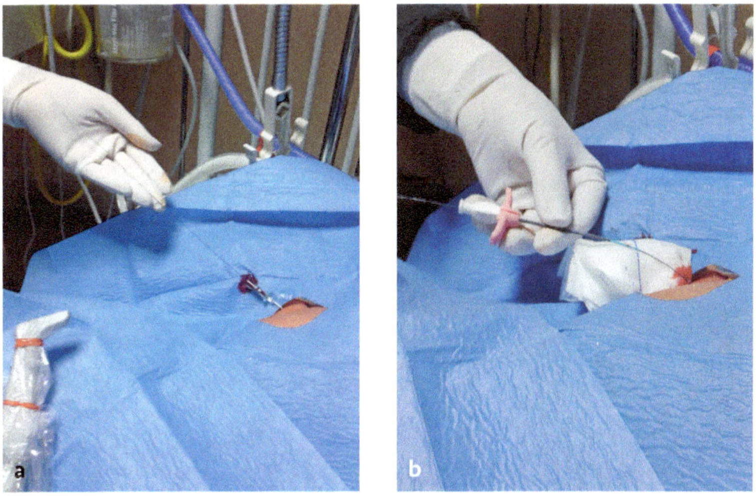

Figure **5.37**

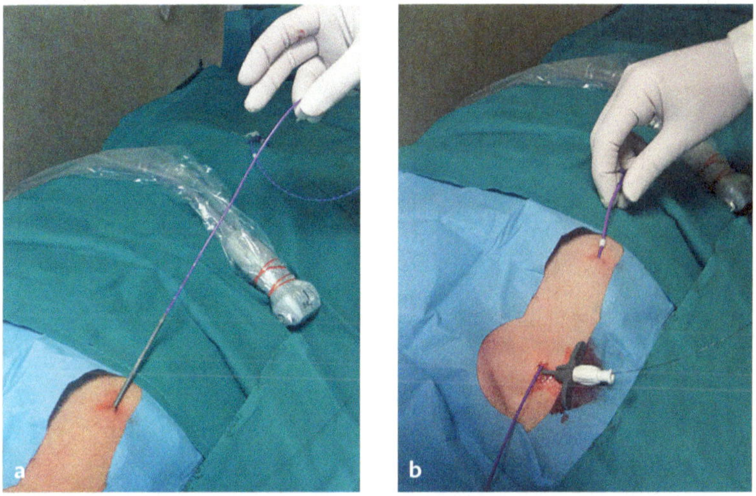

Figure **5.38**

of efficacy of the valve (present in cuffed Groshongs). On the contrary, the valve may increase the risk of malfunctions. It is therefore advisable to use these cuffed PICCs not only for long-term brachial access, but also for long-term "central" (such as cuffed CICCs) or femoral access (such as cuffed FICCs).

It is important to underline that cuffed, tunneled external catheters are not appropriate for long-term access (more than 4-6 months) if the access is expected to be used infrequently (less frequently than once a week). In such conditions, it is generally indicated to use totally implantable systems, such as central ports or PICC-ports.

Table 5.4 summarises the indications for the use of cuffed PICCs.

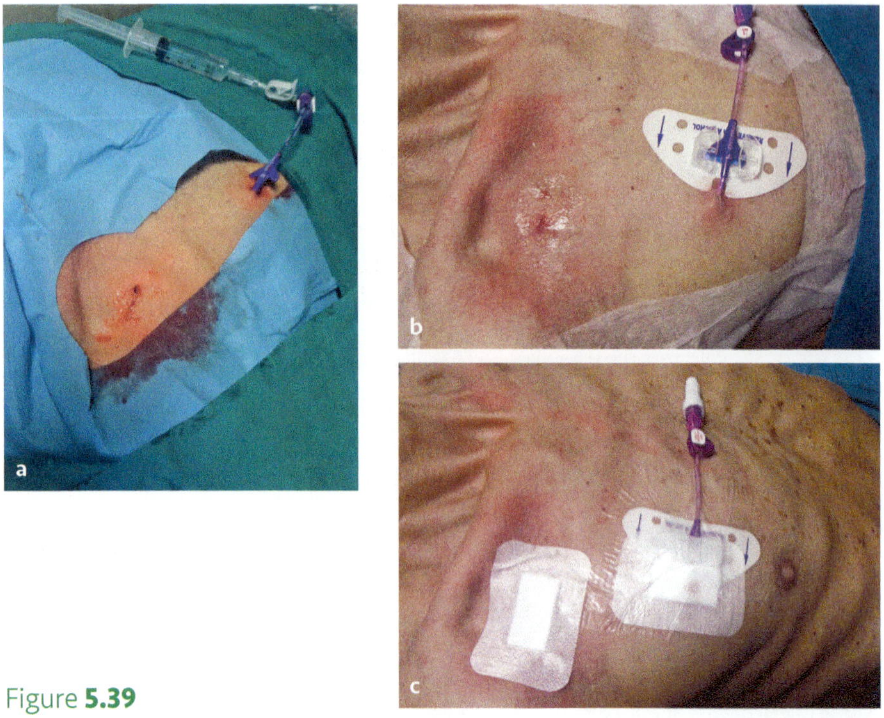

Figure **5.39**

Table 5.4 Indications for cuffed PICCs
• Frequent venous access (>once a week) for an extended period of time (>4-6 months) – for example: long-term home parenteral nutrition
• Patients at high risk of infection and displacement in extra-hospital care – pediatric patients – uncooperative patients

PICC-ports

PICCs (tunneled or otherwise), tunneled CICCs and tunneled FICCs (see Table 1.4) are considered appropriate as medium-term central venous access. For long-term central venous access, tunneled-cuffed catheters (CCT) and totally insertable systems (ports) are used. Long-term access systems are generally reserved for patients with an expected duration of treatment longer than 4-6 months; if frequent use is needed (once a week or more) external cuffed catheters are ideal, whereas totally implantable systems are required for infrequent use (less than once a week). The latter, also called "ports", include centrally inserted ports (chest ports) and brachially inserted ports (PICC-ports).

PICC-ports have been extensively used and may have different names (brachial ports, arm ports, etc.), especially in Europe and Japan. The use of the term "PICC-port" is particularly appropriate because it makes clear that it refers to brachial ports in which the catheter is inserted with the same technique applied for PICC insertion (ultrasound identification of a deep vein of the arm of sufficient calibre; ultrasound-guided venipuncture and cannulation, use of micro-introduction kits and indirect Seldinger technique, verification of tip location by means of the intracavitary ECG method). In the 1990s, ports were sometimes inserted in the arm applying techniques and methods that are now obsolete (puncture of the vein in the crease of the elbow by direct visualisation or palpitation of the vein using large calibre needles, insertion of the catheter with the "*catheter through cannula*" method that does not include guidewires, rough estimation of the catheter length based exclusively on surface landmarks, radiological verification of tip location only after completing the procedure).
Various German, French and Japanese studies carried out in the last 10 years have shown that the insertion of PICC-ports has various advantages compared to the insertion of chest ports: minimal to no risk of complications as well as optimal patient compliance.
The indication for PICC-ports is basically the same as chest ports: prolonged but episodic use of the venous access. Moreover, the use of PICC-ports is recommended when chest ports are difficult or impossible to use (Table 5.5):

- planned irradiation of the thoracic area;
- planned reconstruction of the neck with pectoral muscle flap after radical neck dissection;
- particularly large bilateral breast implants;
- patients who cannot maintain a supine position during the procedure, because of cardiorespiratory problems (indeed, a PICC-port can easily be inserted in sitting position);
- radiodermatitis or other skin abnormalities of the chest;
- tracheostomy with surrounding skin alterations;
- morbid obesity (expected difficulties in puncturing a chest port);
- patients who are candidate for cetuximab treatment (an antiblastic drug potentially associated with micropustules of the skin in the thoracic region);
- patient preference (for cosmetic, psychological or, sometimes, even religious reasons).

Table 5.5 Indications for PICC-ports
Infrequent venous access (<once a week) for an extended period of time (>4-6 months) in patients with an absolute or relative contraindication for a chest port • cosmetic/psychological concerns • skin alterations of the thoracic area • regional radiotherapy • difficulties with the supine position during insertion • complicated tracheotomy, etc.

Table 5.6 Contraindications for PICC-ports

- Bilateral contraindications for the insertion of a PICC in the veins of the arm
  - small calibre veins or local venous thrombosis
  - osteoarticular alterations of the arm
  - previous dissection of the axillary lymph nodes
  - chronic renal failure in haemodialysis
  - etc.
- Need for chemotherapy infusion >12 hours
- Uncooperative patient

Contraindications for PICC-ports are (Table 5.6):

- standard contraindications for PICCs: small arm veins or local venous thrombosis, arterio-venous fistula for haemodialysis, significant skin or bone alterations of the arm, previous dissection of the axillary lymph nodes;
- patients requiring chrono-infusion for more than 12 hours (it is not safe to keep Huber's needles inserted in the brachial port at night);
- uncooperative patients.

The initial phases for inserting a PICC-port (Figure 5.40-5.44) is the same as those needed for PICC insertion:

- ultrasound scan of the veins of the arm and vein selection;
- aseptic technique (hand hygiene, skin antisepsis with 2% chlorhexidine, maximum barrier precautions);
- ultrasound-guided puncture and cannulation of a deep vein of the arm;
- using the modified Seldinger technique and a micro-introducer/dilator, insertion of a catheter in polyurethane and silicone, 4 Fr/5 Fr or appropriate for the calibre of the vein;
- verification of tip position by intracavitary ECG method (this procedure is simplified as the catheter is to be trimmed proximally, without exception).

At this point, the skin incision at the puncture site is enlarged laterally and a subcutaneous pocket is created expanding the tissue with local anaesthetic. The catheter is connected to the reservoir, which is embedded in the subcutaneous tissue. The skin incision is closed with a layer of interrupted intradermal reabsorbable stitches and an layer of cyanoacrylate glue. To minimise complications, it is advisable to follow these recommendations:

- use small reservoirs and embed them above the bicep muscle;
- avoid any tunnel between the puncture site and the pocket of the reservoir: locate the pocket for the reservoir close to the puncture site, in the third proximal or the middle of the arm;
- do not suture the reservoir to the muscle;
- adopt the same methods used for PICC insertion (ultrasound-guidance, micro-introduction kits, intracavitary ECG method);
- close the skin with cyanoacrylate glue.

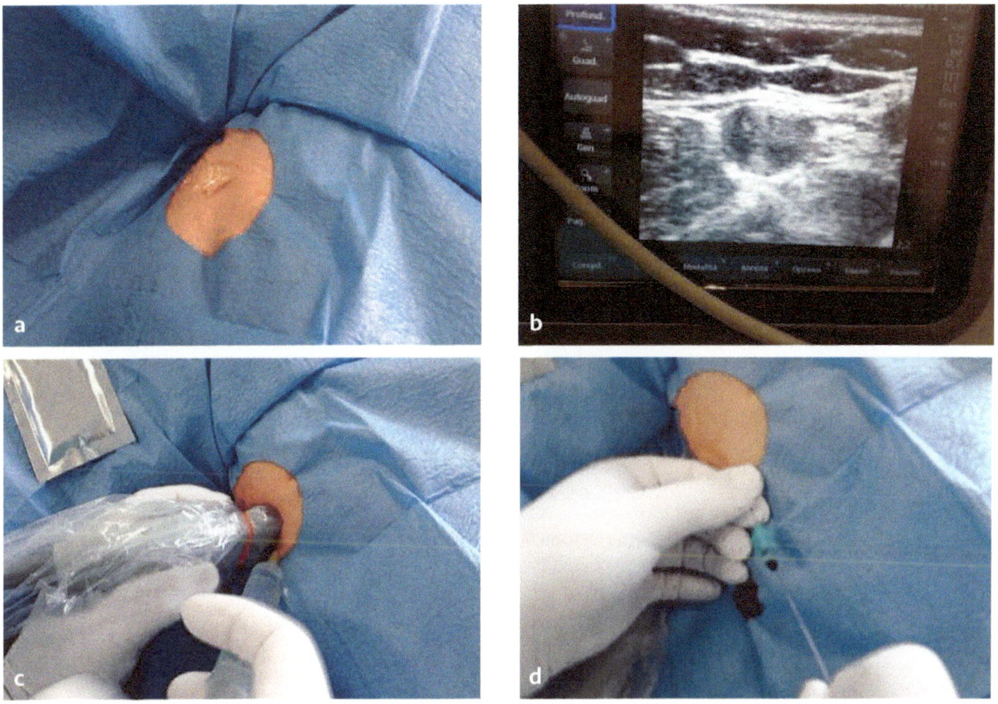

Figure **5.40**

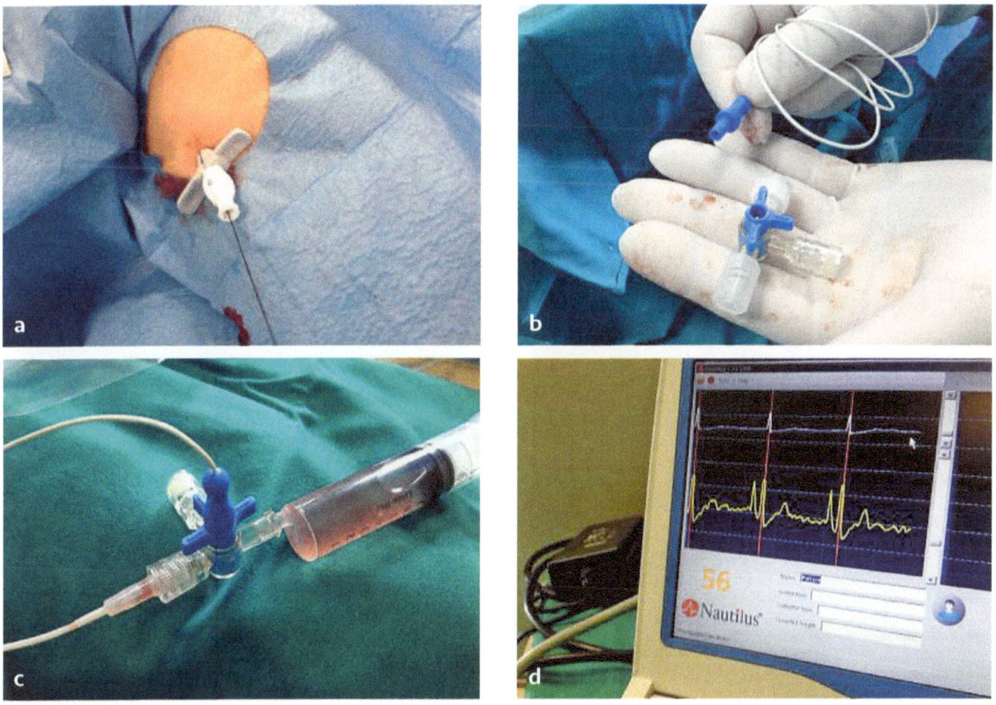

Figure **5.41**

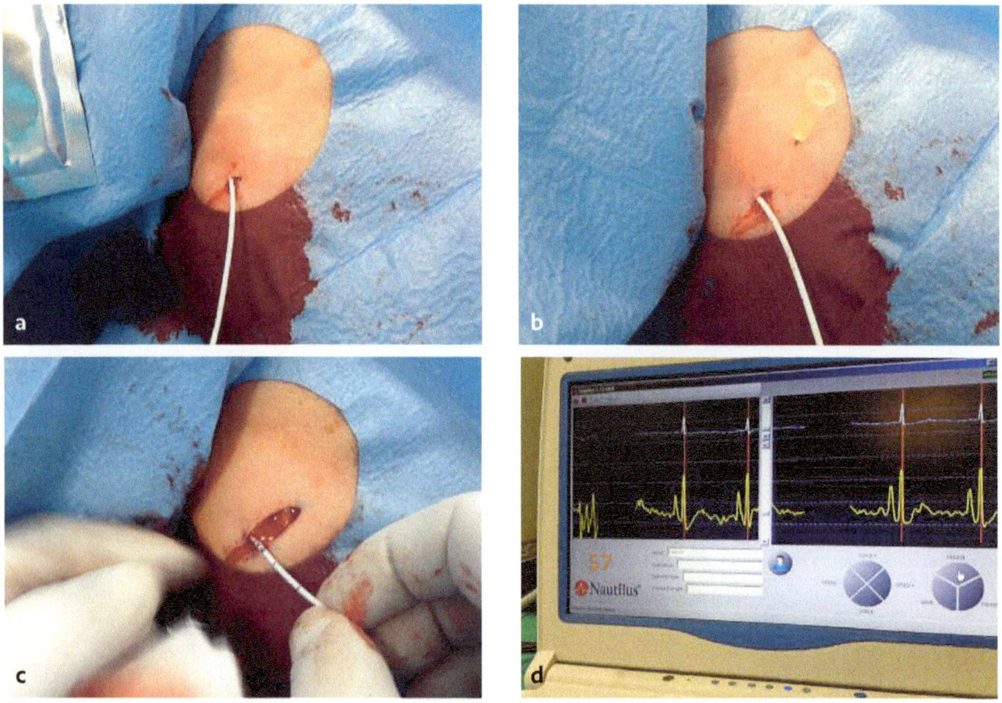

Figure **5.42**

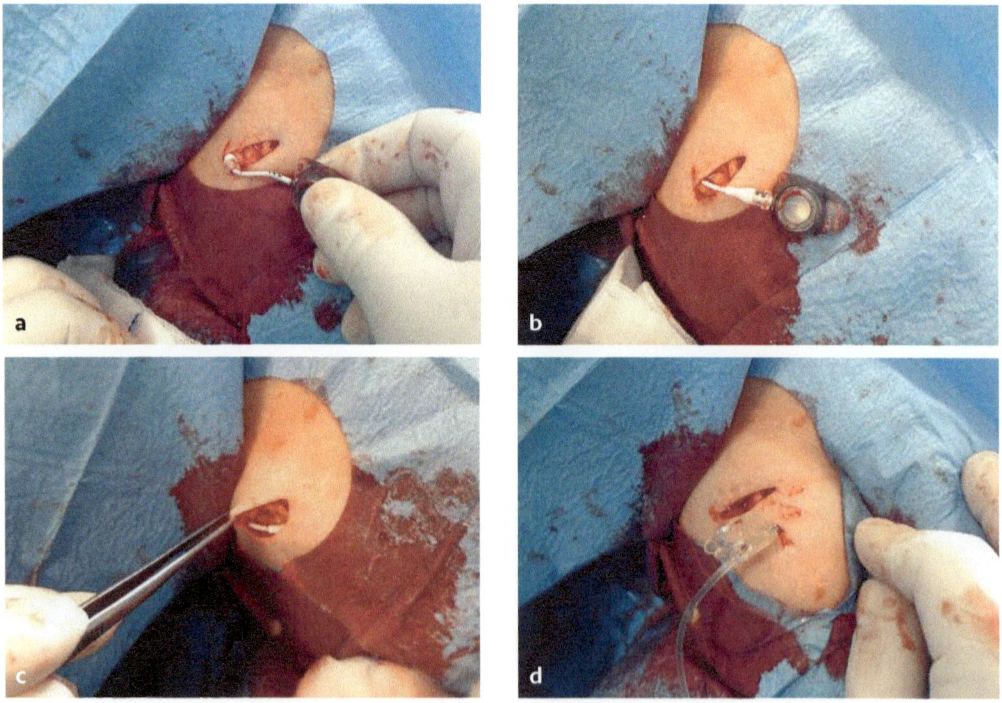

Figure **5.43**

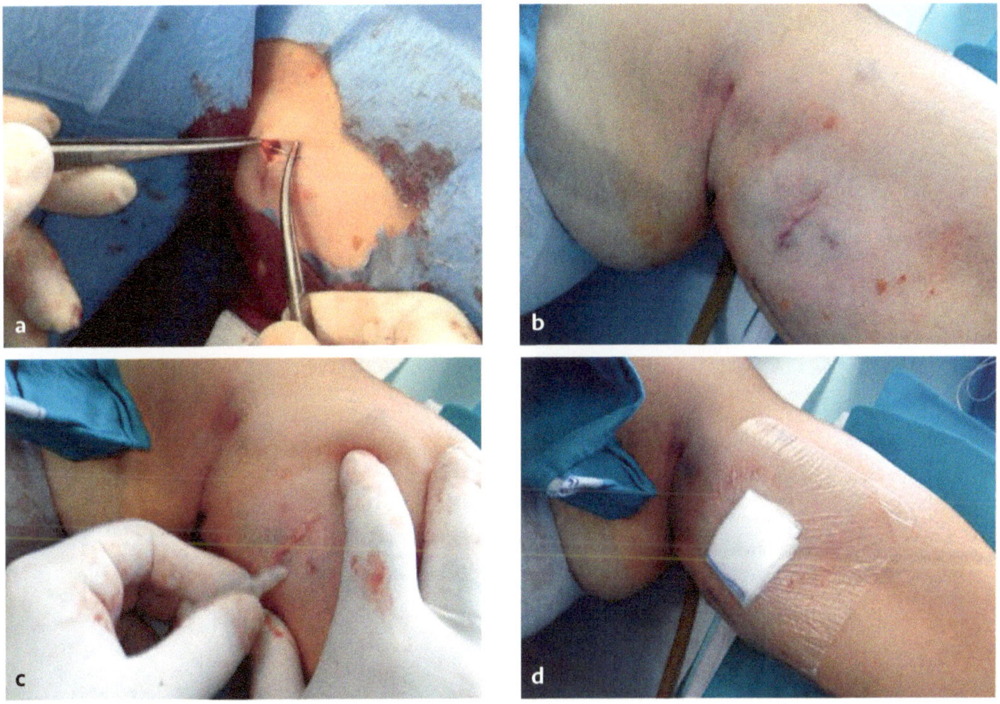

Figure **5.44**

CONCLUSIONS

Recommendations for the correct use of PICCs

PICCs are the most important development in the last decade in the field of venous access devices and are destined to become the central venous catheter of reference for any in-hospital or extra-hospital patient who needs intravenous treatment at home or in outpatient or day hospital setting.

This does not mean that PICCs can replace all types of venous accesses used for in-hospital (like CICCs) or extra-hospital (TCCs and ports) infusions, but that their safety and cost-effectiveness will be the benchmark to assess the safety and cost-effectiveness of all other devices for central venous access. CICCs will continue to have a role in emergencies and in special clinical cases with contraindications for brachial insertion. In extra-hospital settings, ports will continue to be the main device for intermittent, medium to long term treatments (such as antiblastic therapy, typically): the expected role for PICC-ports in this area may cover no more than 15-20% of the indications. Finally, while we wait for further technological developments which could be introduced very rapidly and unexpectedly in this field, the role of PICCs for exchange procedures (hemodialysis, apheresis, diafiltration, etc.) will remain marginal for the time being.

To fully benefit from the versatility, safety and efficacy of this device, it is advisable to define a series of conditions of appropriateness in terms of indication, insertion and management methods, that are necessary to avoid the risk of PICC misuse and the increase in complications potentially associated with them (primarily, venous thrombosis and infections).

Implementing the use of PICCs in a given in-hospital or outpatient operative unit cannot simply be the outcome of individual healthcare operator initiatives, but must be framed within a specific project for the optimisation of venous access.
This implies, above all, the definition of proper indications for PICCs and Midlines compared to other devices. This result may be best obtained by defining an operating unit protocol (or hospital policy) providing an algorithm to guide the most appropriate venous access selection for each individual case, based on the type of solution to be infused, the expected treatment times and the operating environment in which these solutions will be administered. Such algorithm must be adequately disseminated in the operating unit (or hospital) by means of various strategies, such as, for example, the distribution of a poster displaying the algorithm with appropriate explanations (including, for example, a table of drugs and conditions that require the central route), as well as educational meetings with doctors and nurses of the operating unit (or representatives of the operating units of the hospital).
In hospital settings, a PICC Team will need to be identified: it must include specifically trained healthcare operators that are expert in placing venous accesses by the peripheral route and able not only to insert the device but also to provide effective expert help *(counseling)* in access selection. The team must be adequately sized to match each hospital's needs. National and international clinical experience has shown that the presence of a PICC Team may optimise not only the use of PICCs but, indirectly, all types of venous accesses.
It will also be necessary to clearly define a hospital-wide procedure for requesting the peripheral placing of central and peripheral accesses (PICCs, Midlines and mini-Midlines) for in-hospital and extra-hospital patients. Such requests forwarded to the PICC Team should be fully traceable (in terms of applicant, patient, indications and schedule) using the hospital intranet, for example.
Once the device selection has been optimised, it is necessary to optimise the quality of PICC and Midline insertion procedures, which include the following steps:

- definition of specific hospital policies that describe in detail the insertion technique of these devices with an operating checklist attached; this insertion protocol must be consistent with those already described in detail in this manual, and include: correct asepsis and antisepsis techniques, mandatory use of ultrasound guidance, use of the Seldinger technique (modified for PICCs and Midlines; simple for mini-Midlines), verification of the tip position with intracavitary ECG method whenever it is possible, and mandatory use of sutureless devices rather than sutures to secure the device to the skin;
- definition of training and education prerequisites for PICC Team members;
- definition of the most appropriate environment for placing individual devices: "*bedside*" for PICCs, Midlines and mini-Midlines in hospitalised patients; a "dedicated" environment, such as a small room in a day-hospital unit, for example, for the insertion of PICCs, Midlines, cuffed PICCs and PICC-ports in extra-hospital patients.

The hardest challenge is management optimisation. While it is true that it is relatively easy to train a small team of healthcare operators to appropriately insert PICCs and Midlines, it is also true that it is a very complex task to train all the healthcare operators in the operating unit (or – worse – the hospital) in the proper management, which requires different strategic interventions:

- the definition of hospital policies that precisely establish the fundamental principles for proper PICC and Midline dressing (scheduled periodic dressing replacement, antisepsis with 2% chlorhexidine, correct technique for replacing the transparent membrane and the sutureless device, etc.) and proper infusion line management (appropriate *flush* and *lock* protocol, proper use of NFCs and *port protectors*, periodic infusion line replacement schedule);
- adequate continuous personnel training programme designed to effectively disseminate the concepts mentioned above and provide a final *audit* and programmed refresher courses;
- dissemination of posters and other teaching materials among the individual operating units that effectively and briefly summarise the maintenance procedures of PICCs and Midlines;
- hostpital-wide implementation of surveillance and monitoring programmes to check for complications (with particular regard to infective complications).

In conclusion, the appropriate definition of hospital procedures, operating unit protocols and *bundles* for the prevention of complications, as well as a dedicated team of healthcare operators and an adequate importance to the quality of the training are the cornerstones for ensuring that the safety and cost-effectiveness of PICCs and Midlines can be fully exploited for the benefit of patients and the efficiency of hospitals.

APPENDIX I

Main drugs for intravenous infusion

pH, OSMOLARITY AND RISK OF PHLEBITIS RELATED TO PERIPHERAL ROUTE INFUSION				
Medicine	**Dilution**	**pH**	**mOsmol/L**	**Phlebitis**
Aciclovir	5 mg/mL in SF	10,5-11,6	316	Yes
Amphotericin B	0,1 mg/mL in SG5%	5,7	256	Yes
AmphotericinB	0,2-0,8 mg/mL in SG5%	5,0-6,0	280	Yes
AmphotericinB	1-2 mg/mL inSG5%	5,0-6,0	280	Yes
Amikacin	5 mg/mL in SF	3,5-5,5	349	
Aminophylline	5 mg/mL in SF	8,6-9	327	
Amiodarone	2 mg/mL in SG5%	4,1		Yes
Ampicillin	100 mL SF	9(8-10)	328-372	Yes
Ampicillin/Sulbactam	100 mL SF	9(8-10)	400	Yes
Amrinone	2,5 mg/mL in SF	3,2-4	300	Yes
Azithromycin 500 mg	2 mg/mL in SF	6,4-6,8	280	Yes
Aztreonam	100 mL SF	6(4,5-7,5)	315-352	
Bleomycin	3 unit/mL	4,5-6	300	
Carboplatin	0,2-2 mg/mL in SG5%	5,0-7,0	250	
Carmustine	250-500 mL SG5%	5,6-6		
Caspofungin	0,28-0,35mg/mL in SF	6,6		Yes
Cefamandole 1 g	10 mL SD	6-8,5	466	
Cefamandole 1 g	100 mL SF	7(6-8,5)	314	
Cefazolin 1-2 g	10 mL SD	4,5-7	293	
Cefazolin 1-2 g	100 mL SF	4,5-7	317-351	

(continue)

pH, OSMOLARITY AND RISK OF PHLEBITIS RELATED TO PERIPHERAL ROUTE INFUSION				
Medicine	**Dilution**	**pH**	**mOsmol/L**	**Phlebitis**
Cefepime 1-2 g	100 mL SF	4,0-6,0	307	
Cefmetazole 2 g	100 mL SF	4,2-6,2	317	
Cefoperazone	10 mL SD	5(4,5-6,5)	290	
Cefoperazone 1 g	100 mL SF	5(4,5-6,5)	307	
Cefotaxime 1 g	10 mL SD	5-7,5	357	
Cefotaxime 1-2 g	100 mL SF	5-6-7,5	344-351	
Cefotetan 1 g	10 mL SD	4,5-6,5	400	
Cefotetan 1 g	100 mL SF	4,5-6,5	380	
Cefotetan 1-2 g	50 mL SG5%	5,0-6,4	270-330	
Cefotetan 2 g	100 mL SF	4,5-6,5	420	
Cefoxitin 1 g	10 mL SD	4,2-8	390	
Cefoxitin 1-2 g	100 mL SF	4,2-8	319-355	
Ceftazidime 1 g	10 mL SD	5,5-8	240	
Ceftazidime 1-2 g	100 mL SF	5,5-8	330	
Ceftazidime 2 g	20 mL SD	5,5-8	240	
Ceftizoxime 1 g	10 mL SD	5,5-8	350	
Ceftizoxime 1 g	100 mL SF	6,0-8,0	320	
Ceftriaxone1 g	10 mL SD	6,6-6,7	423	
Ceftriaxone 1-2 g	100 mL SF	6,6-6,7	350	
Cefuroxima 0,75-1,5 g	100 mL SF	6,-8,5	300	
Cefuroxime 1 g	10 mL SD	6-8,5	357	
Cyclophosphamide	250 mL SF	6,9(3-7,5)	300	
Cidofovir	100 mL SF	7,4	300	
Cimetidine	50 mL SF	3,8-6,0	314	
Ciprofloxacin 200 mg	100 mL SG5%	3,3-4,6	285	Yes
Ciprofloxacin 400 mg	200 mL SG5%	3,3-4,6	285	Yes
Cisplatin	0,05-2 mg/mL in SF	3,5-6	300	
Cytarabine	100 mg/mL in SF	5(4,0-6,0)	300	
Cytarabine	500 mL SF	5,7-8,0	300	Yes
Clindamycin 600 mg	100 mL SF	6,3(5,5-7,0)	294	
Clindamycin900 mg	100 mL SF	6,3(5,5-7,0)	294	
Chloramphenicol 1 g	10 mL SD	6,4-7,0	344	
Chloramphenicol1 g	100 mL SF	6,4-7,0	330	
Dacarbazine	10 mg/mL in SD	3,0-4,0	109	
Dacarbazine	250 mL SF in SD	3,0-4,0	300	
Daclizumab 5 mg/mL	50 mL SF	6,9	300	
Dactinomycin	0,5 mg/mL in SD	5,5-7,0	189	
Dactinomycin	50 mL SF o SG5%	5,5-7,0	300	
Daunorubicinhydrochloride	15 mL SF	4,5-6,5	300	
Daunorubicinhydrochloride	100 mL SF	4,5-6,5	300	
Deferoxamine	250 mg/mL in SD	4,0-6,0		
Dexrazoxane	5 mg/mL in SF	3,5-5,5		Yes
Dobutaminehydrochloride	4 mg/mL in SF	3,5(2,5-5,5)	280	Yes
Docetaxel	0,3-0,9 mg/mL in SF	4-4,3	503	Yes
Dolasetron	20 mg/mL in SD	3,2-3,8	285	Yes

pH, OSMOLARITY AND RISK OF PHLEBITIS RELATED TO PERIPHERAL ROUTE INFUSION				
Medicine	**Dilution**	**pH**	**mOsmol/L**	**Phlebitis**
Dopamine	in SG5%	3,3(2,5-4,5)	277	Yes
Doxycycline 100 mg-200 mg	1 mg/mL in SF	1,8-3,3	310	
Doxorubicin	2 mg/ml in SD	2,5-4,5	280	
Doxorubicin	2 mg/mL in SF	3,8-6,5		
Heparinsodium	1000 units/mL in SF	5-8,0	283-384	
Epirubicin	2 mg/mL in SD	3		Yes
Erythromycin 500 mg	100 mL SF	7(6,5-7,7)	291	Yes
Erythromycin1 g	250 mL SF	7(6,5-7,7)	290	Yes
Etoposide	0,2-0,4mg/mL in SF	3,0-4,0		Yes
Etoposidephosphate	10 mg/mL in SF	3,0-4,0	290	Yes
Famotidine	50 mL SF	5-5,6	290	
Phenytoin	5 mg/mL in SF	12	312	Yes
Irondextran	0,1 mg/mL in SF	5,2-6,5		Yes
Irondextran	50 mg/mL in SF	5,2-6,5	2000	Yes
Floxuridine	10 mg/mL in SF	4,0 - 5,5	355	
Fluconazole 100 mg	50 mL SF	4,0-8,0	315	
Fluconazole 200 mg	100 mL SF	4-8,0	315	
Fludarabine	100 mL SF	7,2-8,2	352	
Fluorouracil	50 mg/mL in SD	9,2	650	
Foscarnet	24 mg/mL in SD	7,4	271	Yes
Fosphenytoin	1,5 - 25 EF/mL in SF	8,6-9		Yes
Ganciclovir <500 mg	100 mL SF	11	320	Yes
Gatifloxacin	10 mg/mL in SG5%	3,5-5,5		Yes
Gemcitabine	40 mg/mL in SF	2,7-3,3		
Gentamicin 100-250 mg	100 mL SF	3-5,5	280-290	
Glucose 5%		4,0(3-6,5)	252	
Glucose 10%		4,0(3-6,5)	505	
Granisetron	1 mg/mL in SD	4,7-7,3	290	
Idarubicin	1 mg/mL	3,5		
Hydrocortisone	50 mg/mL in SD	7-8,0	360	
Hydromorphone	10 mg/mL in SD	4-5,5	333	
Ifosfamide	0,6-20 mg/mL in SF	6		
Imiglucerase	20 unit/mL in SF	6,1	310	Yes
Imipenem/Cilastatin	5 mg/mL in SF	6,5-7,5	310	Yes
Immunoglobulin	3%-12%	4-7,2	300	
Infliximab	0,4-4 mg/mL in SF	7,2	300	
Irinotecan	0,12-1,1 mg/mL in SG5%	3-3,8		
Itraconazole	3,3 mg/mL in SF	4,8		Yes
Leucovorin	10 mg/mL in SD	8,1	274	
Levofloxacin 250 mg	50 mL SG5%	3,8-5,8	250	Yes
Levofloxacin 500 mg	100 mL in SG5%	3,8-5,8	250	Yes
Linezolid	2 mg/mL in SG5%	4,8	290	
Meperidine	50 mg/mL in SD	3,5-6	302	
Meropenem	5 mg/mL in SF	7,3-8,3	300	Yes
Methotrexate	25 mg/mL in SD	8,5	300	

(continue)

pH, OSMOLARITY AND RISK OF PHLEBITIS RELATED TO PERIPHERAL ROUTE INFUSION				
Medicine	**Dilution**	**pH**	**mOsmol/L**	**Phlebitis**
Meticillin 1 g	10 mL SD	7,6(6-8,5)	510	Yes
Meticillin 2-3 gm	100 mL SF	7,6(6-8,5)	371-415	
Methylprednisolone 500 mg	100 mL SG5%	7-8,0	301	
Methylprednisolone1 g	250 mL SG5%	7-8,0	319	
Metoclopramide	1,25 mg/mL in SF	4,4	285	
Metoclopramide	5 mg/mL in SD	4,5-6,5	280	
Metronidazole	5 mg/mL in SF	5-7,0	310	
Milrinone	200 mg/mL in SG5%	3,2-4		
Minocycline	0,1-0,2 mg/mL in SF	2-2,8	300	
Mitomycins	0,5 mg/mL in SD	6-8,0	333	
Mitoxantrone	0,2 mg/mL in SF	3-4,5	300	Yes
Morphinesulphate	10 mg/mL in SF	4(2,5-6,0)	295	Yes
Nafcillin 1-3 g	100 mL SF	6-8,5	361-398	Yes
Nicardipine	0,1 mg/mL in SF	3,5	300	
Parenteralnutrition	Amino acids + glucose	5,3-6,3	>800	Yes
Nutrizione parenterale	Amino acids + glucose+ lipids	5,5	>600	Yes
Octreotide	0,5 mg/mL in SD	3,9-4,5	279	
Ofloxacin	4 mg/mL in SG5%	3,8-5,8	252	
Ondansetron	32 mg/50 mL in SG5%	3,3-4	270	
Oxacillin 1 g	10 mL SD	6-8,5	398	Yes
Oxacillin 1-2 g	100 mL SF	6-8,5	321-356	Yes
Paclitaxel	0,3-1,2 mg/mL in SG5%	4,4-6,5		
Pamidronate	0,09 mg/mL in SF	6-7,4	300	Yes
Pantoprazole 40 mg	100 mL SF	9,0-10	295	
Penicillin	50 unit/mL in SF	7(6-8,5)	420	
Pentamidine	<3 mg/mL in SG5%	4-4,4	455	Yes
Piperacillin	40 mg/mL in SF	5,5-7,5	404	
Piperacillin	163 mg/mL in SD	5,5-7,5	439	
Piperacillin/Tazobactam 3,375 g	100 mL SF	5,1-5,4	445	
Plicamycin	1000 mL SF	7	300	
Potassiumchloride	0,1 mEq/mL	5	200	
Potassiumchloride	0,2 mEq/mL	5	400	
Potassiumchloride	0,3 mEq/mL	5	600	Yes
Potassiumchloride	0,4 mEq/mL	5	800	Yes
Quinupristin/Dalfopristin	2 mEq/mL in SG5%	4,5-5		Yes
Ranitidine 50 mg	50 mL SF	6,7-7,3	302	
Rifampicin <600 mg	100 mL SG5%	7,8-8,8		
Rituximab	1-4 mg/mL in SG5% o SD	6,5		
Sargramostim	10 mg/mL in SF	7,1-7,7	300	
Sodiumchloride 0,45%		5,0(4,5-7,0)	154	
Sodiumchloride0,9%		5,0(4,5-7,0)	308	
Streptozocin	100 mg/mL in SG5%	3,5-4,5		
Sulfamethoxazol/Trimetoprim 80 mg + 400 mg/5 mL	100 mL in SG5%	10	541	Yes
Teniposide	0,4 mg/mL	5(4-6,5)		

pH, OSMOLARITY AND RISK OF PHLEBITIS RELATED TO PERIPHERAL ROUTE INFUSION				
Medicine	**Dilution**	**pH**	**mOsmol/L**	**Phlebitis**
Ticarcillin 3 g	100 mL SF	6-8,0	442	
Ticarcillin/Clavulanic acid3,1 g	86 mg/mL in SD	6-8,0	573	
Ticarcillin/Clavulanic acid3,1 g	100 mL SF	5,5-7,5	450	
Thiotepa	1 mg/mL in SF	5,5-7,5	269	
Tobramycin 100-250 mg	100 mL SF	3-6	290	
Topotecan	50 mL SG5%	2,5-3,5		
Trastuzumab	250 mL SF	6	300	
Trimetrexate	0,25-2 mg/mL in SG5%	3,5-5,5		
Vancomycin 500 mg	100 mL SF	2,5-4,5	291	
Vancomycin1-1,25 g	250 mL SF	2,5-4,5	290	
Vancomycin1,5 g	250 mL SF	2,5-4,5	300	
Vinblastine	1 mg/mL in SF	3,5-5	278	
Vincristine	1 mg/mL in SD	3,5-5,5	610	
Vindesine	1 mg/ml in SF	4,2-4,5		
Vinorelbine	1,5-3 mg/mL in SG5%	3,5		Yes
Zidovudine	4 mg/mL in SG5%	5,5	260	Yes

EF = equivalent to phenytoinSD = solution of distilled water
SF = saline solution
SG5% = glucose solution 5%

APPENDIX II

Algorithm for intravascular access selection in adults

PERIPHERAL VENOUS ACCESS
pH 5-9
Drugs with osmolarity <600
Non-vesicant drugs
Non-irritating drugs

→ **Needle cannula**
Superficial veins of the arm available
Peripheral access <1 week
Exclusive in-hospital use

→ **Long peripheral cannula**
Superficial veins of the arm not available
Peripheral access >1 week

→ **Midline catheter**
Peripheral access >3 weeks
Peripheral access for extra-hospital use

(continue)

CENTRAL VENOUS ACCESS

pH >9 o <5
Drugs with osmolarity >600
Vesicant drugs
Irritating drugs
Parenteral nutrition with osmolarity>800
Need for repeated and frequent sampling
Need for haemodynamic monitoring

IN-HOSPITAL USE

PICC peripherally inserted catheter
Deep veins of the arm available
Exclusively elective procedure

CICC centrally inserted catheter
Deep veins of the arm not available
Insertion under emergency conditions
Requires "coated" catheter
Requires >3 lumina

Femoral insertion catheters
Not tunneled
In emergency situations
Tunneled
Obstruction of superior vena cava

EXTRA-HOSPITAL USE

Day hospital, home, hospice

MEDIUM TERM ACCESS (<4 MONTHS)

PICC
Deep veins of the arm available
Tunneled CICC
Deep veins of the arm not available

LONG TERM ACCESS (>4 MONTHS)

Episodic use: <1/week
Port

Frequent use: >1/ 1/week
Tunneled cuffed catheter (TCC) with peripheral/central/femoral insertion

APPENDIX III

Dawson's Zone Insertion Method (ZIM)

As mentioned several times in this manual, the definition of the Zone Insertion Method (ZIM) by Robert Dawson is one of the most interesting innovations in PICC and Midlines insertion method introduced into clinical practice after ultrasound-guided venipuncture and the modified Seldinger technique.
The "zone" method, first published by Dawson in 2011 on JAVA, enables a clear, measurable and repeatable definition of the most appropriate point at which to plan the exit site of a PICC in the arm. More recently, the "zone" has also enabled to standardise the indication for tunneling PICCs and the length of such tunneling, where indicated.
The method could be virtually applied to any short, medium or long term catheter (PICC, Midline, long peripheral cannula, needle cannula) that exits the skin in the zone of the upper arm, from the axilla to the elbow. It was predominantly developed for basilic vein or brachial vein puncturing, but can also be extended to the puncture of other veins in this area (cephalic, axillary). Substantially, the method divides this area into three zones, corresponding to three different colours – red, green and yellow – one of which (green) is indicated as the ideal zone for the catheter exit site. The method begins by measuring the distance from the elbow (medial epicondyle) to the axillary line (the imaginary line running across the axillary cavity): this distance obviously varies from patient to patient, but is usually between 18 and 24 cm, and typically between 20 and 22 cm. This distance is divided into three equal parts, which define three different areas of the arm, each formed by a circumferential band and corresponding to distal third (close to the elbow: red zone), middle third (green zone) and proximal third (close to the axilla:

yellow zone). The red zone corresponds to an unfavourable area both for venipuncture and exit site dressing, as the veins here have limited diameters and very variable courses and the characteristic movements of the muscles and layers of muscles in this zone are inevitably transmitted to the skin, making the exit site quite unstable. In other words, even in the era of ultrasound-guided puncture, it is always advisable to avoid the venous approach in this area. Catheters with exit sites in this zone are associated with a prohibitive risk of insertion complications (failure of cannulation or ecchymosis in what was defined by Dawson as the "triangle of the elbow", located on the medial side of the arm, immediately above the antecubital fossa), late complications (thrombosis and infections) and poor patient tolerance.

The green zone corresponds to the middle third of the arm: the zone defined by Dawson as "ideal" is the proximal half of the green zone, which corresponds to a 3-4 cm long band, given that the entire length of the green zone is normally around 7 cm. In this zone, the basilic vein is particularly large, sufficiently far from the neuro-vascular bundle formed of the brachial vessels and the median nerve, as well as very stable since it is below the band of muscles of the arm. An exit site in this region is ideal since it is not subject to the movements transmitted by the bicep contraction, and the skin is usually dry and glabrous, characteristic that gradually disappears as it approaches the axillary cavity.

The yellow zone, on the other hand, corresponds to the medial third of the arm and includes the brachial portion of the axillary cavity as well. The basilic vein here merges with one or more brachial veins, forming the large-calibre axillary vein. This offers easier ultrasound-guided venipuncture and also the possibility of using catheters with larger calibres: bearing in mind the rule mentioned on several occasions in this manual, catheters should be inserted in veins whose internal diameter is at least three times the external diameter of the catheter. The basilic/axillary vein in this region can be up to 6-8 mm, thus enabling the safe positioning of catheters of 6 Fr and above. On the other hand, any exit site in this area presents a high risk of complications, due to the skin characteristics (thicker, moister skin, richer in sebaceous and sweat glands) and due to the inevitable movement of the dressing (linked to the mobility of the skin of the axillary cavity). An exit site in the yellow zone should therefore always be avoided. Whereas Dawson's original work also advised against venipuncture in this site, in more recent times, with the advent of tunneling techniques for PICCs, the yellow zone has been seen as an excellent site for venipuncture, as long as the exit site is moved distally in the green zone.

For ultrasound-guided venipuncture, it is therefore currently recommended to consider the basilic vein as first option or one of the brachial veins as a second option in any site within the green or yellow zone. The venipuncture site should be selected according to vein diameter (in proportion to the desired catheter according with the aforementioned rule) and depth (ideally within 2.5 cm), and allowing a sufficient distance from "dangerous" structures such as the brachial artery or the median nerve. This can lead, in extreme cases, to puncturing the axillary vein in its brachial tract (considering, on the other hand, that the transition between the real brachial vein and what is properly called the axillary vein is not clearly defined in Anatomy literature). If the venipuncture site

lies in the yellow zone, there is clear and definite indication for subcutaneous catheter tunneling in order to move the exit site entirely within the green zone.
The "zone" method therefore not only reduces the risk of immediate and late complication but when associated with the tunneling technique also increases PICC positioning indications, as well as the safe use (that is, with reduced risk of thrombosis) of catheters of greater diameters and with a greater number of lumina.
As strongly emphasised by Dawson in the conclusions of his 2011 work, we now have all the instruments needed to minimise infective, thrombotic and mechanical complications that are potentially associated with the PICC positioning: such methods include the ultrasound-guided method, the modified Seldinger technique, the "zone" method, the possibility of tunneling, etc. We are therefore ethically responsible for using these instruments in the best way possible, bearing in mind that every patient has the right to the greatest comfort and safety.

APPENDIX IV

Guidelines for the prevention of complications with PICCs and Midlines

The guidelines and general agreements cited in this manual are listed below in alphabetical order. These are the most authoritative among the works published in recent years that are of specific interest for the prevention of complications with PICC and Midline catheters. Some guidelines were omitted since they were not particularly original or were outdated. For those who wish to stay up to date, new evidence-based documents are produced annually by many scientific societies and those of greatest significance for the field of venous access are regularly inserted in the Guidelines section of the GAVeCeLT website (www.gavecelt.info) and can be freely downloaded.

ACCP – 2012 guidelines on the prevention and treatment of thrombosis
Guyatt GH, Akl EA, Crowther M et al.: Executive summary: antithrombotic therapy and prevention of Thrombosis. 9th edition: American College of Chest Physicians evidence-based clinical practice guidelines. Chest 2012;141(2) (suppl):7S-47S.
These guidelines of the American College of Chest Physicians (ACCP) cover all aspects of venous thrombosis, but contain helpful recommendations in the specific sector of thrombosis from intravascular catheter.

AIEOP - 2014 consensus on central venous access in paediatric oncology patients
Crocoli A, Tornesello A, Pittiruti M et al.: Central venous access devices in pediatric malignancies: a position paper of the Italian Association of Pediatric Hematology and Oncology. J Vasc Access 2015;16(2):130-6.
The Italian Association of Haematology and Paediatric Oncology (AIEOP) recently published this updated position paper that discusses indications, insertion and management of central venous access in the field of paediatric oncology. Available on the GAVeCeLT website (www.gavecelt.info).

AVA – 2015 guidelines on central venous catheter in paediatrics
Best practice guidelines in the care and maintenance of pediatric central venous catheters – 2nd edition.
These guidelines were developed by the Paediatric Special Interest Group of AVA – Association for Vascular Access. They are available on the official AVA website (www.avainfo.org) and on the GAVeCeLT website (www.gavecelt.info).

BCSH – 2007 guidelines on venous access in haematology
Bishop L, Dougherty L, Bodenham A et al.: Guidelines on the insertion and management of central venous access devices in adults. IntJnl Lab Hem 2007;29:261-78.
Guidelines produced by the British Committee for Standards in Haematology (BCSH): although they are not very up to date on many aspects regarding the types of devices and materials, they do still contain interesting elements. They are available on the GAVeCeLT website (www.gavecelt.info).

CDC – 2011 guidelines on the prevention of infections from intravascular catheters
O'Grady NP, Alexander M, Burns LA et al.: Guidelines for the prevention of intravascular catheter-related infections. Clin Infect Dis 2011;52(9):e162-93.
These are the best-known guidelines on the subject, issued periodically by the US Centres for Disease Control. They are available both in English and translated into Italian by GAVeCeLT on the website www.gavecelt.info.

CVAA – 2013 guidelines on the treatment of occlusions of central venous catheters
Occlusion management guideline for central venous access devices. Vascular Access (Journal of the Canadian Vascular Access Association), 2013; volume 7 (suppl. 1).
Perhaps the only guidelines dedicated specifically to the problem of occlusion of the lumen of central venous access. They are available on the Canadian Vascular Access Association (CVAA) website (www.cvaa.info) and on the GAVeCeLT website (www.gavecelt.info).

EPIC – 2014 guidelines for the prevention of infections from venous catheter
Loveday HP, Wilson JA, Pratt RJ et al.: EPIC3 – National evidence-based guidelines for preventing healthcare-associated infections in NHS hospitals in England. J Hosp Infect 2014; 86:S1-70.
Currently, one of the strictest and most up to date guidelines on the issue, alongside the SHEA-IDSA 2014 (see later in this Appendix). They contain important recommendations for the

prevention of hospital infections, issued by EPIC – Evidence-based Prevention and Infection Control: the section dedicated to the prevention of infections from venous access (S38-S51) is also available translated into Italian (by GAVeCeLT) on the website www.gavecelt.info.

ESPEN – 2009 guidelines on venous catheters in parenteral nutrition
Pittiruti M, Hamilton H, Biffi R et al.: ESPEN Guidelines on Parenteral Nutrition: central venous catheters (access, care, diagnosis and therapy of complications). ClinNutr 2009; 28(4):365-77.
Still up to date even though published in 2009, these official guidelines of the European Society of Parenteral and Enteral Nutrition (ESPEN) tackle the problems of indication, insertion and management, but are limited to venous access used for parenteral nutrition.

GAVeCeLT – 2007 consensus on thrombosis from central venous catheter
Campisi C, Biffi R, Pittiruti M et al.: Catheter-related central venous thrombosis: the development of a nationwide consensus paper in Italy. JAVA 2007; 12(1):38-46.
An important consensus on the issue of catheter-related thrombosis, whose recommendations – although issued many years ago – are still valid. It was also published on Nutritional Therapy & Metabolism *(2007;25:173-82) and it is available on the website www.gavecelt.info.*

GAVeCeLT – 2011 consensus on the use of ports in radiology
Bonciarelli G, Batacchi S, Biffi R et al.: GAVeCeLT consensus statement on the correct use of totally implantable venous access devices for diagnostic radiology procedures. J Vasc Access 2011;12(4):292-305.
Although specifically focused on problems connected to the high-pressure infusion of long-term, port-type systems, this GAVeCeLT consensus also contains many clarifications on the concept of power injectability, *applicable to every venous access.*

GFTC – 2013 guidelines on thrombosis from venous catheter in oncology patients
Debourdeau P, Farge D, Beckers M et al.: International clinical practice guidelines for the treatment and prophylaxis of thrombosis associated with central venous catheters in patients with cancer. J ThrombHaemost 2013;11:71-80.
These guidelines were drawn by the GTFC (Groupe Francophone Thrombose et Cancer) in association with French and Dutch oncology centres, and with the participation of many international experts. The basic recommendations are no different from those of previous guidelines and consensus on the same topic (see SOR 2008 guidelines and GAVeCeLT 2007 Consensus in this Appendix).

IDSA – 2009 guidelines on the diagnosis and treatment of catheter-related infections
Mermel LA, Allon M, Bouza E et al.: Clinical practice guidelines for the diagnosis and management of intravascular catheter-related infection: 2009 update by the Infectious Diseases Society of America. Clin Infect Dis 2009;49:1-45.
The most important reference guidelines for the diagnosis and treatment of catheter-related infections, produced by the Infectious Diseases Society of America (IDSA) in 2009 and still very current.

INS – 2011 guidelines on the management of infusion treatment
Infusion Nursing Society: Infusion Nursing Standards of Practice. J InfusNurs 2011; 34(1S):S1-109.
Important USA nursing guidelines, produced periodically by the Infusion Nursing Society (INS) and dedicated to all aspects of infusion treatment, including management of venous access. They are available on the INS website (www.ins1.org;) and on the GAVeCeLT website (www.gavecelt.info).

NWS Health – 2013 guidelines on the insertion and management of peripheral access
Ministry of Health, New South Wales Government: Peripheral Intravenous Cannula (PIVC) Insertion and Post Insertion Care in Adult Patients (update Dec 2013).
Excellent and up to date, even if focused almost exclusively on short needle cannulas. Available at http://www.health.nsw.gov.au/policies/e on the GAVeCeLT website (www.gavecelt.info).

RCN – 2010 guidelines on the management of infusion treatment
The RCN IV Therapy Forum: Standards for Infusion Therapy. 3rd edition, January 2010. *Available on the RCN (Royal College of Nursing) website (www.rcn.org.uk) and on the GAVe- CeLT website (www.gavecelt.info).*
They contain recommendations on all aspects of infusion treatment management, obviously with a particular emphasis on venous access management.

SHEA-IDSA – 2016 guidelines on the prevention of catheter-related infections
Marshall J, Mermel, LA, Fakih M et al.: Strategies to prevent Central Line-Associated Bloodstream Infections in acute care hospitals: 2014 Update. Infect Contr Hosp Epidemiol 2014; 35(7):753-71.
Currently, one of the strictest and most up to date guidelines on the issue, alongside the EPIC 2014 (see later in this Appendix). Drawn up by the Society for Healthcare Epidemiology of America (SHEA) and by the Infectious Diseases Society of America (IDSA), they are also available translated into Italian (by GAVeCeLT) on the website www.gavecelt.info.

SOR – 2008 guidelines on thrombosis from venous catheter in oncology patients
Debourdeau P, KassabChahmi D, Le Gal G et al.: 2008 SOR guidelines for the prevention and treatment of thrombosis associated with central venous catheters in patients with cancer:report from the working group. Ann Oncol 2009;20:1459-71.
Guidelines issued by a multidisciplinary group of experts of the French Federation of Oncological Centres within the framework of the SOR national ministerial project (Standards, Options and Recommendations).

WoCoVA – 2012 consensus on the use of ultrasound-guidance in vascular access
Lamperti M, Bodenham AR, Pittiruti M et al.: International evidence-based recommendations on ultrasound-guided vascular access. Intensive Care Med 2012;38(7):1105-17.
Probably the most complete and thorough document on ultrasound use for vascular access positioning developed by WoCoVA (World Conference on Vascular Access) in collaboration with CAVeCeLT and WINFOCUS (World Interactive Network Focused On Critical UltraSound).

WoCoVa – 2013 consensus on training for ultrasound-guided positioning of venous access

Moureau N, Lamperti M, Kelly LJ et al.: Evidence based consensus on the insertion of central venous access devices: definition of minimal requirements for training. Br J Anaesth 2013;110(3):347-56.

An important document issued by the WoCoVA Foundation (World Conference on Vascular Access) that for the first time defines the criteria for suitable training for positioning of ultrasound-guided venous access, both in adults and children.

APPENDIX V

GAVeCeLT and the dissemination of PICCs in Italy

The introduction of ultrasound-guided PICCs (in the early years of the 21st century) coincided with the start of the spread of PICCs in Italy. Until the early 2000s, only a few centres in our country used PICCs: these were Oncology Centres that used them in selected patients and only for short-term chemotherapy, or Artificial Nutrition Centres that implanted PICCs for a limited period in candidate patients for parenteral nutrition who had strong contraindications for traditional CICCs. At that time, in all cases, these devices was obviously implanted without using ultrasound guidance and only by performing venipuncture in the antecubital zone. On one hand, this led to a remarkable percentage of insertion failures (just think of patients with depleted peripheral venous resources due to long and repeated hospitalisation or non-essential infusions, as in the case of drug addicts) and, on the other, several local complications (*kinking*, displacement, thrombophlebitis). These reasons led to a limited diffusion of PICCs in clinical units.

Around 2004, the first ultrasound placing of PICCs in Italy was performed at Fondazione Policlinico Universitario "A. Gemelli" – Roma, on the initiative of a group of doctors and nurses with long, established experience in the field of vascular access and active members of GAVeCeLT. In the following years, insertion numbers gradually increased in the various departments of this hospital, following a gradual adoption plan that was applied first to Oncology (day hospital, department, hospice, home assistance) and Infectious Disease (day hospital, department, home assistance) and then was spreaded to all operating units. Local PICC inserters that were already connected through a long estab-

lished professional collaboration with Policlinico "A. Gemelli" – Roma and GAVeCeLT, gradually came together to form a proper, dedicated team for vascular access and, in particular, PICC insertion. This team, whose initial core was made up of two surgeons, an expert in infectious diseases and eight nurses, began to systematically and jointly focus its activity, depending on different responsibilities of members, to all areas regarding venous access: from indication assessment to device selection, from insertion to *counseling* on ordinary management, from complication management to device removal. Its activity was extremely complex, both from the operational point of view since it was virtually extended to all hospital departments, and from the educational perspective in particular. This first Italian PICC Team was therefore established as practical application of the indications suggested by international guidelines and recommendations, and included certain touches of originality in multi-professional and multidisciplinary terms (for example, the permanent presence of an expert in infectious diseases and nurses with different areas of expertise).
For the first time, therefore, the outlines of a vascular access plan to obtain acknowledged international quality standards in this field were drawn including important innovations, all framed within a wider project of risk management for safeguarding patient and operator safety, as well as corporate cost-effectiveness.
Indeed, in 2005, an important study by K. Kokotis identified the following causes of ineffectiveness and inefficiency in the field of vascular accesses:

- absence of a dedicated vascular access team;
- the lack of training of hospital nursing staff;
- the reduction of the nursing personnel with the consequent increase in work and decrease in the time dedicated to training;
- the increasingly compromised integrity of patients' venous resources, as a result of the increase in survival rates, the chronic nature of diseases and numerous co-morbidities;
- an increase in the number of diabetic patients, patients undergoing steroid treatment and chemotherapy patients, all causes of venous resources being compromised;
- the existence of more than 500 injectable drugs with very basic or very acidic pH and high osmolarity, responsible for the phlebitis, infiltrations and extravasation that often occur in the first 48 hours after the start of the infusion;
- the growing number of patients who receive multiple and often incompatible treatments on the same day;
- the lack of *vascular access planning* when the patient is admitted.

On the basis of the above considerations, it was appropriate for the first point of the GAVeCeLT project to address the establishment of a dedicated and specifically trained vascular access team. As expected, besides increasing and improving the insertion activity and the consolidated management of long-term venous access, the presence of a dedicate team gradually led to the growing success of PICCs. The advantages of these devices became so clear over the years that the number of annual PICC insertions at Policlinico "A. Gemelli" – Roma rose from around 600 in 2006 to more than 4,000 in 2015. As months passed by and a highly standardised technique was applied, the success rate for PICC and Midline insertion came close to 100% and the incidence of complications was reduced considerably and almost eliminated.

Given the remarkable improvement of the insertion technique and the exceptional improvement in PICC and Midline performance, it was even more surprising that these devices were not more widely used in our country. Following a survey in 2005, GAVeCeLT identified four possible causes that were potentially obstructing the diffusion of PICCs and Midlines in Italy:

- the lack of knowledge among doctors and nurses about the correct indications for these devices;
- the lack of training and refresher courses focused on PICC and Midline insertion and management;
- the lack of diffusion of the ultrasound-guidance technique: in other words, in the 1990s whenever health professionals showed a certain curiosity and openness to PICCs and Midlines, they inevitably encountered opposition or the impossibility of insertion in patients with exhausted peripheral venous resources (at least the visible and/or palpable peripheral veins) or with the numerous complications that arose after insertion;
- the erroneous conviction on the part of nurses that the insertion of PICCs did not come within their professional profiles, since they are central venous catheters.

In consideration of these factors, the "PICC Team" organised at Policlinico "A. Gemelli" – Roma, was the first of its kind in Italy, and developed a national implementation strategy of awareness concerning PICCs and Midlines made up of various actions, all more or less developed in GAVeCeLT scientific and didactic activities.

- Precise definition of PICC and Midlines indications at the National GAVeCeLT Conferences as well as courses and other educational events organised or sponsored by GAVeCeLT starting from 2005, during dedicated sessions or symposia.
- Participation of GAVeCeLT members to national conferences, meetings, workshops and other cultural events in which essential knowledge about PICCs was disseminated.
- Definition of PICC training offer, including:
  - an on-site GAVeCeLT dissemination 1-day course that deals with PICCs (the so-called "GAVeCeLT 7" module) in an original and largely practical way, that was carried out and is still carried out in several hospitals throughout the country;
  - a residential 3-day PICC that is organised periodically at Policlinico Universitario "A. Gemelli" – Roma, including theory, laboratory practice and clinical practice;
  - a specialist university 60-hour course on PICCs, established at Policlinico Universitario "A. Gemelli" – Roma and dedicated to those who have already been trained in PICC positioning but wish to explore all the issues linked to indications, prevention and management of complications;
  - a specific course for PICC instructors, aimed at operators who are already experts in PICC positioning but wish to become PICC course instructors;
  - finally, the implementation of PICC-related activities as part of University Master's degrees of first and second level dedicated to venous access, which have been held at Università Cattolica del Sacro Cuore – Roma every academic year since 2003-2004.

- Implementing the use of PICCs in hospitals where GAVeCeLT members may be present.
- Original contribution to the definition of training *standards*, a particularly sensitive issue that is constantly developing, both nationally and internationally.
- GAVeCeLT collaboration with the most authoritative international associations dedicated to vascular access (AVA, INS, RCN, WoCoVA, etc.) and many international experts on various issues regarding PICCs, in order to maintain our country's high cultural level in this area.
- Clinical studies presented as an Italian contribution to the international community, some having great importance, such as those dedicated to the application of the intracavitary ECG technique for the verification of the correct positioning of PICC tip.
- Publishing of many educational and scientific documents on various aspects of PICCs and Midlines (indications, insertion technique documented by photos and videos, ordinary complication management) on the GAVeCeLT website (www.gavecelt.info) and on the European Vascular Access Network (www.evanetwork.info) website.

The first and most authoritative training courses ever organised in Italy in the field of PICCs – especially on the ultrasound-guided technique for their positioning – arose out of the clinical experience acquired by the PICC Team at Università Cattolica del Sacro Cuore – Roma and GAVeCeLT educational initiatives.
Between 2005 and 2015, GAVeCeLT promoted activities to disseminate PICCs in Italy through the aforementioned strategies and instruments, and received utterly astounding results and triggered a cultural process of real transformation and innovation in the field of vascular access. The participation of GAVeCeLT members at diverse cultural events has enabled thousands of health operators already active and with consolidated experience in the field of vascular access to receive correct information about PICCs in terms of their indications, possible applications, advantages and correct insertion technique. Such informative activities were able to spark actual interest at the local level, to the point that several Italian hospitals have decided to include the use of these devices in their practice. Thanks to the enormous training effort conducted in this field from 2005 onwards, the number of centres where PICCs are inserted (and correctly managed) rose from very few centers ten years ago to more than a hundred today, along with the establishment of teams dedicated to the insertion of PICCs or, more generally, vascular access, due also to the constant consultancy and supervisory work carried out by GAVeCeLT.
This growing interest at the national level was confirmed by the great success of an unique annual scientific event dedicated exclusively to PICC culture, called "PICC Day". This convention is organized by GAVeCeLT, with the participation and assistance of dozens of national and international experts, its first edition was held in Rome in November 2007 and, since then, has been held annually in different cities.

Recommended reading

Books

Central venous access devices – Care and management, by Lisa Dougherty, Blackwell 2006 (Italian translation "Cateteri venosi centrali", McGraw-Hill Education 2007).

Central venous catheter, by Helen Hamilton and Andrew Bodenham, Wiley-Blackwell 2009. Critical care ultrasound, by Philip Lumb and DimitriosKarakitsos, Elsevier 2014.

Vascular access – Basic information for doctors and nurses by Mario Vigneri, Percorsi Meridiani 2012. Infusion nursing: an evidence-based approach, by Mary Alexander, Ann Corrigan et al., Saunders 2010.

Peripherally inserted central venous catheters, by Sergio Sandrucci and BaudolinoMussa, Springer-Verlag 2014.

Articles

Bellesi S, Chiusolo P, DePascale G et al.: Peripherally inserted central catheters (PICCs) in the management of oncohematological patients submitted to autologous stem cell transplantation. Support Care Cancer 2013;21(2):531-5.

Cotogni P, Barbero C, Garrino C et al.: Peripherally inserted central catheters in non-hospitalized cancer patients: 5-year results of a prospective study. Support Care Cancer 2015;21(2):403-9.

Cotogni P, Pittiruti M.: Focus on peripherally inserted central catheters in critically ill patients. World J Crit Care Med 2014;3(4): 80-94.

Cotogni P, Pittiruti M, Barbero C et al.: Catheter-related complications in cancer patients on home parenteral nutrition: a prospective study of over 51,000 catheter days. J Parenter Enteral Nutr 2013;37(3):375-83.

Davidson IJ, Lok C, Dolmatch B et al.: Virtual reality: emerging role of simulation training in vascular access. Semin Nephrol 2012;32 (6):572-81.

Davidson IJ, Yoo MC, Biasucci DG et al.: Simulation training for vascular access interventions. J Vasc Access 2010;11(3):181-90.

Dawson RB: PICC Zone Insertion Method (ZIM) – a systematic approach to determine the ideal insertion site for PICCs in the upper arm. JAVA 2011;16(3):156-65.

Di Giacomo M: Comparison of three peripherally inserted central catheters – a pilot study. Brit J Nursing 2009;18(1):8-16.

Di Nardo M, Tomasello C, Pittiruti M et al.: Ultrasound-guided central venous cannulation in infants weighing less than 5 kilograms. J Vasc Access 2011;12(4):321-4.

Emoli A, Cappuccio S, Marche B et al.: The SIP (Safe Insertion of PICCs)Protocol: a bundle of eight recommendations to minimise complications linked to the peripheral insertion of central venous catheters (PICC). Assist InfermRic 2014;33(2):82-9.

Gallieni M, Pittiruti M, Biffi R: Vascular access in oncology patients. Ca Cancer J Clin 2008;58(6): 323-46.

Hadaway L: Needleless connectors for IV catheters. Am J Nurs 2012;112(11):32-44.

Hadaway L, Dalton L, Mercanti-Erieg L: Infusion teams in acute care hospitals. J Inf Nurs 2013;36(5):356-60.

Kaler W, Chinn R: Successful disinfection of needleless access port: a matter of time and friction. JAVA 2007;12(3):140-2.

Kokotis K: Cost containment and infusion services. J Inf Nurs 2005;28(3S):S22-32.

Mitidieri A, Pittiruti M, Silva Santos SI et al.: The intracavitary ECG method in the positioning of PICC central venous catheters in a coronary intensive care unit. Scenario 2014;31(2):22-6.

Pittiruti M: Ultrasound guided central vascular access in neonates, infants and children. Curr Drug Targets 2012;13(7):961-9.

Pittiruti M, Bertollo D, Briglia E et al.: The intracavitary ECG method for positioning the tip of central venous catheters: results of an Italian multicenter study. J Vasc Access 2012;13(3):357-65.

Pittiruti M, Brutti A, Celentano D et al.: Clinical experience with power-injectable PICCs in intensive care patients. Crit Care 2012;16(1):R21.

Pittiruti M, Emoli A, Porta P et al.: A prospective, randomized comparison of three different types of valved and non-valved peripherally inserted central catheters. J Vasc Access 2014;15(6):519-23.

Pittiruti M, LaGreca A, Emoli A, Scoppettuolo G. The ISALT 2 for the insertion of long-term central venous access: a GAVeCeLT proposal for a safer and more cost-effective approach. Osp Ital Chir 2010;16:359-68.

Pittiruti M, LaGreca A, Scoppettuolo G: The electrocardiographic method for positioning the tip of central venous catheters. J Vasc Access 2011;12(4):280-91.

Pittiruti M, Lamperti M: Late cardiac tamponade in adults secondary to tip position in the right atrium:an urban legend? A systematic review of the literature. J Cardiothorac Vasc Anesth 2015;29(2):491-5.

Pittiruti M, Scoppettuolo G, LaGreca A et al.: The EKG method for positioning the tip of PICCs: results from two preliminary studies. JAVA 2008;13(4):112-9.

Pronovost P, Needham D, Berenholtz S et al.: An intervention to decrease catheter-related bloodstream infections in the ICU. N Engl J Med 2006;355(26):2725-32.

Quian SY, Horn MT, Barnes R, Armstrong D: The use of 8 cm 22G Seldinger catheters for intravenous access in children with cystic fibrosis. J Vasc Access 2014;15(5):415-7.

Rossetti F, Pittiruti M, Lamperti M et al.: The intracavitary ECG method for positioning the tip of central venous access devices in pediatric patients: results of an Italian multicenter study. J Vasc Access 2015;16(2):137-43.

Shekelle PG, Pronovost PJ, Wachter RM et al.: The Top Patient Safety Strategies that can be encouraged for adoption now. Ann Intern Med 2013;158:365-8.

Simcock L: No going back – Advantages of ultrasound-guided upper arm PICC placement. JAVA 2008;13(4):191-7.

Spaziani S, Micheli T, Vincenzi B, Campisi C: Groshong PICC and home care: an opportunity. Clinical experience after the first 200 implants. J Vasc Access 2000;1:108-11.

Internet sites

www.avainfo.org
AVA – Association for Vascular Access (USA) website

www.evanetwork.info
EVAN – European Vascular Access Network website

www.gavecelt.info
GAVeCeLT – "Long-term Venous Access" Open Group website

www.ivteam.com
IV Team (UK) group website

www.nivas.org.uk
NIVAS – National Infusion and Vascular Access Society (UK) website

www.vascular-access.info
Journal of Vascular Access website, official GAVeCeLT and WoCoVA Foundation journal

www.wocova.com
WoCoVA – World Conference on Vascular Access website

Index